The Chicago Review Press

NCLEX
RN

Practice Test and Review

The Chicago Review Press

NCLEX
RN

Practice Test and Review

Linda Waide, MSN, MEd, RN
and Berta Roland, MSN, RN

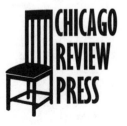

CHICAGO
REVIEW
PRESS

Library of Congress Cataloging-in-Publication Data

The Chicago Review Press NCLEX-RN practice test and review / [edited by] Linda Waide and Berta Roland. — 3rd ed.
   p.: cm.
   ISBN 1-55652-529-X
1. Practical nursing—Examinations, questions, etc. 2. National Council Licensure Examination for Registered Nurses.
[DNLM: 1. Nursing,—Examination Questions. WY 18.2 C532
2004] 1. Title: NCLEX-RN practice test and review. II. Waide, Linda.
III. Roland, Berta.
RT62.C455 2004
610.73'076—dc22

2004013697

100-Item Practice Test CD © 2004 Contemporary Health Systems
Software developed by Vories Pittman

Published by Chicago Review Press, Incorporated
814 North Franklin Street
Chicago, Illinois 60610

ISBN-13:978-1-55652-529-2
ISBN-10:1-55652-529-X
Printed in the United States of America
5   4   3   2

Contents

Practice Test 11

Practice Test 12

Acknowledgments

The authors are grateful to Linda Matthews, Publisher, Chicago Review Press, for her suggestions and advice on how to make this book a quick and efficient way to prepare for the National Council Licensure Examination (NCLEX).

We are grateful as well to the nurse educators who submitted test questions and provided consultation: Joanne Brown, MSN, MPH, RN; Jane Case, MSN, FNP, RN; Amy Chrapliwy, BSN, MS, RN; Judith Cooper, MSN, RN; Mary Ann Dell, EdD, RN; Cathy Horton, BSN, RN; Phillis Horton, MSN, RN; Joyce Jenkins, MSN, RN; Margaret Lyles, MSN, RN, and Sandra Rakestraw, BSN, PNS, RN.

Thanks to Missy Horne and Linda Waide, who created the drawings for the text, and to Loretta Moore for her tireless and tenacious efforts in preparing the many revisions that came across her desk in the preparation of this study guide. She exemplifies professionalism on a daily basis.

Introduction

This review and study guide is designed to prepare you, the candidate, for the NCLEX-RN so that you can pass the examination and receive your license as a registered nurse. It has been written by nursing educators with many years of experience in the classroom as well as in the clinical area. Careful consideration has been given to every topic in the book to bring you greater understanding of nursing content, provide a brief yet comprehensive review, and enable you to prepare for this all-important examination both quickly and efficiently.

Each nursing area that you will be tested on is introduced by way of a brief Overview. Following the Overview, a series of questions are asked in a Practice Test. At the end of the Practice Test, rationales and explanations as to the correct response and why the other options are incorrect will further help you to prepare for the NCLEX-RN.

Reviewing nursing content in preparation for the NCLEX can be time-consuming, difficult, and sometimes overwhelming. This study guide has been created for the express purpose of providing graduates with a quick and efficient way to assure their success on the NCLEX-RN. It will be invaluable in furnishing the knowledge and the confidence needed, by preparing candidates in three fundamental ways.

First, this book increases the graduate's knowledge of the subject matter with carefully written practice tests that include answers and rationales for every question, plus a 100-question practice test on CD, also with answers and rationales. All questions conform to the latest NCLEX test plan and format. The answers and rationales at the end of each practice test are designed to teach the graduate why the correct answer is right and why the three distractors are incorrect. All phases of Client Need are identified for every question: Health Promotion and Maintenance, Physiological Integrity, Psychosocial Integrity, and Safe, Effective Care Environment. Graduates can easily determine their competence in all of these areas.

Second, this book gives each graduate an opportunity to practice and learn test-taking skills and strategies that are vital for success on the NCLEX-CAT (Computerized Adaptive Testing). Becoming familiar with the CAT format and practicing how to select answers using the critical thinking process will improve test scores. Graduates who possess good test-taking skills and are able to apply knowledge correctly are more likely to experience success on the NCLEX the first time they take it.

Third, this book decreases test-taking anxiety. Many graduates tell us they study for tests but are too anxious to remember the subject matter being tested. By preparing for the NCLEX using this approach, graduates can feel confident because they have prepared appropriately. The authors have provided you with an efficient strategy for study, and we wish you well.

About the Examination for Nursing Licensure

Entry into the practice of nursing is regulated by your state board of nursing for the purpose of protecting the public from persons who are unable to practice safely and effectively. The NCLEX asks candidates to provide evidence of their ability to give competent nursing care. Candidates apply directly to their board of nursing to take the NCLEX-RN. For your convenience, a list of all the boards of nursing with their addresses and phone numbers is provided at the end of the introduction. The board of nursing will send you a candidate bulletin containing a registration form and information about the examination.

Basics of NCLEX-RN (CAT)

The licensure examination uses Computerized Adaptive Testing, or CAT, to measure a graduate's knowledge. Questions will appear on the computer screen in several different forms. Most will continue to be the familiar multiple-choice question with four answer options. However, the testing agency has added several innovative formats that take advantage of up-to-date computer technology. You will answer some fill in the blank questions and some select all that apply questions, where there is more than one appropriate answer. Some items may ask you to identify an area (a "hot spot") on a picture or drawing. Charts, tables, and diagrams may also be presented on the computer screen. The following examples show four ways that questions may appear on the NCLEX-RN.

1. Traditional multiple choice

Which type of chemical compound would you use to prevent the growth of bacteria?

1. bactericidal
2. bacteriolytic
3. bacteremia
4. bacteriostatic

Answer: 4

2. Fill in the blank

Lipids are a group of organic compounds that are insoluble in water and are commonly referred to as:

Answer: _____

Fill in the blank

Answer: Fats

3. More than one answer (select all that apply)

When assessing your client's neck, you will check for:

Select all that apply:

☐ 1. Range of motion (ROM)
☐ 2. Lymph nodes
☐ 3. Venous distention
☐ 4. Thyroid size and consistency

Answer: All the above

4. "Hot spot" (graphic image)

Your are taking your client's apical pulse.
At which location will you place your stethoscope?

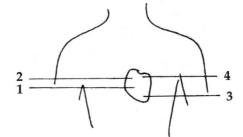

Answer: Click on #3

Before taking the NCLEX, candidates should read the booklet provided by their institution to nursing graduates. This booklet gives detailed explanations of licensure requirements and how to apply for and obtain a license to practice nursing.

Directory of State and Territorial Boards of Registered Nursing

Alabama
Alabama Board of Nursing
770 Washington Avenue
RSA Plaza, Suite 250
Montgomery, AL 36130-3900
Phone: (334) 242-4060

Alaska
Alaska Board of Nursing
550 W. Seventh Avenue, Suite 1500
Anchorage, AK 99501-3567
Phone: (907) 269-8196

Arizona
Arizona State Board of Nursing
1651 E. Morten Avenue, Suite 210
Phoenix, AZ 85020
Phone: (602) 331-8111

Arkansas
Arkansas State Board of Nursing
University Tower Building
1123 S. University Street, Suite 800
Little Rock, AR 72204-1619
Phone: (501) 686-2700

California
California Board of Registered Nursing
400 R Street, Suite 4030
Sacramento, CA 95814-6239
Phone: (916) 322-3350

Colorado
Colorado Board of Nursing
1560 Broadway, Suite 880
Denver, CO 80202
Phone: (303) 894-2430

Connecticut
Connecticut Board of Examiners for Nursing
Dept. of Public Health
410 Capitol Avenue, MS #13PHO
PO Box 340308
Hartford, CT 06234-0328
Phone: (860) 509-7624

Delaware
Delaware Board of Nursing
862 Silver Lake Boulevard
Cannon Building, Suite 203
Dover, DE 19904
Phone: (302) 739-4522

District of Columbia
District of Columbia Board of Nursing
Department of Health
825 N. Capitol Street N.E., 2nd Floor
Room 2224
Washington, DC 20002
Phone: (202) 442-4778

Florida
Florida Board of Nursing
Capital Circle Officer Center
4052 Bald Cypress Way
Room 120
Tallahassee, FL 32399-3252
Phone: (850) 488-0595

Georgia
Georgia State Board of Registered Nurses
237 Coliseum Drive
Macon, GA 31217-3858
Phone: (478) 207-1620

Guam
Guam Board of Nurse Examiners
PO Box 2816
Agana, Guam 96932
Phone: (670) 475-0251

Hawaii
Hawaii Board of Nursing
Professional & Vocational Licensing Division
PO Box 3469
Honolulu, HI 96801
Phone: (808) 586-3000

Idaho
Idaho Board of Nursing
280 N. 8th Street, Suite 210
PO Box 83720
Boise, ID 83720
Phone: (208) 334-3110

Illinois
Illinois Department of Professional Regulation
James R. Thompson Center
100 W. Randolph, Suite 9-300
Chicago, IL 60601
Phone: (312) 814-2715
320 Washington Street, 3rd Floor
Springfield, IL 62786
Phone: (217) 782-8556

Indiana
Indiana State Board of Nursing
Health Professions Bureau
402 W. Washington Street, Room W041
Indianapolis, IN 46204
Phone: (317) 232-2960

Iowa
Iowa Board of Nursing
River Point Business Park
400 S.W. 8th Street, Suite B
Des Moines, IA 50309-4695
Phone: (515) 281-3255

Kansas
Kansas State Board of Nursing
Landon State Office Building
900 S.W. Jackson, Suite 1051
Topeka, KS 66612
Phone: (785) 296-4629

Kentucky
Kentucky State Board of Nursing
312 Whittington Parkway, Suite 300
Louisville, KY 40222
Phone: (502) 329-7000

Louisiana
Louisiana State Board of Nursing (RN)
3510 N. Causeway Boulevard, Suite 501
Metairie, LA 70002
Phone: (504) 838-5332

Maine
Maine State Board of Nursing
158 State House Station
Augusta, ME 04333
Phone: (207) 287-1133

Maryland
Maryland Board of Nursing
4140 Patterson Avenue
Baltimore, MD 21215
Phone: (410) 585-1900

Massachusetts
Massachusetts Board of Registration in Nursing
Commonwealth of Massachusetts
239 Causeway Street
Boston, MA 48933
Phone: (617) 727-9961

Michigan
Michigan CIS/Bureau of Health Services
Ottawa Towers North
611 W. Ottawa, 4th Floor
Lansing, MI 48933
Phone: (517) 373-9102

Minnesota
Minnesota Board of Nursing
2829 University Avenue S.E., Suite 500
Minneapolis, MN 55414

Mississippi
Mississippi Board of Nursing
1935 Lakeland Drive, Suite B
Jackson, MS 39216-5014
Phone: (601) 987-4188

Missouri
Missouri State Board of Nursing
3605 Missouri Boulevard
PO Box 656
Jefferson City, MO 65102-0656
Phone: (573) 751-0681

Montana
Montana State Board of Nursing
301 S. Park Street
PO Box 200513
Helena, MT 59620-0513
Phone: (406) 841-2340

Nebraska
Nebraska Health and Human Services System
Dept. of Regulation & Licensure,
Nursing Section
301 Centennial Mall South
Lincoln, NE 68509-4986
Phone: (402) 471-4376

Nevada
Nevada State Board of Nursing
License Certification and Education
4330 S. Valley View Boulevard, Suite 106
Las Vegas, NV 89103
Phone: (702) 486-5800

New Hampshire
New Hampshire Board of Nursing
PO Box 3898
78 Regional Drive, Bldg B
Concord, NH 03302
Phone: (603) 271-2323

New Jersey
New Jersey Board of Nursing
PO Box 45010
124 Halsey Street, 6th Floor
Newark, NJ 07101
Phone: (973) 504-6586

New Mexico
New Mexico Board of Nursing
4206 Louisiana Boulevard N.E., Suite A
Albuquerque, NM 87109
Phone: (505) 841-8340

New York
New York State Board of Nursing
Education Bldg.
89 Washington Avenue
2nd Floor, West Wing
Albany, NY 12234
Phone: (518) 474-3817

North Carolina
North Carolina Board of Nursing
3724 National Drive, Suite 201
Raleigh, NC 27612
Phone: (919) 782-3211

North Dakota
North Dakota Board of Nursing
919 S. 7th Street, Suite 504
Bismarck, ND 58504
Phone: (701) 328-9777

Ohio
Ohio Board of Nursing
17 S. High Street, Suite 400
Columbus, OH 43215-3413
Phone: (614) 466-3947

Oklahoma
Oklahoma Board of Nursing
2915 N. Classen Boulevard, Suite 523
Oklahoma City, OK 73106
Phone: (405) 962-1800

Oregon
Oregon State Board of Nursing
800 N.E. Oregon Street, Box 25, Suite 465
Portland, OR 97232
Phone: (503) 731-4745

Pennsylvania
Pennsylvania State Board of Nursing
P.O. Box 2649
124 Pine Street
Harrisburg, PA 17101
Phone: (717) 783-7142

Puerto Rico
Commonwealth of Puerto Rico Board of Nurse
Examiners
800 Roberto H. Todd Avenue
Room 202, Stop 18
Santurce, PR 00908
Phone: (787) 725-7506

Rhode Island
Rhode Island Board of Nurse Registration and
Nursing Education
105 Cannon Bldg
Three Capitol Hill
Providence, RI 02908
Phone: (401) 222-5700

South Carolina
South Carolina State Board of Nursing
110 Centerview Drive, Suite 202
Columbia, SC 29210
Phone: (803) 896-4550

South Dakota
South Dakota Board of Nursing
4300 S. Louise Avenue, Suite C-1
Sioux Falls, SD 57106-3124
Phone: (605) 362-2760

Tennessee
Tennessee State Board of Nursing
426 Fifth Avenue N.
1st Floor, Cordell Hull Bldg.
Nashville, TN 37247
Phone: (615) 532-3202

Texas
Texas Board of Nurse Examiners
William P. Hobby Bldg., Tower 3
333 Guadalupe Street, Suite 3-460
Austin, TX 78701
Phone: (512) 305-8100

Utah
Utah State Board of Nursing
Heber M. Wells Bldg., 4th Floor
160 E. 300 South
Salt Lake City, UT 84111
Phone: (801) 530-6628

Vermont
Vermont State Board of Nursing
109 State Street
Montpelier, VT 05609-1106
Phone: (802) 828-2396

Virgin Islands
Virgin Islands Board of Nurse Licensure
Veterans Drive Station
St. Thomas, VI 00803
Phone: (340) 776-7397

Virginia
Virginia Board of Nursing
6603 W. Broad Street, 5th Floor
Richmond, VA 23230-1712
Phone: (804) 662-9909

Washington
Washington State Nursing Care
Quality Assurance Commission
Department of Health
1300 Quince Street S.E.
Olympia, WA 98504-7864
Phone: (360) 236-4700

West Virginia
West Virginia State Board of Examiners for
Registered Professional Nurses
101 Dee Drive
Charleston, WV 25311
Phone: (304) 558-3572

Wisconsin
Wisconsin Department of Regulation and
Licensing
1400 E. Washington Avenue
PO Box 8935
Madison, WI 53708
Phone: (608) 266-0145

Wyoming
Wyoming State Board of Nursing
2020 Carey Avenue, Suite 110
Cheyenne, WY 82002
Phone: (307) 777-7601

The Chicago Review Press

NCLEX
RN

Practice Test and Review

Practice Test 1

Cardiocirculatory and Peripheral Circulatory Systems

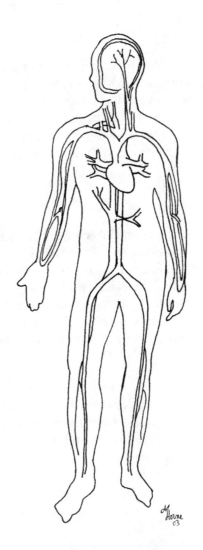

The Cardiocirculatory System

OVERVIEW

The cardiocirculatory system consists of blood, vessels to transport the blood, and a four-chambered muscular pump called the heart. The cardiocirculatory system is responsible for transporting food and oxygen to all the cells and organs of the body.

Blood vessels in the lungs absorb oxygen that is inhaled from the air, and blood vessels in the small intestine absorb food materials from the digestive tract. Blood also provides a means whereby cellular wastes, i.e., carbon dioxide and urea, are transported to the lungs and kidneys, where they are eliminated from the body.

BLOOD VESSELS

There are three types of blood vessels: arteries, veins, and capillaries.

Arteries

Arteries are large vessels that carry oxygenated blood away from the heart. In order to withstand the high pressure of the heart's pumping action, arteries are made of connective tissue, elastic fibers, and inner walls of epithelial cells. As the heart forces blood into the arteries, their elastic qualities enable them to expand and contract. Some of the arteries in the body are very large compared to their smaller branches, called arterioles. The walls of arterioles are much thinner than the walls of the larger arteries. The thin walls of arterioles allow them to carry blood to the smallest of vessels, which are known as capillaries.

Capillaries

The walls of capillaries are very thin (just one epithelial cell thick). Because they are so small (microscopic), they are capable of allowing oxygen and nutrients to pass out of the bloodstream and into the tissue fluid (interstitial fluid) that surrounds all body cells. Once nutrients and oxygen are inside the cells, the nutrients are burned (catabolized) and needed energy is released within the cells. At the same time that oxygen and nutrients are passing into the interstitial fluid, the waste products of catabolism, namely, carbon dioxide and water, pass out of the cells and into the thin-walled capillaries. These waste products flow back to the heart via small veins known as venules, which branch to form larger vessels known as veins.

Veins

Veins do not have to withstand the pressures that arteries do. Therefore, vein walls are thinner than arterial walls, and veins are less elastic and have less connective tissue than arteries. Compared to arteries, blood pressure in the veins is low. To keep blood flowing toward the heart, veins have small valves on their inner walls that prevent blood from flowing backward. In addition to these valves, muscular action also helps to "milk" blood flow along in the veins.

THE HEART

The four chambers of the heart actually form two pumps. The right side of the heart pumps blood from the heart into the lungs, where it gives off carbon dioxide and picks up oxygen; the left side of the heart pumps the oxygenated blood from the lungs into the body.

Pulmonary Circulation

Pulmonary circulation consists of the flow of blood through the vessels from the heart to the lungs and then back to the heart again.

When blood goes into the heart, the top two chambers (the right and left atria) relax and deoxygenated blood flows from the veins into the right atrium. This is known as venous return. At the same time, oxygenated blood coming from the lungs flows into the left atrium. At this point the blood-filled atria contract and the blood pushes open the heart valves (the bicuspid and tricuspid valves). This allows oxygenated blood from the left atrium to pass into the left ventricle, and deoxygenated blood from the right atrium to pass into the right ventricle.

When blood leaves the heart, the right and left ventricles contract and deoxygenated blood in the right ventricle flows into the lung (via the pulmonary artery), where it will give off its carbon dioxide and pick up oxygen, and oxygenated blood in the left ventricle flows out of the heart (via the coronary arteries and aorta), where it begins its travels into the body.

DISEASES/DISORDERS OF THE CARDIOCIRCULATORY SYSTEM INCLUDE

Acquired Inflammatory Heart Disease

ENDOCARDITIS Other names for endocarditis are infective or bacterial endocarditis. The infection affects the endocardium, heart valves, or cardiac processes and is characterized by bacteria or fungi creating vegetative growths on the heart valves and on the endocardial lining of the heart chambers. These growths may also be located on the endothelium of a blood vessel, where they may embolize to organs such as the spleen, kidneys, central nervous system, and lungs. An organism commonly associated with endocarditis is *Streptococcus viridans*.

MYOCARDITIS Myocarditis is associated with diffuse inflammation of the cardiac muscle (the myocardium). This condition is caused by viral infections, bacterial infections, immune reactions, radiation therapy, chemical poisons, parasitic infestations, and helminthic infestations.

PERICARDITIS Pericarditis is the inflammation of the pericardium (the membranous fibroserous sac that encloses the heart and the bases of the great vessels). Common causes include infections with bacteria, viruses, or fungi; also neoplasms, radiation to the chest, and postcardiac injury.

RHEUMATIC FEVER/HEART DISEASE Rheumatic fever is a consequence of infection with a group of beta-hemolytic streptococcal bacteria. Rheumatic heart disease refers to the sequelae, or aftereffects, of rheumatic fever, and may include: Myocarditis, pericarditis, endocarditis, and eventually, valvular disease.

Cardiac Complications

CARDIAC ARRHYTHMIAS/DYSRHYTHMIAS Cardiac arrhythmias/dysrhythmias are faulty electrical conductions that change the rate and rhythm of the heart. Types of arrhythmias include: Sinus arrhythmia, sinus tachycardia, sinus bradycardia, sinoatrial arrest/block, premature atrial contraction, ventricular tachycardia, and ventricular fibrillation.

CARDIAC TAMPONADE Cardiac tamponade is a sequela of pericarditis or injuries to the heart or great blood vessels that cause an accumulation of blood in the pericardial sac. The classic signs of cardiac tamponade are increased venous pressure with neck vein distention, reduced arterial blood pressure, muffled heart sounds, and pulsus paradoxus (an abnormal inspiratory drop in systemic blood pressure greater than 15 mm Hg.)

CARDIOGENIC SHOCK Cardiogenic shock occurs when cardiac output diminishes and severe tissue ischemia takes place. Cardiogenic shock is associated with left-sided heart failure and is seen in approximately 15% of clients experiencing a myocardial infarction (MI).

HYPOVOLEMIC SHOCK Hypovolemic shock is best described as lack of tissue perfusion due to insufficient blood volume. Untreated, this condition may cause irreversible cerebral and renal damage, cardiac arrest, and death. Typical causes of this condition are gastrointestinal bleeding and accidental or surgical trauma, severe burns, or ascites resulting in significant blood loss..

VENTRICULAR ANEURYSM An aneurysm is an abnormal ballooning or dilatation of a blood vessel (usually an artery) due to either a congenital defect or weakness in the vessel wall. A ventricular aneurysm is a ballooning or out-pouching of the left ventricle. Untreated, this condition may lead to arrhythmias, systemic embolization, and heart failure, including sudden death.

Congential Acyanotic Defects

ATRIAL SEPTAL DEFECT (ASD) An atrial septal defect is a congenital heart defect that allows blood to flow through an opening between the right and left atria.

COARCTATION OF THE AORTA This is a localized malformation that results in the narrowing of the aorta. Untreated, it may lead to left-sided heart failure and possibly cerebral hemorrhage and aortic rupture.

PATENT DUCTUS ARTERIOSUS (PDA) In PDA, the lumen of the ductus remains open following birth, allowing blood to flow from the aorta to the pulmonary artery and causing recirculation of arterial blood through the lungs. Respiratory distress and signs of heart failure are the two most common symptoms.

VENTRAL SEPTAL DEFECT (VSD) This is the most common congenital heart disorder. The defect (a septum between the left and right ventricles of the heart) allows blood to be shunted between the ventricles, and may cause left atria and right ventricle hypertrophy. Untreated, the condition leads to biventricular heart failure and cyanosis.

Congenital Cyanotic Defects

TETRALOGY OF FALLOT As the name implies, this condition is created by four cardiac defects, namely: ventricular septal defect (VSD), right ventricular outflow tract obstruction (pulmonary stenosis), right ventricular hypertrophy, and dextroposition of the aorta with an overriding of the ventricular septal defect. These defects allow unoxygenated blood to mix with oxygenated blood, causing cyanosis.

Degenerative Cardiovascular Disorders

CORONARY ARTERY DISEASE (CAD) CAD is associated with narrowing of the coronary arteries sufficient to prevent an adequate supply of blood to the myocardium (heart muscle). The usual cause is atherosclerosis, the most common form of arteriosclerosis, which is marked by cholesterol-lipid-calcium deposits in the linings of the arteries.

DILATED CARDIOMYOPATHY In this condition, the striated muscle fibers of the myocardium (heart muscle) suffer extensive damage, interfering with myocardial metabolism and causing gross dilatation of all four chambers of the heart.

HEART FAILURE This condition results from failure of the heart to maintain adequate circulation to the heart. As a consequence, failure of the right, left, or both ventricles may occur.

HYPERTENSION Hypertension is a condition in which a person has greater than normal blood pressure. A person is said to have hypertension if the systolic pressure is persistently above 140 mm Hg, if the diastolic pressure is persistently above 90 mm Hg, and when either the systolic pressure is 160 or above, or the diastolic pressure is 115 or above.

HYPERTROPHIC CARDIOMYOPATHY This is a primary disease of cardiac muscle. Another name for it is idiopathic hypertrophic subaortic stenosis. It is associated with thickening of the interventricular septum (especially in the free wall of the left ventricle). If low cardiac output occurs, the condition may lead to fatal heart failure.

MYOCARDIAL INFARCTION (MI) Myocardial infarction is commonly known as a heart attack. It is a consequence of prolonged myocardial ischemia due to reduced blood flow through one of the coronary arteries. MI is the leading cause of death in the United States and Western Europe.

RESTRICTIVE CARDIOMYOPATHY Characterized by restricted ventricular filling, this condition is the result of left ventricular hypertrophy as well as endocardial fibrosis and thickening. In some cases, it may be irreversible.

Vascular Disorders

ABDOMINAL ANEURYSM An abdominal aneurysm is a localized dilatation (ballooning) of the wall of the abdominal aorta. This disorder may be asymptomatic; however, symptoms may include generalized abdominal pain, low back pain that is unaffected by movement, a feeling of gastric fullness, and a pulsating mass in the periumbilical area.

ARTERIAL OCCLUSIVE DISEASE This disease is characterized by the narrowing of the lumen of the aorta and the major branches of the aorta. This narrowing affects blood flow to the legs and feet. Occlusions may cause ischemia, skin ulcerations, and gangrene.

BEURGER'S DISEASE This disease is associated with chronic recurring inflammation and vascular occlusion. It typically affects the peripheral arteries and veins of the extremities. Smoking tobacco is thought to be the main cause. Treatment includes the discontinuation of tobacco in any form.

FEMORAL AND POPLITEAL ANEURYSMS Also known as peripheral arterial aneurysms, these are the result of progressive atherosclerotic changes in the walls of the major peripheral arteries. Symptoms include pain in the legs and feet due to ischemia.

RAYNAUD'S DISEASE This is a peripheral vascular disorder found almost exclusively in women between 18 and 40 years of age. It is characterized by severe vasoconstriction in the extremities when exposed to cold or vasoconstriction associated with emotional stress. Symptoms include intermittent attacks of pallor or cyanosis in the digits (typically the fingers). Other symptoms include numbness and tingling in the fingers. Rarely, gangrene necessitating amputation of the affected digits may occur.

THORACIC AORTIC ANEURYSM This condition is characterized by widening (ballooning) of either the ascending, transverse, or descending parts of the aorta. The most common cause is atherosclerosis, which weakens the wall of the aorta and slowly distends the lumen. Pain is the most common symptom.

THROMBOPHLEBITIS An acute condition associated with inflammation and thrombus formation in deep or superficial veins, this disease is usually progressive and may lead to pulmonary embolism. Superficial thrombophlebitis is generally self-limiting and rarely leads to pulmonary embolism.

Valvular Heart Diseases

All of these conditions interfere with the normal flow of blood into, through, and out of the heart. They include

- Mitral insufficiency
- Mitral stenosis
- Mitral valve prolapse (MVP)
- Aortic insufficiency
- Aortic stenosis
- Pulmonic insufficiency
- Pulmonic stenosis
- Tricuspid insufficiency

Practice Test 1

Questions

1 - 1

A client is admitted to the Coronary Care Unit complaining of chest pain and nausea. Six hours after admission, the client tells the nurse, "I need to have a bowel movement." The most appropriate response by the nurse would be:

1. "You need to walk slowly to the bathroom. I will assist you."
2. "I will see that a commode chair is brought to your bedside."
3. "You should avoid straining while having a bowel movement."
4. "Wait until a prescription can be obtained for a Fleet enema."

1 - 2

A client is admitted to the Intensive Cardiac Care Unit (ICCU) with a diagnosis of superventricular tachycardia. The client complains of dizziness and fatigue. In the presence of a rapid heart rate, the nurse will assess the client first for the development of:

1. fluid in the lungs.
2. pallor.
3. increasing urinary output.
4. unstable angina.

1 - 3

Your client is hypertensive and has been taking an angiotensin-converting enzyme inhibitor for several days. Today's medication prescriptions include a loop diuretic. The expected outcome of this therapy is:

1. excretion of calcium with no diuretic effect.
2. an increase in diastolic blood pressure.
3. a decrease in blood pressure.
4. hypotension.

1 - 4

A client diagnosed with acute myocardial infarction develops acute pericarditis 4 days after admission to the hospital. Nursing assessment on the fifth day of hospitalization reveals client complaints of chest pressure, shortness of breath, increasing anxiety, and restlessness. Physical findings show diminished heart sounds and a mild friction rub. The nurse recognizes these symptoms as evidence of:

1. cardiac tamponade.
2. pericardial effusion.
3. increased cardiac output.
4. cardiomyopathy.

1 - 5

Your 55-year-old client is unresponsive and has a pulse that is barely palpable. The electrocardiogram has identified a supraventricular tachycardia of 180 beats per minute (BPM). You will anticipate cardioversion by defibrillation with:

1. 20 joules.
2. 50 joules.
3. 200 joules.
4. 500 joules.

1 - 6

Which of the following statements are correct regarding coronary artery disease (CAD) in women?

Select all that apply by placing a ✔ in the square:

❑ 1. Diabetes mellitus is a predictor of CAD in women.

❑ 2. Estrogen replacement in post-menopausal women reduces the risk of CAD.

❑ 3. Smoking cigarettes contributes to CAD in women.

❑ 4. Hypertension is not a risk factor for CAD in women.

❑ 5. CAD is the number-one cause of death in American women.

1 - 7

A client with generalized arteriosclerosis approaches the nurse and says, "I don't sleep well at night because my feet get cold. What should I do?" Which of the following responses by the nurse would be the most effective and safest recommendations?

1. "Rub your feet briskly to improve circulation."
2. "Place a light blanket over your feet at night."
3. "Place your feet on a covered hot-water bottle."
4. "Put a covered heating pad on your feet with the dial on the lowest setting."

1 - 8

A client with esophageal varices is experiencing hematemesis. A balloon tamponade has been inserted. The nurse recognizes that the primary purpose of this intervention is to:

1. apply pressure to the affected area.
2. prevent paralytic ileus.
3. provide a means for irrigating the stomach.
4. prevent vomiting of blood.

1 - 9

A 3-year-old was hospitalized with congestive heart failure. The child has been digitalized and is now receiving a maintenance dose of digoxin 0.08 mg po bid. The available medication contains 0.05 mg digoxin per 1 cc of solution. How much of the solution will the nurse administer?

1. 0.06 cc
2. 0.6 cc
3. 1.6 cc
4. 2.6 cc

1-10

The most distinctive electrocardiogram change associated with hyperkalemia is:

1. absence of P waves.
2. atrial fibrillation.
3. heightened QRS complexes.
4. peaked T waves.

1-11

Which assessment should be completed frequently on clients receiving Tridil?

1. blood pressure
2. blood glucose
3. breath sounds
4. urine output

1-12

Atrial flutter may best be described as:

1. an irregular, chaotic ventricular rhythm.
2. an irregular rhythm with little wave formation between QRS complexes.
3. an atrial rhythm characterized by a sawtooth pattern between QRS complexes.
4. a barely discernible rhythm, not associated with any heart muscle activity.

1-13

A client is receiving a continuous drip of nitroprusside sodium (Nitropress) to decrease cardiac afterload. What special precaution will the nurse take when administering this medication?

1. Use special intravenous tubing.
2. Protect the solution from light.
3. Put medication in glass bottles only.
4. Do not allow solution to hang for more than 4 hours.

1-14

Your client has an asymptomatic abdominal aortic aneurysm. Ultrasonographic examination indicates the aneurysm is 3.5 centimeters. You anticipate:

1. administration of an antihypertensive medication.
2. excision of the aneurysm with replacement of the excised segment with a synthetic graft.
3. a gastrointestinal bleed that may progress to shock.
4. a complaint by the client of intense back and flank pain with awareness of a pulsating mass in the abdomen.

1-15

You are concerned that your client is getting too much digoxin. What signs and symptoms are indicative of digitalis toxicity?

1. convulsions
2. yellow-green halo vision
3. muscle cramping
4. orthostatic hypotension

1-16

The nurse routinely obtains a client's central venous pressure readings. Should interventions become necessary based on the central venous pressure readings, they would be implemented for the purpose of:

1. maintaining a normal range of pressure in the right atrium.
2. lowering the pressure in the pulmonary artery.
3. detecting dysrhythmias in the left ventricle.
4. promoting circulation through the aorta.

1-17

A client is diagnosed with Raynaud's phenomenon. When assisting the client to manage activities of daily living, the nurse should include which of the following in the teaching plan?

1. Moving to a warmer climate.
2. Taking pain medication when exposed to cold or cold objects.
3. Wearing gloves when exposed to cold or cold objects.
4. Limiting activity to decrease metabolic demands upon the body.

1-18

The foot of your client's casted leg is mottled and warmer than the unaffected leg. You notify the physician immediately because you suspect:

1. arterial insufficiency.
2. venous insufficiency.
3. compartmental syndrome.
4. fat emboli.

1-19

Which of the following symptoms is characteristic of intermittent claudication?

1. extensive discoloration
2. dependent edema
3. pain associated with activity
4. petechiae

1-20

A client experiencing stage II hypertension may be treated with which of the following medications?

1. levothyroxine
2. phenytoin
3. cefprozil
4. metoprolol

1-21

Your client has thromboangiitis obliterans. You are teaching the client how to participate in the treatment of this condition. Which statement by the client indicates a need for further teaching?

1. "It will be helpful if I can find employment that allows me to sit most of the time."
2. "I know it's essential that I quit smoking."
3. "I intend to walk 30 minutes twice daily."
4. "I'll need to be careful that I don't injure my legs."

1-22

The nurse is observing a client for symptoms of postoperative shock. The earliest symptom of postoperative shock would be obtained by monitoring the:

1. pulse rate.
2. pulse pressure.
3. temperature.
4. respirations.

1 - 2 3

A client with hypertension is receiving the angiotensin-converting enzyme inhibitor enalapril to decrease blood pressure. The nurse understands that this medication lowers blood pressure by:

1. promoting vasodilation.
2. blocking beta-adrenergic impulses.
3. inhibiting angiotensin-converting enzyme.
4. preventing reabsorption of sodium chloride.

1 - 2 4

A 65-year-old takes 0.125 mg of digoxin po qid. Which condition could predispose the client to develop digitalis toxicity?

1. pneumonia
2. hyperkalemia
3. hypothyroidism
4. hypocalcemia

1 - 2 5

A client complaining of severe substernal pain is presently being seen in the emergency department. An acute anterior myocardial infarction is suspected. An elevation of which enzyme would confirm the diagnosis at this time?

1. creatine kinase (CK) and its isoenzyme (CK-MB)
2. creatine kinase (CK) and its isoenzyme (CK-MM)
3. lactic dehydrogenase (LDH2)
4. serum glutamic-oxaloacetic transaminase (SGOT)

1 - 2 6

Which of the following laboratory value combinations is most likely to represent the client with the least risk of heart disease?

1. a high-density lipoprotein of 70 mg/dl and a low-density lipoprotein of 110 mg/dl
2. a high-density lipoprotein of 30 mg/dl and a low-density lipoprotein of 110 mg/dl
3. a high-density lipoprotein of 30 mg/dl and a low-density lipoprotein of 140 mg/dl
4. a high-density lipoprotein of 70 mg/dl and a low-density lipoprotein of 140 mg/dl

1 - 2 7

Your client is experiencing an evolving myocardial infarction and is being evaluated for thrombolytic therapy. Which statement made by the client would constitute a possible contraindication for this treatment?

1. "I've been having chest pain for 2 hours."
2. "I feel really nauseated right now."
3. "I've been taking blood pressure medicine for years."
4. "I'm still taking medicine for my stomach ulcers."

1 - 2 8

A client experiencing coronary artery disease may be treated with all of the following medications. Which medication will the nurse recognize as a calcium channel blocker?

1. metoprolol
2. nifedipine
3. nitroglycerin
4. aspirin

1-29

A 7-month-old infant with tetralogy of Fallot is in the recovery room following a right heart catheterization. Which of the following assessment findings should be reported immediately?

1. an apical pulse of 74 beats per minute
2. the left foot cool to the touch
3. mild clubbing of fingers and toes
4. irritable when dressing is changed

1-30

A client is returned to the unit following an angiocardiography. Which nursing action is appropriate at this time?

1. Discourage fluid intake and place the client in a prone position.
2. Apply heat to the puncture site and passively exercise the involved extremity.
3. Limit motion of the affected extremity and assess the puncture site.
4. Restrict fluid intake and encourage ambulation.

1-31

An adult client was admitted to the coronary care unit following a subendocardial myocardial infarction. A balloon-tipped pulmonary artery catheter was inserted when the client began to exhibit signs of cardiogenic shock. The nurse measures the client's pulmonary capillary wedge pressure and finds it to be 18 mm Hg. The nurse knows this pressure is:

1. within normal limits.
2. elevated above normal.
3. less than normal.
4. life threatening.

1-32

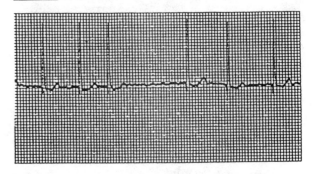

Your client's cardiac monitor displayed the above dysrhythmia. The client's blood pressure is 110/70 mm Hg, the pulse rate is between 120 and 140 beats per minute, and the respiratory rate is 18 breaths per minute. The client is alert, oriented, and complaining of palpitations and fatigue. The nurse will anticipate the administration of:

1. lidocaine.
2. atropine.
3. digitalis.
4. pronestyl.

1-33

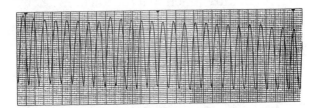

A 64-year-old client in the Intensive Coronary Care Unit is experiencing the above dysrhythmia. The client is hemodynamically stable. You will anticipate the administration of:

1. digoxin.
2. inderal.
3. lidocaine.
4. verapamil.

1 - 3 4

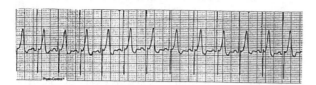

The nurse will recognize the above rhythm strip as an example of:

1. normal sinus rhythm.
2. sinus tachycardia.
3. ventricular tachycardia.
4. atrial fibrillation.

1 - 3 5

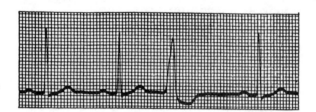

The above rhythm strip is an example of:

1. second-degree AV block, type II.
2. premature junctional contractions.
3. premature ventricular contractions.
4. third-degree AV block.

1 - 3 6

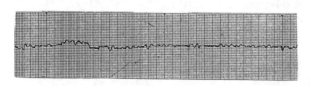

A client in the Intensive Coronary Care Unit converts to the above dysrhythmia. What should be done immediately?

1. cardioversion
2. defibrillation
3. administration of lidocaine
4. administration of sodium bicarbonate

1 - 3 7

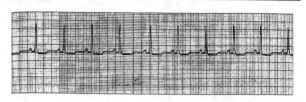

The above rhythm strip is an example of:

1. sinus tachycardia.
2. sinus bradycardia.
3. first-degree block.
4. normal sinus rhythm.

1 - 3 8

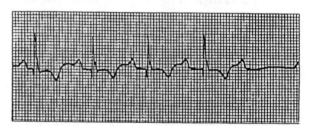

The above rhythm is an example of which dysrhythmia?

1. first-degree AV heart block
2. second-degree AV heart block, type I
3. second-degree AV heart block, type II
4. third-degree AV heart block

1 - 3 9

Sinus tachycardia may best be described by which of the following?

1. a chaotic rhythm with no discernible pattern that is not associated with cardiac output
2. a regular rhythm with rate greater than 100 beats per minute
3. a ventricular rapid rhythm that may or may not produce a palpable pulse
4. a regular rhythm with rates between 60 and 100 beats per minute

1 - 4 0

Sinus bradycardia is best described as:

1. an irregular rhythm of ventricular origin with faint, if any, palpable pulse.
2. an irregular, slow ventricular rate with variable numbers of P waves between complexes.
3. a normal rhythm with a rate of less than 60 beats per minute.
4. a normal rhythm with a rate of more than 100 beats per minute.

1 - 4 1

Which of the following instructions should be given to a client who has Nitrostat on hand for the treatment of angina?

1. "Keep your medication in the refrigerator at all times."
2. "Replace your tablets every 8 months."
3. "Swallow your pill with a big glass of water, not milk."
4. "If your angina is not relieved after 3 pills, come to the emergency department."

1 - 4 2

Nursing measures that include instructing clients in the prevention of coronary artery disease are referred to as:

1. primary interventions.
2. acute-care interventions.
3. secondary interventions.
4. tertiary interventions.

1 - 4 3

A client who is taking daily digoxin says to you, "I have been experiencing nausea." Upon further inquiry, it is discovered that the client's pulse rate is 52 beats per minute. The nurse should instruct the client to:

1. double the digoxin dose.
2. take an antacid 1 hour prior to today's digoxin dose.
3. take the digoxin on an empty stomach, but with a full glass of water.
4. hold the digoxin dose and come to the clinic for evaluation.

1 - 4 4

A client who has had a 12-lead electrocardiogram tells you there was a premature ventricular contraction noted by the technician taking the electrocardiogram. Your response to your client's concern about this is based on the knowledge that:

1. premature ventricular contractions may be benign.
2. there are no lifestyle changes to decrease their incidence.
3. premature ventricular contractions are a prelude to lethal arrhythmias.
4. premature ventricular contractions indicate myocardial infarction.

1 - 4 5

Risk factors in primary (essential) hypertension include:

Select all that apply by placing a ✔ in the square:

☐ 1. age
☐ 2. low serum lipids
☐ 3. race
☐ 4. diabetes mellitus
☐ 5. active lifestyle

1 - 4 6

Your client was brought to the emergency department following a myocardial infarction. Morphine sulfate IV has been prescribed. You understand this medication will decrease the cardiac workload by:

Select all that apply by placing a ✔ in the square:

- ❑ 1. increasing myocardial oxygen consumption.
- ❑ 2. reducing contractility.
- ❑ 3. lowering blood pressure.
- ❑ 4. increasing the heart rate.
- ❑ 5. decreasing pain.

1 - 4 7

Which of the following do you recognize as risk factors associated with sudden cardiac death (SCD)?

Select all that apply by placing a ✔ in the square:

- ❑ 1. hypercholesterolemia
- ❑ 2. coronary artery disease
- ❑ 3. hypotension
- ❑ 4. cigarette smoking
- ❑ 5. female gender

1 - 4 8

The contraction phase of the cardiac cycle is referred to as the:

_____.

Fill in the blank

Practice Test 1

Answers, Rationales, and Explanations

1 - 1

③ The client should be told that straining at stool is discouraged. Straining initiates the Valsalva's maneuver, which increases pressure in the large vein in the thorax and can interfere with the return of blood flow to the heart. The client should be provided with a bedpan to conserve energy.

1. Clients admitted to a Coronary Care Unit (CCU) are placed on bed rest and should not walk to the bathroom.

2. Until a definitive diagnosis is made, the client should not use a bedside commode chair.

4. There is no indication that the client needs an enema.

Client Need: Health Promotion and Maintenance

1 - 2

① The nurse will assess the client for the development of fluid in the lungs, which may be manifested by the presence of crackles (formerly referred to as rales). Rapid heart rhythms may cause heart failure along with accumulation of fluid in the lungs.

2. Pallor (paleness of skin) may be present. However, the nurse will assess the client for the most life-threatening possibilities, such as fluid accumulation in the lungs.

3. Urinary output will be decreased in the presence of heart failure, not increased. Diminished cardiac output prevents an adequate supply of blood from reaching the body tissues and organs (low perfusion). Low perfusion of the kidneys causes an abnormal reduction in urinary output (oliguria).

4. Rapid heart rates are not always associated with unstable angina. However, fluid in the lungs is likely and life threatening.

Client Need: Physiological Integrity

1 - 3

③ **An expected outcome of loop diuretic therapy is a decrease in blood pressure. Loop diuretics are often administered with angiotensin-converting enzyme (ACE) inhibitors to manage hypertension. A diuretic reduces circulatory volume by increasing renal excretion of water, sodium, chloride, magnesium, hydrogen, and calcium. An ACE inhibitor prevents the production of angiotensin II, a potent vasoconstrictor. Therefore, by reducing circulatory volume and preventing vasoconstriction, the blood pressure can be lowered.**

1. When a loop diuretic is administered, it inhibits reabsorption (the absorbing of sodium and chloride by the nephron after they have been through the glomerulus). The client will receive the benefit of the diuretic without the excretion of calcium.

2. Loop diuretics cause a decrease in diastolic blood pressure, not an increase.

4. Hypotension is a side effect of ACE inhibitors and diuretics, not an expected therapeutic outcome.

Client Need: Health Promotion and Maintenance

1 - 4

② **Chest pressure, shortness of breath, anxiety, restlessness, diminished heart rate, and friction rub are all classic manifestations of pericardial effusion (the accumulation of an abnormally large amount of pericardial fluid in the pericardium). Other symptoms of pericardial effusion include hypotension and elevated jugular vein distension (JVD).**

1. Cardiac tamponade may follow pericardial effusion. Symptoms of cardiac tamponade include increased intracardiac pressure, limitation of ventricular filling, reduction in stroke volume, jugular vein distention, a decrease in cardiac output, and increase in heart rate. The usual complaint is dyspnea.

3. Chest pressure, shortness of breath, anxiety, restlessness, diminished heart sounds, and friction rub would cause a decrease in cardiac output, not an increase in cardiac output.

4. Cardiomyopathy is a disease of the myocardium (the middle layer of the walls of the heart). Cardiomyopathy is characterized by impaired contractility and pumping ability of the heart.

Client Need: Physiological Integrity

1 - 5

② **Cardioversion by defibrillation with 50 joules is anticipated. Treatment for symptomatic supraventricular tachycardia is cardioversion. Defibrillation with 50 joules is the appropriate dosage.**

1. Defibrillation with 20 joules is a pediatric defibrillation dose.

3. Defibrillation with 200 joules is indicated for ventricular fibrillation or pulseless ventricular tachycardia.

4. Defibrillation with 500 joules is an inappropriately excessive dosage of current.

Client Need: Physiological Integrity

1 - 6

① Women with diabetes mellitus are 5 to 7 times more likely to develop CAD than women who do not have diabetes mellitus.

② Estrogen replacement in postmenopausal women may reduce the risk of CAD by 50%. Estrogen replacement lowers LDL and raises HDL cholesterol.

③ Smoking cigarettes is the biggest contributor to CAD in women under 50 years old. Nicotine causes vasoconstriction and can increase blood pressure.

⑤ CAD is the number-one cause of death in American women.

4. Hypertension is a risk factor in the development of CAD in women.

Client Need: Health Promotion and Maintenance

1 - 7

② The nurse should recommend that the client cover the feet with a light blanket. This is the most effective and safest way to keep the feet warm.

1. Clients with arteriosclerosis are susceptible to thrombi formation. Therefore, rubbing the feet is dangerous since it could cause the release of thrombi.

3 and 4. Clients with poor circulation may experience paresthesia (numbness and tingling) of the extremities. For this reason it would be unsafe to suggest the use of a hot-water bottle or a heating pad.

Client Need: Physiological Integrity

1 - 8

① The primary purpose for the balloon tamponade is to apply pressure at the site of the bleeding. Esophageal varices are dilated, tortuous veins that may bleed easily. This condition is usually caused by portal hypertension and is life threatening.

2. A paralytic ileus is characterized by lack of bowel sounds and lack of peristalsis, accompanied by distention of the abdomen. The client may experience nausea and vomiting. Fecal material may be vomited because of the potential for reverse peristalsis. This condition is treated with a nasogastric tube, not a balloon tamponade. Paralytic ileus may occur following abdominal surgery or with the administration of certain psychotropic drugs.

3. Balloon tamponade does allow for gastric suctioning. However, this is not the primary purpose. Gastric suctioning is usually done to monitor bleeding.

4. Balloon tamponade will not prevent vomiting of blood. However, to prevent the aspiration of blood, an endotracheal tube is sometimes inserted.

Client Need: Physiological Integrity

1 - 9

③ The nurse will administer 1.6 cc of the solution. The following equation may be used:

$$\frac{0.05 \text{ mg}}{1 \text{ cc}} = \frac{0.08 \text{ mg}}{X}$$

$$0.05X = 0.08$$

$$X = \frac{0.08}{0.05} = 1.6 \text{ cc}$$

1, 2, and 4. are incorrect dosages.

Client Need: Physiological Integrity

1 - 1 0

④ The most distinctive electrocardiogram (ECG) change associated with hyperkalemia is an elevated T wave.

1. The P wave represents atrial muscle depolarization. Absence of the P wave is associated with conditions such as atrial flutter and ventricular fibrillation.

2. Atrial fibrillation is a dysrhythmia in which minute areas of the atrial myocardium are in uncoordinated stages of depolarization and repolarization. This is due to multiple reentry circuits within the atrial myocardium. When this occurs, the atria quivers continuously in a chaotic pattern.

3. Heightened QRS complexes are associated with ventricular hypertrophy. Ventricular hypertrophy is due to chronic pressure overload.

Client Need: Physiological Integrity

1 - 1 1

① Clients receiving nitroglycerin (Tridil) intravenously should have their blood pressure monitored frequently. Tridil is the intravenous form of nitroglycerin. Because of its vasodilating effects, the blood pressure should be monitored frequently for the frequent side effect of hypotension.

2. Tridil does not affect blood glucose.

3. The respiratory system is not directly affected by Tridil.

4. The genitourinary system is not directly affected by Tridil.

Client Need: Health Promotion and Maintenance

1 - 1 2

③ **Atrial flutter is best described as an atrial rhythm characterized by a sawtooth pattern between QRS complexes. Atrial flutter occurs when the sinoatrial node is no longer the primary atrial pacemaker and an ectopic pacemaker resumes pacing. This ectopic pace-maker may have a very high rate, which is represented as a sawtooth pattern on the electrocardiogram (ECG). The QRS complexes appear normal.**

1. An atrial flutter is not a ventricular rhythm.
2. An atrial flutter has a very definite pattern between the QRS complexes.
4. An atrial flutter is associated with heart muscle activity and there is a discernible rhythm.

Client Need: Health Promotion and Maintenance

1 - 1 3

② **When administering nitroprusside sodium (Nitropress), the nurse will need to protect the fluid from light by wrapping the infusion bottle in aluminum foil. Nitropress is a potent arterial/venous vasodilator that increases or decreases cardiac output depending on the extent of preload and afterload reduction.**

1. Unlike Tridil, Nitropress does not require special intravenous tubing. However, Nitropress should only be mixed with distilled water.
3. Unlike Tridil, Nitropress does not require a glass bottle.
4. Nitropress should not be left hanging for more than 24 hours.

Client Need: Physiological Integrity

1 - 1 4

① **The nurse will anticipate administering an antihypertensive medication and scheduling ultrasonographic examinations every 6 months to determine any changes in the size of the aneurysm.**

2. Surgery is not generally performed when an abdominal aortic aneurysm is less than 4 to 5 cm.
3. Gastrointestinal bleeding that produces shock is the presenting sign when an abdominal aortic aneurysm ruptures into the duodenum.
4. Clients do not have complaints if their abdominal aortic aneurysm is asymptomatic.

Client Need: Health Promotion and Maintenance

1 - 1 5

② Signs and symptoms of digoxin toxicity include headaches, yellow-green halo vision, blurred vision, drowsiness, restlessness, muscle weakness, anorexia, nausea, vomiting, diarrhea, and cardiac dysrhythmias.

1. Convulsions are not among the side effects of digoxin administration.

3. Muscle cramps are not among the side effects of digoxin administration.

4. Orthostatic hypotension is not among the side effects of digoxin administration. However, anti-hypertensive agents may cause orthostatic hypotension.

Client Need: Physiological Integrity

1 - 1 6

① The goal of any interventions based on central venous pressure (CVP) reading would be maintaining normal pressure in the right atrium. The CVP is an estimate of the pressure within the right atrium and provides information concerning the function of the right side of the heart. Changes in CVP represent changes in blood volume and in the venous return to the right side of the heart.

2. Central venous pressure (CVP) readings estimate the pressure in the right atrium. CVP does not pertain to pressure in the pulmonary artery.

3. Central venous pressure (CVP) readings will not detect dysrhythmias in the left ventricle.

4. Central venous pressure (CVP) readings will not promote circulation through the aorta.

Client Need: Physiological Integrity

1 - 1 7

③ The nurse would recommend that the client who is experiencing Raynaud's phenomenon wear gloves when exposed to cold or cold objects. Raynaud's phenomenon is initiated by exposure to cold. (Occasionally it is initiated by emotional disturbance.) Raynaud's phenomenon is characterized by intermittent attacks of pallor followed by cyanosis; then the digits become red and return to normal.

1. Moving to a warmer climate, although desirable, may not be beneficial since symptoms may continue to occur in the cooler weather of that climate.

2. The medications used are focused on vasodilatation, not relief of pain. Medications include Nifedipine (Procardia) and isoxuprine (Vasodilan).

4. Raynaud's phenomenon is a vasospastic disorder of small cutaneous arteries that is self-limiting. Episodes last about 15 minutes, frequently involving the fingers, toes, and ears. Limiting activities is not necessary.

Client Need: Health Promotion and Maintenance

1-18

(2) **The nurse will suspect venous insufficiency and will notify the physician. With venous insufficiency, the casted limb feels warmer than the uncasted limb and appears bluish or mottled in color.**

1. The hallmark of arterial insufficiency is intermittent claudication, experienced as sharp, unrelenting, constant pain.

3. Compartmental syndrome occurs when a structure such as a nerve or tendon is constricted in a space, as in carpal tunnel syndrome. Symptoms include throbbing pain out of proportion to the original condition or injury, pain that is not relieved by analgesics, pain experienced when flexing or extending the affected body part.

4. A fat embolus produces symptoms that include hypoxia, tachycardia, dyspnea, and pallor.

Client Need: Safe, Effective Care Environment

1-19

(3) **Pain associated with activity is characteristic of intermittent claudication. The pain is caused by inadequate arterial circulation to contracting muscle. Severe pain occurs when walking and subsides with rest. The inadequate blood supply may be due to arterial spasms, atherosclerosis, arteriosclerosis, or an occlusion.**

1, 2, and 4. Extensive discoloration, dependent edema, and petechia are not characteristic of intermittent claudication.

Client Need: Physiological Integrity

1-20

(4) **A client with stage II hypertension may be treated with metoprolol (Lopressor). Metoprolol inhibits a portion of the sympathetic nervous system and reduces myocardial contractility, heart rate, and blood pressure. This medication belongs in the group of medications called beta-blockers, used to treat hypertension and arrhythmias. Stage II hypertension is hypertension with blood pressures of 160–170 mmHg systolic and 100–109 mmHg diastolic. These pressures are typically treated medically.**

1. Levothyroxine (Synthroid) is a thyroid hormone replacement and does not impact hypertension.

2. Phenytoin (Dilantin) is an anticonvulsant and does not impact hypertension.

3. Cefprozil (Cefzil) is an antibiotic and does not impact hypertension.

Client Need: Physiological Integrity

1 - 2 1

① **The nurse will teach the client that sitting or standing in one position for long periods of time is not recommended, since this contributes to venous stasis. Thromboangiitis obliterans (Buerger's disease) is characterized by inflammation of the small and intermediate arteries and veins. It results in the formation of thrombi and eventually occlusion of vessels.**

2. Clients with Buerger's disease should absolutely not use tobacco in any form. Research indicates that heavy smoking is either a causative or a contributive factor. Cigarette smoking causes arterial constriction and increases platelet adhesion, which leads to thrombus formation.

3. Walking is advisable and helps prevent stasis of blood flow.

4. Clients with Buerger's disease should avoid injury to the extremities because of the likelihood of infection due to poor circulation.

Client Need: Health Promotion and Maintenance

1 - 2 2

① **The nurse would monitor the client's pulse rate for signs of postoperative shock. The earliest sign of shock is a pulse rate that steadily increases over time. An increase in the heart rate is an attempt to compensate for a decrease in cardiac volume.**

2. Pulse pressure is the difference between the diastolic and systolic pressures. The pulse pressure would drop if a client were in shock. However, a drop in pulse pressure would not be the earliest sign of shock.

3. Body temperature refers to the balance between the heat produced by the body and the heat lost by the body. A drop in body temperature would not be the first sign of shock.

4. Respiration would increase in response to postoperative shock, but this would not be the first sign of shock.

Client Need: Health Promotion and Maintenance

1 - 2 3

③ **Ace inhibitors such as enalapril (Vasotec) decrease blood pressure by inhibiting the angiotensin-converting enzyme. Therefore, angiotensin (a potent vasoconstrictor) is not released.**

1. Vasodilators such as hydralazine hydrochloride (Apresoline) and diazoxide (Hyperstat) act primarily on the smooth muscle of arterioles to cause vasodilation.

2. Beta-adrenergic blockers such as propranolol hydrochloride (Inderal) decrease the blood pressure by blocking the beta-adrenergic impulses.

4. Diuretics such as furosemide (Lasix) block the reabsorption of sodium and chloride and thus decrease fluid volume and blood pressure.

Client Need: Physiological Integrity

1 - 2 4

③ **Hypothyroidism affects the body's ability to metabolize digitalis and predisposes a client to digitalis toxicity.**

1. Pneumonia does not affect the body's ability to metabolize digoxin.

2. Hypokalemia, not hyperkalemia, predisposes a client to digitalis toxicity.

4. Hypercalcemia, not hypocalcemia, predisposes a client to digitalis toxicity.

Client Need: Physiological Integrity

1 - 2 5

① **An elevation of the CK (creatine kinase) MB (isoenzyme of creatine kinase associated with the cardiac muscle) is the best indication of myocardial damage within the first 2 to 4 hours following the acute ischemic event. The enzyme CK (MB) is found almost exclusively in the myocardium.**

2. An elevation of CK (creatine kinase) MM (isoenzyme of creatine kinase associated with skeletal muscle) is an indicator of skeletal muscle damage, not myocardial damage.

3. An elevation of LDH1 and LDH2 is indicative of myocardial necrosis. Approximately 80% of clients show an increase of these enzymes within 48 hours after a myocardial infarction.

4. The enzyme SGOT (serum glutamic-oxaloacetic transaminase) is found in the liver, and to some extent, in the skeletal muscle. Therefore, an elevated SGOT is not helpful in confirming damage to the myocardium.

Client Need: Physiological Integrity

1 - 2 6

① **Laboratory values with the least risk for heart disease would be a high-density lipoprotein (HDL) of 70 mg/dl and a low-density lipoprotein (LDL) of 110 mg/dl. High-density lipoproteins, although a form of cholesterol, tend to bind with low-density lipoproteins, thereby lowering total cholesterol levels. HDL levels above 35 mg/dl are desirable. Low-density lipoproteins contribute to elevated total cholesterol levels, and levels < 130 mg/dl are most desirable. The combination of an elevated HDL and low LDL will have the least risk for heart disease.**

2, 3, and 4. All are associated with heart disease. An HDL of 30 mg/dl is too low and LDL levels of >130 mg/dl are too high.

Client Need: Health Promotion and Maintenance

1 - 2 7

④ Clients with stomach ulcers may not receive thrombolytic therapy. Thrombolytic therapy is the administration of medications specifically designed to dissolve blood clots. Muscle damage associated with arterial blockage by blood clots has been completely avoided with the use of these medications. Because these medications affect blood viscosity and clotting mechanisms, possible contradictions include disorders that are hemorrhagic in nature. Bleeding ulcers, recent surgeries, blood dyscrasias, and aneurysms are examples of disorders that may contraindicate such treatment.

1. Antithrombolytic therapy has been found to be very successful if administered early on in the course of the event.

2. Nausea is not an uncommon symptom associated with an evolving myocardial infarction and would not prevent a client from receiving antithrombolytic therapy.

3. Persons who take antihypertensive medications may receive thrombolytic therapy.

Client Need: Physiological Integrity

1 - 2 8

② Nifedipine (Procardia) is a calcium channel blocker. Calcium channel blockers tend to inhibit the flow of calcium ions across cell membranes. This class of drugs is specific for cardiac tissue and decreases excitability of cardiac tissue. As a result, the heart rate decreases and blood pressure drops.

1. Metoprolol (Lopressor) belongs in the group of drugs called beta-blockers.
3. Nitroglycerine (Nitrostat) is an antianginal vasodilatory medication.
4. Aspirin is an antipyretic analgesic with antiplatelet activity.

Client Need: Safe, Effective Care Environment

1 - 2 9

① An apical pulse of 74 beats per minute (BPM) is too low for an infant 7 months old and should be reported immediately. Cardiac catheterization can result in dysrhythmia or rates that are too slow or too fast. This may occur because of temporary or permanent damage to the conduction system.

2. Access to the vessels would have been in the right femoral area. Coolness of the left foot is most likely related to environmental temperature, not the catheterization.

3. Clubbing is not related to catheterization. It is related to the cardiac defect and usually develops slowly as a result of hypoxia to the distal tissues.

4. An infant 7 months old may experience anxiety in the presence of strangers and in connection with a new procedure.

Client Need: Health Promotion and Maintenance

1-30

③ **The nurse will limit the motion of the affected extremity and assess the puncture site. The client is at risk for hemorrhage from the puncture site following an angiocardiography.**

1. Fluid intake should be encouraged to flush out the radiopaque dye used in the angiocardiography. However, the client should be placed in a supine position with the affected leg straight and the head elevated no more than 30 degrees.

2. Application of heat would facilitate hemorrhage, as would passive exercise to the affected extremity.

4. The client should be encouraged to drink plenty of fluids to flush out the dye used in the angiocardiography. Ambulation is contraindicated due to the likelihood of hemorrhage at the puncture site. The site needs time to heal.

Client Need: Health Promotion and Maintenance

1-31

② **The nurse will recognize a capillary wedge pressure of 18 mm Hg as elevated. The normal pulmonary capillary wedge pressure is 5 to 12 mm Hg. The higher the pressure, the more severe the heart failure. Pressures that exceed 25 to 30 mm Hg are associated with pulmonary edema.**

1. This client's pulmonary capillary wedge pressure is 18 mm Hg (normal is 5 to 12 mm Hg).

3. The capillary wedge pressure is above normal, not less than normal.

4. At this point, the pulmonary capillary wedge pressure is 18 mm Hg and is considered elevated. However, if the pressure should continue to rise, it would become life threatening.

Client Need: Physiological Integrity

1-32

③ **The nurse will anticipate the administration of digitalis. The rhythm shown on the client's monitor depicts atrial fibrillation. It is characterized by an irregular rhythm with no identifiable P waves.**

1. Lidocaine (Zylocaine) is administered to treat ventricular tachycardia.

2. Atropine (Atropair) increases the heart rate. Therefore, it would not be administered, since the client's heart rate is already fluctuating between 120 and 140 beats per minute (BPM). Atropine is administered to clients who have slow rhythms.

4. Procainamide (Pronestyl) is frequently indicated for ventricular dysrhythmia, not atrial dysrhythmia.

Client Need: Physiological Integrity

1 - 3 3

③ **Lidocaine (Xylocaine) is the drug of choice for clients who experience ventricular tachy-cardia and are hemodynamically stable.**

1. Digoxin (Lanoxin) is the drug of choice for atrial fibrillation.

2 and 4. Propranolol (Inderal) and verapamil (Calan) are administered for supraventricular tachy-cardia.

Client need: Physiological Integrity

1 - 3 4

② **The nurse will recognize the rhythm strip as an example of sinus tachycardia. There is a P wave for every QRS, the rhythm is regular, and the PR interval and QRS intervals are within normal limits. The only abnormality is the rate.**

1. The rate of a normal sinus rhythm is between 60 and 100 beats per minute (BPM). Sinus tachy-cardia has a rate between 100 and 150 BPM.

3. Ventricular tachycardia is characterized by 3 or 4 consecutive premature ventricular contrac-tions.

4. Atrial fibrillation is characterized by an irregular rhythm with no identifiable P wave.

Client Need: Physiological Integrity

1 - 3 5

③ **The rhythm strip is an example of premature ventricular contractions. The PVCs are characterized by wide, bizarre QRSs, no associated P waves preceding the QRS com-plex, and the T waves are in the opposite direction from the QRS deflection.**

1. Second-degree AV block type II results in intermittently dropped QRS complexes with normal-appearing P waves occurring at regular intervals.

2. Premature junctional contractions are characterized by upward impulses from the AV junction to the atria; thus in lead II, the P waves are inverted and the PR interval shortens to 0.12 sec-onds.

4. In third-degree AV block, all impulses from the atria are blocked, resulting in complete disasso-ciation of the atria and ventricles and causing differences in heart rate and QRS durations.

Client Need: Physiological Integrity

1 - 3 6

② The immediate treatment is defibrillation. The dysrhythmia depicted is ventricular fibrillation. This is characterized by a bumpy line of unidentifiable waves. This is a life-threatening dysrhythmia, and without prompt treatment, death will occur.

1. Cardioversion cannot be performed because it requires that the electric shock be correlated with the QRS complex. There are no QRS complexes with ventricular fibrillation. Therefore, the machine would never fire if it is programmed for cardioversion.

3. Lidocaine (Xylocaine) is utilized for ventricular tachycardia and frequent PVCs. After defibrillation and restoration of a rhythm, a lidocaine drip will probably be initiated to decrease the irritability of the myocardium, but first the rhythm must be converted out of ventricular fibrillation.

4. Sodium bicarbonate is administered to correct the acidosis that occurs with cardiac arrest. It will probably be given to a client with ventricular fibrillation, but again, the client needs to be defibrillated first. If the client is not converted, the client will die.

Client Need: Physiological Integrity

1 - 3 7

④ The electrocardiograph will be documented as normal sinus rhythm. A normal electrocardiograph consists of a series of waveforms designated by the letters P, Q, R, S, and T. The P waves represent depolarization (contraction) of the atria.

1, 2, and 3. All are incorrect electrocardiograph rhythms.

Client Need: Physiological Integrity

1 - 3 8

② This strip depicts second-degree AV block, type I. This dysrhythmia is characterized by a PR interval that progressively lengthens until a P wave is not followed by a QRS complex.

1. First-degree AV block is characterized by a PR interval greater than 0.20 seconds.

3. Second-degree AV block, type II is characterized by nonconducted sinus impulses despite constant PR intervals.

4. In third-degree AV Block the entire sinus or atrial impulses are blocked and the atria and ventricles are forced to beat independently.

Client Need: Physiological Integrity

1 - 3 9

② Sinus tachycardia may best be described as a regular rhythm with a rate greater than 100 beats per minute. Sinus tachycardia originates in the sinus node and follows the normal conduction pathways through the ventricles. In the adult client, the parameters of sinus tachycardia are generally considered to be between 100 and 150 beats per minute (BPM). Rates greater than 150 beats per minute are not thought to originate from the sinoatrial node, but from an ectopic site above the ventricles; hence the term supraventricular tachycardia.

1. A chaotic rhythm with no cardiac output is most likely a ventricular fibrillation.
3. A ventricular rhythm with variable output is most likely ventricular tachycardia.
4. A regular rhythm with rates between 60 and 100 beats per minute is usually considered normal sinus rhythm in the adult client.

Client Need: Physiological Integrity

1 - 4 0

③ Sinus bradycardia is best described as a normal rhythm with a rate of less than 60 beats per minute (BPM). Sinus bradycardia originates from the sinus node and follows the regular conduction pathways through the ventricles. In the adult client, rates of less than 60 beats per minute (BPM) are considered to be bradycardic. This term does not define pathology; it defines a rhythm that may be completely benign.

1. An irregular ventricular rhythm would describe an idioventricular or ventricular rhythm.
2. An irregular ventricular rate with variable numbers of P waves between complexes describes a complete, or third-degree, heart block.
4. A normal rhythm with a rate of greater than 100 BPM describes sinus tachycardia.

Client Need: Physiological integrity

1 - 4 1

④ As a rule, chest pains that are not relieved by 3 doses of nitroglycerin should be evaluated by a physician. Anginal pain is often managed well and without complications. However, angina not relieved by repeated doses of nitroglycerin should be evaluated for myocardial ischemia or infarction.

1. Nitroglycerin should be kept with the client who experiences angina and should be accessible; protecting the medication from extreme temperatures is usually adequate for storage.
2. Nitroglycerin is usually replaced 6 months after opening to maintain potency.
3. This medication is to be taken via the sublingual route, not swallowed.

Client Need: Physiological Integrity

1 - 4 2

① **Primary interventions contribute to the prevention of a disease process. Examples of primary intervention include immunizations against disease and teaching wellness.**

2 and 3. Acute and secondary interventions focus on the diagnosis and treatment of a disease process.

4. Tertiary interventions focus on rehabilitation from a disease process.

Client Need: Health Promotion and Maintenance

1 - 4 3

④ **Clients who experience nausea and have a pulse rate of 52 beats per minute (BPM) should be instructed to withhold their morning dose of digoxin and come to the office or hospital for evaluation. Digoxin is a cardiac antiarrhythmic with positive inotropic qualities (it regulates and strengthens the heart's contractions). Digoxin toxicity is a risk for anyone taking this medication because it has a relatively narrow therapeutic range. Signs and symptoms of digoxin toxicity include nausea, dizziness, visual disturbances, bradycardia, and other arrhythmias.**

1. This client may be experiencing digoxin toxicity. Therefore, the client should not take any more digoxin until further evaluation.

2. Antacids are not recommended in this situation because they could mask symptoms.

3. When digoxin is taken, it is recommended that it be taken on an empty stomach.

Client Need: Physiological Integrity

1 - 4 4

① **Premature ventricular contractions (PVCs) may be benign contractions that originate from the ventricles, rather than the atria, and are early in the cycle. They are usually wide and rather bizarre in their morphology. It is not uncommon to notice rare PVCs on a monitored client who has no cardiac pathology; they may be completely benign.**

2. PVCs may be caused by substances that increase sympathetic tone, such as caffeine and nicotine.

3. PVCs do not necessarily indicate a pending lethal arrhythmia, although frequent premature ventricular contractions, symptomatic PVCs, or coupled PVCs may indicate an arrhythmia disorder.

4. Clients experiencing myocardial infarctions may have numerous arrhythmias, including PVCs; however, all persons having PVCs are not necessarily experiencing myocardial infarctions.

Client Need: Physiological Integrity

1 - 4 5

① Approximately 50% of people over the age of 65 are experiencing hypertension.

③ African Americans are 50% more likely to experience hypertension than Caucasians.

④ Clients who have diabetes are more likely to become hypertensive.

2. High serum lipid levels are associated with hypertension, not low lipid levels.

5. A sedentary lifestyle is associated with hypertension, not an active lifestyle. Regular exercise helps to control weight and decrease hypertension.

Client Need: Health Promotion and Maintenance

1 - 4 6

② Morphine sulfate administered IV will decrease cardiac workload by reducing contractility.

③ Morphine sulfate administered IV will lower blood pressure and thereby decrease cardiac workload. It is very important to monitor the vital signs of clients receiving morphine because hypotension and bradycardia are adverse reactions.

1. Morphine sulfate administered IV reduces myocardial oxygen consumption. By reducing myocardial oxygen consumption, the cardiac workload will be decreased.

4. Morphine sulfate administered IV will reduce the heart rate. Reducing the heart rate will decrease cardiac workload.

5. Morphine sulfate is an analgesic. However, reducing pain does not directly lower myocardial oxygen consumption. Reducing pain will lower the client's anxiety level.

Client Need: Physiological Integrity

1 - 4 7

① Hypercholesterolemia is a risk factor associated with sudden cardiac death (SCD).

② Coronary artery disease (CAD) is the most common cause of sudden cardiac death (SCD).

④ Cigarette smoking is a risk factor associated with sudden cardiac death (SCD).

3. Hypertension, not hypotension, is associated with sudden cardiac death (SCD).

5. Male gender, in particular among African Americans, is among the risk factors associated with sudden cardiac death (SCD).

Client Need: Physiological Integrity

1 - 4 8

Fill in the blank correct answer:

Contraction of the heart chambers is known as <u>systole</u>. During systole, the myocardial fibers shorten, making the heart chambers smaller and causing blood to be forced out.

Practice Test 2

Endocrine System and Diabetes

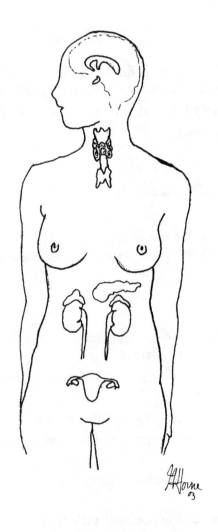

The Female Endocrine System

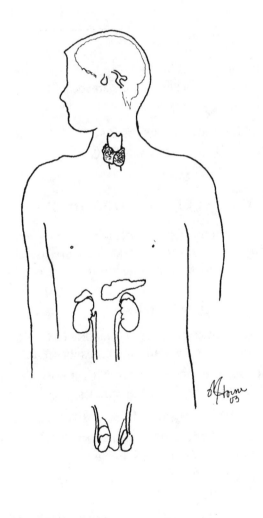

The Male Endocrine System

OVERVIEW

The endocrine system acts in concert with the nervous system to control activities in the body and maintain physiological equilibrium (homeostasis). There is a great difference as to how each system accomplishes its tasks. The nervous system transmits nerve impulses to muscles and glands, which cause them to respond immediately. The glands in the endocrine system secrete hormones, which are transmitted in body fluid to the tissues they influence. The process may take several minutes, hours, or days.

The body contains a second type of glands, the exocrine glands, which secrete chemical substances through ducts to (a) the surface of the body, i.e., tear and sweat glands; (b) body cavities, i.e., salivary glands, which empty into the mouth; and (c) body organs. For instance, the liver, gall bladder, and pancreas empty bile, enzymes, and digestive juices into the duodenum, and mucus-producing glands empty their secretions into the respiratory passages of the lungs. The exocrine glands do not constitute a body system. They will be discussed individually when they are relevant to other body systems that are reviewed in this book.

ENDOCRINE GLANDS

The glands specific to the endocrine system are the pituitary, the thyroid, the parathyroids, the adrenals, and the pancreas. These glands are located in various parts of the body. The hormones they secrete regulate

- Bone growth
- Maturation of sex organs
- Maturation of reproductive cells
- Metabolic rate within all the individual cells of the body
- Endocrine activity overall

PITUITARY GLAND (HYPOPHYSIS)

The pituitary gland is located at the base of the brain. It is small in size and attaches to the hypothalamus by the pituitary stalk. There are two distinct areas of the pituitary gland: the anterior lobe and the posterior lobe. Each lobe has its own secretions.

Anterior Lobe Secretions

ADRENOCORTICOTROPIC HORMONE (ACTH) The adrenocorticotropic hormone stimulates the growth of the adrenal cortex and increases its secretion of steroid hormone, mainly cortisol.

GONADOTROPIC HORMONE This stimulates the development of the reproductive organs: the testes in males and the ovaries in females.

GROWTH HORMONE (GH, SOMATOTROPIN) Growth hormone acts on bones to stimulate growth.

THYROID-STIMULATING HORMONE (TSH, THYROTROPIN) This stimulates the growth of the thyroid gland and the secretion of thyroxine.

PROLACTIN (PRL) Prolactin promotes the growth of breast tissue and stimulates and sustains milk production after birth.

MELANOCYTE-STIMULATING HORMONE (MSH) The melanocyte-stimulating hormone (MSH) influences the formation of melanin and causes pigmentation of the skin.

POSTERIOR LOBE SECRETIONS These hormones are formed in the hypothalamus. However, the secretion comes through the posterior pituitary gland.

ANTIDIURETIC HORMONE (ADH, VASOPRESSIN) The antidiuretic hormone stimulates reabsorption of water by the kidney tubules. Also, the antidiuretic hormone can raise blood pressure by constricting the arterioles.

OXYTOCIN Oxytocin stimulates the uterus to contract during childbirth in order to maintain labor. Oxytocin is secreted when an infant sucks and thereby facilitates the production of milk from the mammary glands.

DISEASES/DISORDERS OF THE PITUITARY GLAND (HYPOPHYSIS) INCLUDE

Dwarfism (Hypopituitary Dwarfism)

This condition is associated with congenital hyposecretion of growth hormone (GH). These children are normal mentally; however, their bones are small and undeveloped.

Gigantism

This condition is associated with oversecretion of the growth hormone and is a chronic progressive disorder that begins before epiphyseal closure. Oversecretion may cause a person's height to exceed 8 feet. This condition is rare and is usually associated with a tumor of the pituitary gland. Hormones other than GH are also likely to secrete excessively. This results in many metabolic disturbances that shorten life expectancy.

Acromegaly

This condition is associated with oversecretion of the growth hormone and is a chronic progressive disease. Acromegaly occurs after epiphyseal closure and results in bone thickening and enlargement of the viscera. The client also has enlarged hands and feet, large tongue and nose, and a protruding jaw.

Diabetes Insipidus (Pituitary Diabetes Insipidus)

This disorder involves faulty or insufficient water reabsorption due to a deficiency of vasopressin (antidiuretic hormone or ADH). ADH is secreted by the posterior lobe of the pituitary gland. Diabetes insipidus can have many causes but is usually due to organic lesions. (Do not confuse pituitary diabetes insipidus with nephrogenic diabetes insipidus, a rare congenital disease of water disturbances resulting from renal tubular resistance to vasopressin).

THYROID GLAND

The thyroid gland is located in the neck. It regulates metabolism in the body cells and stimulates the passage of calcium into the bones and blood; it also regulates calcium levels in the blood.

The thyroid gland secretes three hormones: Thyroxin (T-4); triiodothyronine (T-3); and calcitonin (thyrocalcitonin). T-3 and T-4 are synthesized (made or manufactured) in the thyroid gland from iodine, which the blood absorbs from food. Calcitonin secretes when blood calcium levels are high. Calcitonin stimulates calcium to leave the blood and pass into the bones. In this manner, blood calcium levels are kept in balance.

DISEASES/DISORDERS OF THE THYROID GLAND INCLUDE

Hypothyroidism

This condition results from low serum (blood) levels of thyroid hormone. It is prevalent in women and also in people 40 to 50 years of age. Hyposecretion of the thyroid gland results in cretinism in children and myxedema in adults.

Cretinism

This disorder affects children and is manifested by lack of physical and mental growth in infancy and early childhood.

Myxedema

This condition occurs due to atrophy of the thyroid gland and lack of hormone production. The client's skin becomes dry and puffy due to a mucus-like material that accumulates under the skin.

Thyroiditis

This form of hypothyroidism is caused by inflammation of the thyroid gland. It is more common in women than men. There are three types of thyroiditis: (1) Autoimmune thyroiditis (Hashimoto's), in which antibodies to thyroid antigens are carried in the blood. (2) Subacute granulomatous (Riedel's), which usually follows mumps, influenza, coxsackie virus, or adenovirus infection. This is a rare condition with unknown etiology. (3) Chronic infective and noninfective (miscellaneous) thyroiditis, resulting from bacterial invasion.

Simple Goiter (Nontoxic)

Simple goiter is an enlargement of the thyroid gland not caused by inflammation or neoplasm (new growth). This condition usually is classified as either endemic or sporadic.

ENDEMIC GOITER This condition is caused by an inadequate dietary intake of iodine, as when crops are grown in iodine-depleted soil or as an effect of malnutrition during pregnancy, adolescence, or menopause, when the body demands more hormones.

SPORADIC GOITER This condition occurs following intake (ingestion) of certain drugs or foods that are goitrogenic. Sporadic goiter affects no specific population segment. Specific foods that are goitrogenic include: Rutabagas, cabbage, soybeans, peanuts, peaches, peas, strawberries, spinach, and radishes. Both drugs and foods containing goitrogenic agents decrease thyroxin (T-4), which is needed to regulate metabolism in cells. Goitrogenic drugs include: Propylthiouracil, iodides, phenylbutazone, para-aminosalicylic acid, cobalt, and lithium. In pregnancy, these substances may cross the placental barrier and affect the fetus.

NOTE: Inherited defects may be responsible for the lack of T-4 synthesis or impaired iodine metabolism.

Hyperthyroidism (Graves's Disease; Basedow's Disease; Thyrotoxicosis)

This is a metabolic disorder resulting from overproduction of thyroid hormone. The metabolic rates in cells increase, causing nodular or adenomatous goiter. Protrusion of the eyeballs results from swelling of tissue behind the eyeballs. Hyperthyroidism may be caused by genetic or immunologic factors.

PARATHYROID GLANDS

The parathyroid glands are four in number and are embedded in the tissue of the thyroid gland. They are small and oval-shaped, measuring approximately 6mm long and 3mm wide.

The parathyroid glands secrete parathyroid hormone (PTH), also known as parathormone. PTH regulates calcium and phosphorus metabolism.

DISEASES/DISORDERS OF THE PARATHYROID GLANDS INCLUDE

Hypoparathyroidism

Hypoparathyroidism (hyposecretion of the parathyroid glands) usually develops as a result of disease or injury. Often the injury is caused by surgery. Congenital malfunction is another cause. As the name implies, hypoparathyroidism is underproduction of parathyroid hormone (PTH), which leads to hypocalcemia, or inability of calcium to enter the bloodstream from the bones. Symptoms include: Muscle weakness, muscle spasms, and tetany (continuous muscle contractions). Usually this condition is correctable with the administration of calcium and vitamin D. However, some complications are not reversible.

Hyperparathyroidism

Hyperparathyroidism is caused by excessive production of PTH, leading to hypercalcemia, or excessive loss of calcium from the bones into the bloodstream. This is followed by an increase in renal and GI absorption of calcium. Bones become decalcified and susceptible to fracture, and kidney stones may develop. Hyperparathyroidism is associated with the growth of parathyroid tumors. Treatment is focused on the resection of these tumors.

ADRENAL GLANDS

These are two triangular-shaped glands, each one attached to the top of a kidney. They are also known as the suprarenal glands. Each weighs about 4 grams and is composed of two parts, the inner, or medulla, and the outer, or cortex. Each part secretes different hormones. The adrenal medulla secretes catecholamines and the adrenal cortex secretes steroids.

Adrenal Medulla

The adrenal medulla is controlled by the sympathetic nervous system and is closely involved in the body's adjustments to stress and emotional changes. The three catecholamines secreted by the adrenal medulla are: Dopamine, norepinephrine (noradrenaline), and epinephrine (adrenaline). The primary function of dopamine is to dilate systemic arteries, increase cardiac output, and increase blood flow to the kidneys. The primary function of norepinephrine is to constrict vessels and raise blood pressure. Epinephrine increases cardiac activity, dilates the bronchial tubes, and stimulates the production of glucose.

Diseases/Disorders of the Adrenal Medulla Include

PHEOCHROMOCYTOMA This is a tumor of the adrenal medulla. The tumor cells produce excess secretion of epinephrine and norepinephrine. Symptoms are: Hypertension, palpitations, severe headaches, sweating, flushing of the face, and muscle spasms. Possible treatments may include surgery to remove the tumor and administration of antihypertensive drugs.

Adrenal Cortex

The adrenal cortex secretes three steroid hormones, or corticosteroids. These are the mineralocorticoids, such as aldosterone; the glucocorticoids, such as cortisol; and the sex hormones, including androgens, estrogens, and progestins.

Mineralocorticoids are essential to life. They regulate the amount of mineral salts (electrolytes) that are retained in the body. Glucocorticoids such as cortisol increase the ability of cells to create new sugars from fats and proteins. They regulate the amount of sugars, fats, and proteins in the blood and cells. Androgens, estrogens, and progestins are among the male and female hormones that produce secondary sex characteristics such as facial hair and the development of breasts. They are essential for reproduction.

Diseases/Disorders of the Adrenal Cortex Include

ADRENAL VERILISM (HYPERSECRETION) This condition is due to excessive output of adrenal androgens and is caused by hyperplasia or tumor in adult women. Symptoms are: Amenorrhea, hirsutism (excessive hair on face and body), acne, and deepened voice. Treatments include drug therapy to suppress androgen production, and adrenalectomy.

CUSHING'S DISEASE (HYPERSECRETION) (HYPERFUNCTION) This condition is caused by hyperfunction of the adrenal cortex with increased glucocorticoid (cortisol) secretion. Due to the overstimulation of ACTH (adrenocorticotrophic hormone) from the pituitary gland and adrenal cortex hyperplasia (excessive growth of normal cells), obesity, moonlike fullness of the face, and excess deposits of fat in the chest and the back (buffalo hump) may occur. Many other conditions result from hypersecretion; namely, hyperglycemia (high blood sugar), hypernatremia (high blood sodium), hypokalemia (low blood potassium), osteoporosis, and hypertension. Treatment consists of hypophysectomy or pituitary irradiation in order to decrease ACTH secretion.

NOTE: Occasionally, a tumor of the adrenal gland may be associated with excessive secretion of cortisol and the same clinical features will be manifested. This is known as Cushing's syndrome and is treated surgically by adrenalectomy.

ADDISON'S DISEASE (HYPOSECRETION) Addison's disease is a rare, gradual, and progressive failure of the adrenal cortex. Persons with Addison's disease do not make adequate amounts of glucocorticoids and mineralocorticoids. Hypoglycemia (low blood sugar) occurs where glucocorticoids are deficient. Hyponatremia (low blood sodium) occurs when large amounts of water and salts accumulate in the body due to insufficient mineralocorticoids. Weakness, weight loss, and dark pigmentation of the skin due to increased blood levels of MSH (melanocyte-stimulating hormone) also occur. Treatment consists of daily replacement of cortisone and salts.

PANCREAS

The pancreas is located behind the stomach and is both an exocrine and an endocrine gland. Its head is attached to the duodenum and its tail reaches to the spleen. The hormone-producing cells of the pancreas are known as the islets of Langerhans. Ten to 30% of these cells produce glucagons and the remaining 60 to 90% produce insulin. The islets of Langerhans carry on the endocrine functions of the pancreas. The remaining pancreatic cells carry on its exocrine functions. The exocrine cells form glands that resemble a cluster of grapes. They have individual ducts that connect to the common bile duct, which then empties into the duodenum. The substances produced by the exocrine cells are known as enzymes and pancreatic juices. They contribute to the digestion of foods in the small intestine.

DISEASES/DISORDERS ASSOCIATED WITH THE EXOCRINE FUNCTIONS OF THE PANCREAS INCLUDE

Pancreatitis

Pancreatitis (inflammation of the pancreas) is a life-threatening disorder caused by pancreatic digestive enzymes attacking and damaging the pancreas. The attacking enzymes cause autodigestion (digestion of tissues by their own secretions), necrosis (tissue death), gangrene, and hemorrhage. Causes include alcoholism, gallstones, abdominal trauma, and certain drugs.

DISEASES/DISORDERS ASSOCIATED WITH THE ENDOCRINE FUNCTIONS OF THE PANCREAS INCLUDE

Diabetes Mellitus

This chronic condition requires insulin replacement, dietary planning, and exercise as treatment. Diabetes is a disorder of carbohydrate, fat, and protein metabolism resulting from impaired beta cell synthesis, impaired release of insulin, or inability of body tissues to metabolize glucose. Diabetes mellitus occurs in four forms:

1. Type 1 diabetes: This condition is due to loss of beta cell function and insulin deficiency. Type 1 diabetes is seen mostly in children and adolescents. Effective treatment is achieved with insulin replacement, diet, and exercise.

2. Type 2 diabetes: This condition results from a deficiency in insulin secretion and is seen mostly in older adults. Effective treatment includes: Diet, exercise, and oral hypoglycemic agents. These oral agents stimulate the release of insulin.

3. Gestational diabetes (GDM): This condition occurs during pregnancy; however, glucose levels usually return to normal after delivery.

4. The "other types": Genetic defects, endocrinopathies (diseases resulting from disorders of an endocrine gland or glands), and exposure to certain drugs or chemicals can result in various forms of diabetes known as "other types."

Practice Test 2

Questions

2 - 1

An emaciated client is to receive NPH insulin 20 units 1 hour before breakfast daily. The insulin should be administered:

1. intramuscularly at 90 degrees.
2. subcutaneously at 90 degrees.
3. intramuscularly at 45 degrees.
4. subcutaneously at 45 degrees.

2 - 2

An adolescent 15 years of age is hospitalized with type 1 insulin-dependent diabetes. Which of the following is essential to teach the client?

1. Insulin dosage will be determined by food intake.
2. Insulin will have to be administered the rest of the client's life.
3. Insulin dosage will be adjusted by the way the client eats.
4. Insulin will be adjusted as the client grows older.

2 - 3

The only insulin that can be administered IV is:

_____.

Fill in the blank

2 - 4

Your client is receiving 30 units of NPH insulin daily at 7:00 a.m. What would the client need to do each day?

1. exercise for 30 minutes prior to lunch
2. consume a snack each day at 4:00 p.m.
3. exercise for 30 minutes prior to bedtime
4. consume a bedtime snack at 9:00 p.m.

2 - 5

A 26-year-old gravida 1 has type 1 insulin-dependent diabetes. Due to a change in insulin requirements during the first trimester, the nurse will carefully observe the client for signs of:

1. hypoglycemia.
2. ketoacidosis.
3. hyperglycemia.
4. pregnancy-induced hypertension.

2 - 6

A client is to receive 12 units of Regular insulin and 26 units of NPH insulin subcutaneously daily. Which procedure is correct?

1. Store all insulin in the refrigerator.
2. Massage the injection site after the injection.
3. Draw up the NPH insulin first, and then the Regular.
4. Roll the NPH insulin bottle between the palms of the hands prior to drawing it up.

2 - 7

Your client was started on 0.1 mg of Synthroid daily. What teaching will the client need in relation to this medication?

1. Take the medication with meals.
2. Do not substitute generic brands.
3. Dosage can be self-adjusted based on energy needs.
4. Expect to lose 10 to 15 pounds within the first 6 months of therapy.

2 - 8

Your client had a bilateral adrenalectomy and Solu-Cortef has been prescribed. You know the purpose of this medication is to:

1. lower serum glucose.
2. relieve postoperative pain.
3. prevent adrenal insufficiency.
4. decrease the risk of postoperative stress ulcers.

2 - 9

A 22-year-old female is admitted to the unit with a blood glucose of 822 mg/dl and an arterial blood pH of 7.02. The client is unresponsive. The insulin type and route you anticipate administering is:

1. Humulin N given intravenously.
2. Humulin R given intravenously.
3. Humulin 70/30 given intravenously.
4. Humulin N given subcutaneously only.

2 - 10

A client is admitted to the nursing unit with a medical diagnosis of chronic hypothyroidism. The nursing assessment reveals a body temperature of 90°F, an apical heart rate of 58, and a respiratory rate of 10 breaths per minute. The nurse immediately recognizes these findings as indicative of:

1. hypercalcemia.
2. hypermagnesemia.
3. metabolic acidosis.
4. myxedema coma.

2 - 11

A client with diabetes has been taking tolazamide 100 mg po daily. The client has just had a hip replacement and is to be on Coumadin 5 mg po daily. You anticipate the following potential changes:

1. an increase in serum glucose levels.
2. a decrease in prothrombin times.
3. a decrease in serum glucose and an increase in prothrombin times.
4. an increase in serum glucose and an increase in prothrombin times.

2 - 12

A client arrives in the emergency department restless, hypotensive, confused, and vomiting. The client's friend states that the client stopped taking betamethasone 4 days ago because it tended to cause heartburn. You anticipate the administration of:

1. large doses of loop diuretics.
2. narcotic analgesics.
3. sodium bicarbonate and Humulin N intravenously.
4. glucocorticoids.

2 - 1 3

Your client is being treated with gluco-corticoids for adrenal insufficiency secondary to abrupt withdrawal of cortisone. You client's friend asks you what happened to the client's adrenal glands. You explain:

1. the adrenal glands were destroyed by the cortisone therapy.
2. the adrenal glands were not really affected and "adrenal insufficiency" is just a loosely applied term.
3. the adrenal glands have probably developed tumors.
4. the adrenal function was suppressed during the cortisone therapy.

2 - 1 4

Your client has been placed on a regime of methylprednisolone because of severe allergies. Your client teaching will include instructions to:

1. taper the medication dose according to the regime.
2. take the medication only on days when allergies flare up.
3. discontinue taking the medication when the symptoms of allergies are no longer noticeable.
4. contact the physician because this is not a recommended therapy for allergic reactions.

2 - 1 5

During a thyroidectomy, a client's parathyroid glands were inadvertently removed. Which of the following laboratory tests must be monitored very closely?

1. urine specific gravity
2. creatine kinase-MB isoenzyme
3. serum calcium
4. amylase

2 - 1 6

The nurse recognizes that clients receiving large dosages of vasopressin (ADH) may experience:

1. facial pallor.
2. headache.
3. flushing.
4. dyspnea.

2 - 1 7

An adolescent with diabetes asks about the use of alcohol. The most appropriate counsel would be:

1. Diabetics require more insulin when they consume alcohol.
2. Alcohol consumption increases blood glucose.
3. Hypoglycemia occurs with alcohol consumption.
4. Diabetics who consume alcohol become intoxicated easily.

2 - 1 8

The physician prescribed 20 units of isophane (NPH) insulin 30 minutes before breakfast daily for a client with diabetes mellitus. The client is to have a midafternoon snack of milk and crackers. The client asks the nurse why the snack is necessary. Which response by the nurse would be best?

1. "It will improve your nutritional status."
2. "It will improve carbohydrate metabolism."
3. "It prevents an insulin reaction."
4. "It prevents diabetic ketoacidosis."

2-19

A client with hypoparathyroidism complains of tingling of the lips, hands, and face. You notify the physician because you suspect the development of which complication?

1. syndrome of inappropriate antidiuretic hormone
2. tetany
3. myxedema
4. Cushing's syndrome

2-20

Hyperthyroidism is suspected in a 28-year-old client. Prescriptions include a radioactive iodine uptake test. The nurse will explain to the client that the chief purpose of a radioactive iodine uptake test is to:

1. ascertain the ability of the thyroid gland to produce thyroxine.
2. measure the activity of the thyroid gland.
3. estimate the concentration of thyrotropic hormone in the thyroid gland.
4. determine the best method of treating the thyroid condition.

2-21

A client develops carpopedal spasms subsequent to a subtotal thyroidectomy. Which of the following medications will the nurse have available for administration?

1. calcium gluconate
2. potassium chloride
3. diazepam
4. phenytoin sodium

2-22

A client undergoes a subtotal thyroidectomy. During the immediate postoperative period, the nurse should assess for laryngeal nerve damage. Which of the following findings would indicate the presence of this problem?

1. facial twitching
2. wheezing
3. hoarseness
4. hemorrhage

2-23

Your client is experiencing acromegaly (hyperpituitarism). You will expect your assessment to reveal:

Select all that apply by placing a ✔ in the square:

☐ 1. enlarged hands and broad feet.
☐ 2. alopecia.
☐ 3. prominent frontal and orbital ridges.
☐ 4. hypertension.
☐ 5. pallor.

2-24

An insulin-dependent diabetic is scheduled for surgery. Administration of Regular insulin is prescribed in lieu of isophane insulin. The client asks why the insulin prescription had to be changed. Which explanation by the nurse would be best?

1. Stress-induced fluctuations in blood glucose can be more adequately managed with Regular insulin.
2. During the first week following recovery from diabetic acidosis, the likelihood of a recurrence is greatest.
3. Diminished activity intensifies the body's response to long-acting insulin.
4. Diabetic acidosis causes a temporary increase in the rate of food absorption.

2-25

A mother makes all of the following comments about her 3-month-old daughter to the nurse. Which comment will indicate to the nurse that the infant may have thyroid hormone deficiency?

1. "My baby smiles a lot."
2. "My baby's good and never cries."
3. "My baby notices toys and knows my voice."
4. "My baby spends a great deal of time watching her hands."

2-26

The physician has prescribed warm saline dressings to be applied to a heel ulcer of a diabetic client. You observe another nurse preparing a clean basin and washcloth to implement the procedure. Which of the following actions should you take?

1. Interrupt the nurse assembling supplies to discuss the procedure.
2. Present the situation for discussion at a staff meeting.
3. Do nothing, as the nurse is following the correct procedure.
4. Do nothing, because nurses are accountable for their own actions.

2-27

A client with Addison's disease is admitted to your unit. What do you expect your assessment to reveal?

1. osteoporosis
2. hirsutism
3. sodium and water retention
4. dark pigmentation of skin

2-28

A client with type 2 non-insulin-dependent diabetes takes 5 mg po daily of glyburide for glucose control. Which statement by the client indicates a need for further teaching?

1. "I will not take an extra pill if I eat too much."
2. "I will eat 3 meals a day."
3. "I will call my physician if I get sick."
4. "I will take my pill every night before I go to bed."

2-29

The physician has written the following prescriptions for a client with myxedema. Which prescription will you question?

1. levothyroxine sodium 0.2 mg intravenously every day
2. nitroglycerin gr 1/150 sublingually prn for chest pain
3. morphine sulfate 4 mg intravenously every 4 hours prn for severe pain
4. monitor capillary blood glucose at 7:00 a.m., 11:00 a.m., 4:00 p.m., and 9:00 p.m.

2-30

A client had a subtotal thyroidectomy. While assessing, the nurse observes that the client swallows frequently and speaks with a twang. The blood pressure is 20 points lower, the pulse is 30 points higher, and respirations are twice as fast as baseline admission assessment. Which of the following is an appropriate nursing action?

1. Continue to monitor vital signs every 30 minutes as prescribed.
2. Record findings; considering the client's postoperative state, vital signs are within normal ranges.
3. Notify the surgeon; the client may be bleeding internally.
4. Report findings to the nursing supervisor.

2 - 3 1

A client with myxedema was admitted to your unit. What do you expect your assessment to reveal?

1. weight loss
2. subnormal temperature
3. tachycardia
4. hirsutism

2 - 3 2

You are planning a teaching program for a 16-year-old who has recently been diagnosed with type 1 diabetes. When planning the program, you understand the greatest influence on its success is:

1. the client's acceptance of the diagnosis.
2. the parents' acceptance of the diagnosis.
3. whether or not the entire teaching plan is implemented by one nurse.
4. whether or not teaching is limited to 1-hour periods.

2 - 3 3

A mother with diabetes mellitus has delivered her baby. Two hours after delivery, the nurse observes that the infant is lethargic and has developed mild generalized cyanosis and twitching. The nurse should recognize that the infant is probably exhibiting symptoms of:

1. hypoglycemia.
2. hypercapnia.
3. hypothermia.
4. hypercalcemia.

2 - 3 4

Which of the following measures is the most effective in achieving normal blood sugar levels in the client with type 2 diabetes?

1. increasing sodium intake
2. decreasing water intake
3. achieving ideal body weight
4. decreasing daily exercise

2 - 3 5

Your client has a closed head injury and is experiencing increased intracranial pressure. You will monitor the client for potential damage to the:

1. adrenal gland.
2. parathyroid gland.
3. thyroid gland.
4. pituitary gland.

2 - 3 6

Your client has acromegaly. You know this condition is caused by the oversecretion of:

_____.

Fill in the blank

2 - 3 7

Increased levels of serum calcium may result in which of the following?

1. increased secretion of growth hormone
2. increased secretion of parathormone
3. decreased secretion of follicle-stimulating hormone
4. decreased secretion of parathormone

2-38

Clients experiencing hypothyroidism are generally treated with thyroid replacement therapy. Which of the following is a potentially serious side effect of the initiation of thyroid replacement?

1. angina
2. increased urination
3. increase in energy level
4. myxedema

2-39

A client is to receive Lugol's solution 0.2 ml tid 12 days prior to a thyroidectomy. The nurse knows to administer this medication:

1. on an empty stomach.
2. immediately before meals.
3. diluted in juice and taken through a straw.
4. with an iodine-rich food.

2-40

An infant is receiving levothyroxine for the treatment of congenital hypothyroidism. The infant's parents should be taught to notify their child's health-care provider if they observe:

1. mottled and cool skin.
2. a pulse rate above 150 beats per minute.
3. feeding difficulty.
4. edema and weight gain.

2-41

The following diagnostic studies have been prescribed: protein-bound iodine, radioactive iodine uptake, and triiodothyronine. Which of the following instructions will the nurse give to prepare the client for these procedures?

1. Food and fluids are restricted prior to these procedures.
2. Proper imaging of the thyroid during these tests requires restricting movement.
3. The tests may take some time because injected dyes travel slowly to the thyroid.
4. Ingestion of iodine is restricted prior to these tests.

2-42

A client has pheochromocytoma. The nurse will monitor the client's:

1. blood pressure.
2. respiratory rate.
3. hemoglobin level.
4. white blood cell count.

2-43

A client who is experiencing manifestations of a pituitary tumor will probably complain of:

1. decrease in peripheral vision.
2. tearing and eye pain with exposure to sunlight.
3. dependent edema.
4. dyspnea.

2 - 4 4

Which of the following medications would most likely be administered to treat the signs and symptoms associated with Graves' disease?

1. epinephrine
2. codeine
3. beta-blockers
4. laxatives

2 - 4 5

Your client is experiencing hypothyroidism. Which of the following comments made by this client do you associate with this condition?

Select all that apply by placing a ✔ in the square:

- ❒ 1. "I don't seem to have an appetite."
- ❒ 2. "I have difficulty sleeping."
- ❒ 3. "I have gained a lot of weight recently."
- ❒ 4. "I take laxatives 2 to 3 times a week for constipation."
- ❒ 5. "My heart feels like it is going to come out of my chest."

2 - 4 6

Your client had a subtotal thyroidectomy. You are teaching the client to prevent postoperative complications by avoiding goitrogenic foods. Which of the following do you recognize as potent goitrogens?

Select all that apply by placing a ✔ in the square:

- ❒ 1. grapes
- ❒ 2. turnips
- ❒ 3. rutabagas
- ❒ 4. pinto beans
- ❒ 5. peanut skins

2 - 4 7

Your client is experiencing Cushing's syndrome. You expect your assessment of the client to reveal:

Select all that apply by placing a ✔ in the square:

- ❒ 1. weight loss
- ❒ 2. moon face
- ❒ 3. hirsutism
- ❒ 4. ecchymosis
- ❒ 5. facial pallor

2 - 4 8

Your client is experiencing hypothyroidism and is constipated due to gastrointestinal hypomotility. You are teaching the client how to avoid constipation. Which comments by the client suggest a need for additional teaching?

Select all that apply by placing a ✔ in the square:

- ❒ 1. "I will drink 2 or 3 liters of fluid daily."
- ❒ 2. "I will consume foods low in bulk and roughage."
- ❒ 3. "I will take a stool softener if needed."
- ❒ 4. "I will cut back on my physician activity."
- ❒ 5. "I will schedule small, frequent meals."

2-49

A client with hyperthyroidism is experiencing exophthalmos. To minimize the risk factors associated with exophthalmos, you will teach the client to:

Select all that apply by placing a ✔ in the square:

- ❑ 1. increase dietary salt intake.
- ❑ 2. sleep with the head of the bed raised.
- ❑ 3. exercise extraocular muscles daily.
- ❑ 4. apply methylcellulose eyedrops.
- ❑ 5. cover the eyes with a mask at night.

2-50

Your client has Addison's disease. You anticipate an assessment of the client's skin to reveal:

Select all that apply by placing ✔ in the square:

- ❑ 1. cyanosis.
- ❑ 2. hyperpigmentation.
- ❑ 3. bluish-black gums and oral mucosa.
- ❑ 4. pallor.
- ❑ 5. ecchymosis.

2-51

The exogenous administration of glucocorticoids is usually given:

1. to promote diuresis.
2. for their anti-inflammatory effects.
3. for their analgesic properties.
4. for their antiarrhythmic properties.

Practice Test 2

Answers, Rationales, and Explanations

---

2 - 1

---

④ **Emaciated clients should have insulin administered at a 45-degree angle into the subcutaneous tissue. The first factor to consider is the emaciated state of this client. Because of the client's emaciated condition, the nurse will give the injection at a 45-degree angle.**

1 and 3. Insulin is administered subcutaneously, not intramuscularly.

2.   Giving the injection at a 90-degree angle would cause the needle to go through the subcutaneous tissue of an emaciated client.

Client Need: Physiological Integrity

---

2 - 2

---

② **Exogenous insulin will need to be administered the rest of the client's life. Persons with type 1 diabetes have little or no endogenous insulin.**

1, 3, and 4. Food intake, eating habits, and growth patterns are important facts regarding insulin dosage; however, it is most essential for the adolescent to know that insulin injections will be required throughout life.

Client Need: Physiological Integrity

---

2 - 3

Fill in the blank correct answer:

<u>Regular insulin</u>

Regular insulin is the only insulin that can be given intravenously. Regular insulin is clear and does not contain any modifying agents.

Client Need: Safe, Effective Care Environment

2 - 4

② Since NPH insulin peaks between 6 and 8 hours after administration, the client should consume a snack at 4:00 p.m. to prevent hypoglycemia. The onset of NPH insulin is 2 hours, peak 6 to 8 hours, and duration 12 to 16 hours.

1 and 3. Daily exercise should be accounted for and adjustments in daily insulin dosages need to be made based on exercise regimens. Additional glucose needs to be consumed if the client exercises more than usual, since exercise has a hypoglycemic effect.

4. Long-acting insulin given at bedtime requires a bedtime snack the next day (onset 2 hours, peak 16 to 20 hours, duration 24+ hours).

Client Need: Health Promotion and Maintenance

2 - 5

① The nurse will observe the client for signs of hypoglycemia. There is a decreased need for insulin in the first trimester. The level of human placental lactogen (HPL) (an insulin antagonist) is low. Also, the client and the developing fetus use more glucose and glycogen.

2 and 3. Ketoacidosis accompanies hyperglycemia, not hypoglycemia.

4. Pregnancy-induced hypertension is not a factor in the first trimester

Client Need: Health Promotion and Maintenance

2 - 6

④ NPH insulin is an intermediate-acting insulin and should be rolled between the palms of the hands to thoroughly mix the dose prior to withdrawal of the dose.

1. Insulin in use may be left at room temperature for up to 4 weeks unless the room temperature is higher than 85°F or below freezing. Extra insulin may be stored in the refrigerator.

2. After injecting insulin, some pressure should be applied to the site while the needle is being withdrawn. The swab should be held in place for a few seconds, but the site should not be massaged because massage may cause bruising.

3. When mixing an intermediate-acting insulin with Regular insulin, the Regular insulin should always be drawn up first.

Client Need: Health Promotion and Maintenance

2 - 7

② **Clients receiving Synthroid (levothyroxine) should not substitute generic brands. Different brands of thyroid preparations may not be the same. To maintain appropriate thyroid levels, no substitutes are allowed.**

1. Synthroid (levothyroxine) does not have to be taken with meals. However, it is recommended that it be taken at the same time each day to establish consistency.

3. The dosage of synthroid can not be self-adjusted. The dosage needs to be adjusted based on serum laboratory values and is adjusted only under the direction of a qualified health care provider.

4. Weight loss may occur as a result of an increase in basal metabolic rate but it may not occur for all clients.

Client Need: Safe, Effective Care Environment

2 - 8

③ **Hydrocortisone (Solu-Cortef) will replace the corticosteriod normally produced in the adrenal gland's cortex and prevent adrenal insufficiency.**

1. Solu-Cortef tends to raise serum glucose levels rather than lower them.

2. Solu-Cortef is not an analgesic and will not relieve postoperative pain.

4. Solu-Cortef causes gastric irritation and should be administered with meals.

Client Need: Health Promotion and Maintenance

2 - 9

② **You will anticipate administering Humulin R intravenously. Humulin R is rapid-acting insulin and is administered to treat high blood glucose levels.**

1. Humulin N is in suspension and cannot be given intravenously.

3. Humulin 70/30 insulin cannot be given intravenously. It is a combination of 70 units of Intermediate insulin and 30 units of Regular insulin.

4. A rapid-acting insulin is needed. Humulin N cannot be given intravenously.

Client Need: Physiological Integrity

2 - 1 0

④ **The nurse will associate the client's symptoms with myxedema coma. A body temperature of 90°F, an apical heart rate of 58 beats per minute (BPM), and respirations of 10 per minute are classical symptoms of myxedema coma seen in clients who have hypothyroidism.**

1. Hypercalcemia (calcium serum levels above 10.1 mg/dl) may be seen in hyperthyroidism, not hypothyroidism.
2. Hypermagnesemia (magnesium serum levels above 2.1 mg/dl) is associated with acute adrenocortical insufficiency and untreated diabetic ketoacidosis.
3. Symptoms of metabolic acidosis include increased respiratory rate and depth, not bradypnea (abnormally slow breathing).

Client Need: Physiological Integrity

2 - 1 1

③ **You will anticipate a decrease in serum glucose and an increase in prothrombin times. Tolazamide (Tolinase) and warfarin (Coumadin) tend to augment each other's actions. Therefore, the prothrombin time will increase and the serum glucose levels will be lowered even more, since the two drugs are being used in combination.**

1. A combination of Tolinase and Coumadin tends to decrease serum glucose levels even more than when administering Tolinase alone.
2. A combination of Tolinase and Coumadin tends to increase the prothrombin time even more than when Coumadin is administered alone.
4. A combination of Tolinase and Coumadin tends to decrease serum glucose levels.

Client Need: Health Promotion and Maintenance

2 - 1 2

④ **You will anticipate the administration of glucocorticoids. This person is exhibiting classic signs of adrenal insufficiency, probably due to the abrupt cessation of glucocorticoid therapy.**

1. Diuretics are usually not given to hypotensive clients because they lower blood pressure by decreasing circulating volume.
2. An analgesic is not anticipated since there is no indication that the client is experiencing pain.
3. There is no indication that the client is experiencing metabolic acidosis and would require sodium bicarbonate.

Client Need: Physiological Integrity

2 - 1 3

④ **You will explain that the function of the adrenal glands is suppressed during glucocorticoid therapy and abrupt cessation of glucocorticoids does not allow time for the adrenal glands to resume normal functioning.**

1. There is no evidence of permanent adrenal damage.
2. The adrenal function was affected by glucocorticoid use.
3. There is no evidence of an adrenal tumor.

Client Need: Physiological Integrity

2 - 1 4

① **The client will be taught to taper the methylprednisolone (Medrol) according to the regime. Tapering the dosage will avoid adrenal insufficiency.**

2. Corticosteroids such as methylprednisolone (Medrol) are to be taken on a regular basis, not just when an allergy is bothersome.
3. Sudden withdrawal of a corticosteroid can precipitate adrenal insufficiency.
4. Methylprednisolone (Medrol) is an appropriate medication for the treatment of allergic reactions.

Client Need: Health Promotion and Maintenance

2 - 1 5

③ **Serum calcium should be monitored carefully. The parathyroid gland's function is to increase calcium absorption and increase blood calcium levels. Serum calcium levels must be scrupulously monitored. Extreme disturbances in calcium levels may lead to tetany or lethal arrhythmias.**

1. Urine specific gravity is not directly affected by parathormone (PTH).
2. Creatine kinase (CK) and its isoenzyme (CK-MB) are monitored to confirm an acute myocardial infarction. CK-MB is not associated with parathormone (PTH).

Client Need: Health Promotion and Maintenance

2 - 1 6

① **When large dosages of vasopressin (Pitressin) are administered, a client may experience facial pallor due to the drug's vasoconstrictive action.**

2. Clients may experience dizziness and a pounding sensation in the head, but not a headache.
3. Clients may experience perspiration, paleness, and perioral blanching, but not flushing.
4. Dyspnea is not associated with the administration of Pitressin.

Client Need: Physiological Integrity

2 - 1 7

③ **Diabetics should be taught that alcohol consumption inhibits the release of glycogen from the liver, which results in hypoglycemia.**

1 and 2. Alcohol does not increase the need for more insulin or increase the blood glucose level. However, it does inhibit the release of glycogen from the liver, which results in hypoglycemia.

4. Diabetics who drink alcohol do not become intoxicated any sooner or later than people who drink alcohol and don't have diabetes. However, diabetics may develop hypoglycemia and fail to get the proper medical help because their symptoms may appear to be those associated with alcohol intoxication.

Client Need: Physiological Integrity

2 - 1 8

③ **A midafternoon snack will prevent an insulin reaction. Isophane insulin is an intermediate-acting insulin with a peak action of 6 to 12 hours. During peak action, maximum insulin effect is expected. To prevent an insulin reaction, appropriate food supplements must be given.**

1. The snack of milk and crackers is given strictly to prevent an insulin reaction. It has nothing to do with improving the client's nutritional status.

2. The crackers are a source of carbohydrates that will prevent an insulin reaction and hypoglycemic rebound.

4. Diabetic ketoacidosis (DKA) is caused by an absence or insufficient amount of insulin.

Client Need: Health Promotion and Maintenance

2 - 1 9

② **The nurse will suspect the development of tetany. Hypoparathyroidism causes a decrease in serum calcium levels due to a lack of parathyroid hormone stimulation. A decrease in calcium ion concentration causes tetany. Signs of tetany syndrome include tingling of the lips, hands, and feet; muscle tension, stiffness, and paresthesia (sensation of numbness).**

1. Syndrome of inappropriate antidiuretic hormone (SIADH) is a complication of conditions such as increased intracranial pressure (ICP) and endocrine and pulmonary disorders. It is associated with an increase in the secretion of antidiuretic hormone (ADH), which causes an extracellular volume overload and a decrease in urine output.

3. Myxedema is a type of hypothyroidism associated with the extreme symptoms of that condition.

4. Cushing's syndrome results from excessive adrenocortical activity, not hypoparathyroidism.

Client Need: Physiological Integrity

2-20

② The purpose of a radioactive iodine uptake test is to measure the activity of the thyroid gland. The thyroid gland cannot distinguish between regular iodine and radioactive iodine. By administering tracer doses of radioactive iodine, the percent of radioactive iodine used by the gland to produce thyroxine provides an indicator of gland activity. In clients with hyperthyroidism, the gland may use up to twice as much iodine as in a euthyroid (normal) state.

1. A radioactive iodine uptake test does not determine the ability of the thyroid gland to produce thyroxine.

3. A radioactive iodine uptake test does not estimate the concentration of thyrotropic hormone (thyroid-stimulating hormone) in the thyroid gland.

4. Treatment will not be addressed until a thorough assessment of the client has been completed. The radioactive iodine uptake test is only one consideration.

Client Need: Safe, Effective Care Environment

2-21

① The nurse will have calcium gluconate available. When a client develops carpopedal spasms (spasms of the hands and feet) subsequent to a thyroidectomy, calcium gluconate should be administered. Muscular twitching and hyperirritability of the nervous system indicates tetany due to hypocalcemia. This condition develops if the parathyroid glands are accidentally removed during thyroid surgery. Calcium replacement therapy is indicated for the treatment of this problem.

2. Potassium chloride (Slow-K) is administered for the treatment of potassium deficiencies and digitalis intoxication. It is not affected by a thyroidectomy.

3. Diazepam (Valium) is a sedative/hypnotic, anticonvulsant, and skeletal muscle relaxant. It does not replace calcium.

4. Phenytoin sodium (Dilantin) is an anticonvulsant and does not replace calcium.

Client Need: Physiological Integrity

2-22

③ Hoarseness and weakness of the voice following a subtotal thyroidectomy is an indication of laryngeal nerve damage. The damage occurs if there is unilateral injury of the pharyngeal nerve during surgery.

1. Facial twitching may occur if the parathyroid glands are damaged or removed during the thyroidectomy.

2. Wheezing could occur as a result of edema, not laryngeal nerve damage.

4. Hemorrhage could occur following a thyroidectomy due to the vascularity of the operative site. However, hemorrhage is not associated with laryngeal nerve damage.

Client Need: Physiological Integrity

2 - 2 3

① ③ and ④ The growth hormone effects associated with acromegaly (hyperpituitarism) include enlarged hands and broad feet, prominent frontal and orbital ridges, and hypertension.

2. Clients experiencing acromegaly (hyperpituitarism) have increased body hair, not alopecia (absence or loss of hair).

5. Clients experiencing acromegaly (hyperpituitarism) have increased skin pigmentation, not pallor.

Client Need: Physiological Integrity

2 - 2 4

① Stress-induced fluctuations in blood glucose can be more adequately managed with Regular insulin. Regular insulin is rapid acting, beginning within 15 minutes after administration. It peaks within 2 to 4 hours and duration is 5 to 8 hours. Regular insulin is the only insulin that may be used intravenously when the client's blood glucose is out of control. Regular insulin may also be used with intermediate- or long-acting insulin to maintain better control. Regular insulin is the only insulin that can be used in the insulin pump. The use of Regular insulin with this client will minimize occurrence of intraoperative and postoperative complications associated with blood glucose levels.

2. There is no indication that the client is experiencing or will experience diabetic acidosis.

3. The long-acting insulin will not be used because it cannot be administered intravenously and is not fast acting. Regular insulin is needed to adequately manage blood glucose levels.

4. There is no indication that the client is experiencing diabetic acidosis. Also, food absorption is not affected by insulin.

Client Need: Physiological Integrity

2 - 2 5

② An early indication that the infant may have thyroid hormone deficiency is the statement by the mother, "My baby is good and never cries." Early manifestations of hypothyroidism are inactivity, excessive sleeping, and minimal crying, which leads a parent to the erroneous conclusion that a baby is quiet and good.

1, 3, and 4. A normal 3-month-old infant should be smiling, vocalizing, and noticing surroundings.

Client Need: Physiological Integrity

2 - 2 6

(1) The nurse assembling the supplies should be interrupted and informed regarding the need for sterile technique. The client is a diabetic with a foot ulcer and is susceptible to infection and gangrene. Sterile technique is an essential factor in the client's recovery.

2. Presenting the situation for discussion at a staff meeting could jeopardize the client's health. Immediate action should be taken to prevent contamination of the client's foot ulcer.

3. Sterile technique is required when applying soaks to a foot ulcer of a client with diabetes.

4. Safe practice should be monitored by any nurse directly or indirectly involved in client care.

Client Need: Safe, Effective Care Environment

2 - 2 7

(4) An assessment of a client with Addison's disease would reveal dark pigmentation of the skin, especially the sun-exposed areas over joints and in creases such as on the palms of the hands. Other assessment findings in the early period of the disease include muscular weakness, hypotension, fatigue, emaciation, anorexia, and low blood glucose. Addison's disease (adrenal insufficiency) results from a deficiency in the secretion of the adrenocortical hormones due to autoimmune influences (75% of cases) and other conditions such as surgical removal, infection, or tuberculosis of the adrenal glands.

1. Adrenocortical insufficiency does not affect reduction in bone mass (osteoporosis).

2. Hirsutism (excessive growth of hair or presence of hair in unusual places) is not associated with adrenocortical insufficiency.

3. Sodium and water retention are not associated with adrenocortical insufficiency.

Client Need: Physiological Integrity

2 - 2 8

(4) Clients who have type 2 non-insulin-dependent diabetes and are taking glyburide (Micronase) for glucose control should take the medication at the same time daily at breakfast or at the first main meal. Following administration, the medication is absorbed within 1 hour, peaks between 2 and 4 hours, and lasts 24 hours.

1. Glyburide (Micronase) po should be taken once daily. Extra doses are contraindicated.

2. Clients receiving glyburide (Micronase) should consume 3 meals a day on a regular schedule.

3. Clients receiving glyburide (Micronase) who become ill should notify the physician. It may be necessary to control blood glucose levels with Regular insulin administered intravenously.

Client Need: Health Promotion and Maintenance

2-29

③ **The nurse will question a prescription for morphine sulfate. Clients who have myxedema (a type of hypothyroidism) are sensitive to sedatives, opiates, and anesthetic agents. The nurse should question any prescription for these medications.**

1. Levothyroxine (Synthroid) is a thyroid hormone replacement and is an appropriate medication.
2. Nitroglycerin is an appropriate medication since clients with myxedema are likely to have elevated serum cholesterol levels and coronary artery disease.
4. Monitoring capillary blood glucose is necessary since Synthroid increases the metabolic rate of body tissue.

Client Need: Physiological Integrity

2-30

③ **The client's behavior and vital signs indicate internal bleeding and the surgeon should be notified. As a result of bleeding, tracheal narrowing has occurred, causing the client to speak with a nasal twang.**

1. Just monitoring the client's vital signs every 30 minutes is inadequate. The nurse must recognize that the client may be hemorrhaging and notify the surgeon.
2. The client's vital signs indicate changes beyond normal postoperative expectations.
3. The surgeon should be notified since internal bleeding is probable.

Client Need: Physiological Integrity

2-31

② **The nurse would expect an assessment of a client with severe hypothyroidism (myxedema) to include a subnormal body temperature, bradycardia, and weight gain. The client's skin becomes thickened, the face expressionless, and mental processes are dulled. Early symptoms of myxedema include fatigue, hair loss, brittle nails, dry skin, numbness and tingling of fingers, and hoarseness.**

1. Weight gain would be expected in clients with myxedema (a type of hypothyroidism).
3. Bradycardia would be expected, not tachycardia.
4. Thinning and dryness of hair is associated with myxedema, not hirsutism (increased growth of hair or hair occurring on unusual places).

Client Need: Physiological Integrity

2 - 3 2

(1) The nurse will recognize that clients' acceptance of their condition will have the greatest influence on the success of the teaching program. When initiating a teaching plan, the nurse will be aware that this client is an adolescent in the process of forming a unique identity as a significant, capable person who is able to assume responsibility.

2. The ultimate success of the program will depend on the client's acceptance of his or her diabetic condition, not the parents' acceptance of their child's condition. Adolescents are usually more concerned about what their peers' attitudes are, not what their parents think.

3. The number of health-care providers involved in the teaching plan should not affect its success.

4. Teaching should not exceed 1-hour periods. Clients who are learning about their condition, dietary restrictions, and medication need time to absorb what is being taught.

Client Need: Health Promotion and Maintenance

2 - 3 3

(1) The nurse will recognize that the neonate of the diabetic mother is experiencing hypoglycemia. Prior to delivery, the fetus was exposed to high levels of maternal glucose. The fetus responded to the high glucose levels by increasing insulin production and hyperplasia of the pancreatic beta cells. Following the birth of the infant, the maternal glucose supply is gone and the infant becomes hypoglycemic as a result of high levels of circulating insulin.

2. There is no reason to suspect hypercapnia (increased amounts of carbon dioxide serum levels.) Hypercapnia is associated with conditions such as chronic obstructive pulmonary disease (COPD).

3. The cyanosis is due to hypoglycemia, not hypothermia.

4. Hypercalcemia (calcium serum levels above 10.0 mg/dl) is not associated with infants born of diabetic mothers.

Client Need: Physiological Integrity

2 - 3 4

(3) Achieving ideal body weight is effective in maintaining normal blood sugar levels. The number of insulin receptors is decreased in the very obese. Many obese persons who experience marked fluctuations in their blood sugar find their blood sugars can be regulated with weight loss. Obese people tend to be insulin resistant.

1. Increasing sodium in the diet may lead to hypertension and electrolyte imbalance.

2. Decreasing water intake may lead to dehydration.

4. Regular daily exercise is encouraged for clients who experience hyperglycemia. Exercise stimulates insulin production.

Client Need: Health Promotion and Maintenance

2-35

④　A client experiencing a closed head injury should be monitored for evidence of damage to the pituitary gland, which is located in the inferior portion (base) of the brain. Pressure may be exerted on the pituitary gland if the brain swells. Fluctuations in blood pressure or diuresis may be evident in the client experiencing an increase in intracranial pressure because of the lack of vasopressin secreted by the pituitary gland. Although all endocrine function may be affected by a head injury, the pituitary gland is especially vulnerable due to the effects of increased intracranial pressure.

1.　The adrenal glands are located near the kidneys.

2 and 4. Both the parathyroid glands and thyroid glands are located in the neck.

Client Need: Physiological Integrity

2-36

Fill in the blank correct answer:

<u>growth hormone</u>

Acromegaly, or enlargement of the viscera, develops as a result of oversecretion of growth hormone (GH). This hormone is secreted by the pituitary gland. Oversecretion of growth hormone developing in early childhood may result in giantism.

Client Need: Physiological Integrity

2-37

④　Elevated serum calcium levels will result in decreased secretion of parathormone. Parathormone is secreted by the parathyroid glands. Parathormone regulates calcium metabolism and is affected by serum calcium levels. A feedback loop causes decreases in parathormone secretion to result in elevated serum calcium levels, and vice versa.

1 and 3.　Neither growth hormone nor follicle-stimulating hormone are directly affected by serum calcium levels.

2.　An increase in serum calcium levels will result in a decrease in parathormone secretion.

Client Need: Physiological Integrity

2 - 3 8

① At the time thyroid replacement therapy is initiated, the client could experience the side effect of angina. Clients who experience hypothyroidism for extended periods often develop elevated cholesterol levels and atherosclerotic changes in their vessels. They also tend to have a slow heart rate and relatively low metabolic demands. With the institution of thyroid replacement therapy, the metabolic rate increases, as does the heart rate. This may precipitate angina or an ischemic cardiac event.

2. A marked increase in urination is not associated with the institution of thyroid replacement therapy.

3. An increase in energy level is a desirable effect of thyroid replacement therapy.

4. Myxedema occurs as a result of hypothyroidism, not thyroid replacement therapy.

Client Need: Health Promotion and Maintenance

2 - 3 9

③ Lugol's solution (a strong iodine solution) should be diluted in fruit juice, water, or milk, and taken through a straw. Iodine may cause nausea and vomiting and will also stain the teeth.

1 and 2. Lugol's solution should be taken at meals to prevent gastric irritation.

4. Iodine-rich foods are not permitted because they interfere with the dosage of the prescribed iodine. High-iodine foods include iodized salts, oysters, spinach, lima beans, beef liver, and navy beans.

Client Need: Health Promotion and Maintenance

2 - 4 0

② A pulse rate above 150 beats per minute (BPM) indicates possible tachycardia and can be a sign of too much levothyroxine.

1, 3, and 4. Mottled and cool skin, feeding difficulty, edema, and weight gain are all signs of hypothyroidism and suggest that the medication has not yet eliminated these symptoms.

Client Need: Physiological Integrity

2-41

④ Ingestion of iodine is restricted prior to tests that utilize iodine. The protein-bound iodine (PBI) and the triiodothyronine (T-3) uptake tests are blood studies. The radioactive iodine uptake shows the percentage of radioactive iodine ingested orally which has been stored in the thyroid gland. No special preparation is needed for any of these tests. However, ingesting iodine in the form of iodized salt, foods, or drugs may alter the results of these tests.

1. There is no need to restrict food or fluids for any of these diagnostic studies.
2. There is no imaging required with any of these tests.
3. No dyes are injected. The client is given a po tracer dose of 131 iodine when being prepared for the radioactive iodine uptake test.

Client Need: Safe, Effective Care Environment

2-42

① Clients with pheochromocytoma should have their blood pressure monitored closely. Pheochromocytoma is a tumor of the adrenal medulla. Functioning tumors of the adrenal medulla cause hypertension and other cardiovascular disturbances. Life-threatening blood pressures as high as 350/200 mm Hg have been recorded.

2, 3, and 4. Pheochromocytoma does not directly affect or impact the client's respiratory rate, hemoglobin level, or white blood cell count.

Client Need: Physiological Integrity

2-43

① Clients who are experiencing manifestations of a pituitary tumor will probably complain of a decrease in peripheral vision. Complaints of visual field disturbance are not uncommon in clients with a pituitary tumor. Growing pituitary tumors may exert pressure on surrounding structures. Visual fields may be affected by the tumor's growth as pressure is exerted on the optic chiasm.

2. Tearing and eye pain with exposure to sunlight is often due to a disorder in the eye itself, such as increased pressure due to glaucoma.

3 and 4. Dyspnea and dependent edema are most likely due to disorders of the cardiovascular or renal systems, such as congestive heart failure or fluid overload, or to respiratory disorders.

Client Need: Physiological Integrity

2 - 4 4

③ **Beta-blockers may be prescribed for clients with Graves' disease. Graves' disease (a form of hyperthyroidism) is associated with signs and symptoms of accelerated metabolism. Tachycardia, nervousness, and tremors are typical signs of this condition. Beta-blockers tend to slow the heart rate and are thus very useful in the adjunct therapy for Graves' disease.**

1. Epinephrine tends to increase, not decrease, the sympathetic nervous system response.
2. Codeine's analgesic effects are not indicated for this typically painless disease.
4. Laxatives are rarely indicated because persons with Graves' disease tend to have hyperactive bowel function.

Client Need: Health Promotion and Maintenance

2 - 4 5

① ③ **and** ④ **Clinical manifestations of hypothyroidism include decreased appetite, weight gain, and constipation.**

2. Insomnia is associated with hyperthyroidism, not hypothyroidism.
5. A bounding, rapid pulse with palpitations is associated with hyperthyroidism, not hypothyroidism.

Client Need: Physiological Integrity

2 - 4 6

② ③ **and** ⑤ **Substances that produce enlargement of the thyroid gland are known as goitrogens. Goitrogens are found naturally in foods. Potent goitrogens include turnips, rutabagas, and peanut skins.**

1. Grapes are not goitrogens.
4. Pinto beans are not goitrogens.

Client Need: Health Promotion and Maintenance

2 - 4 7

② ③ **and** ⑤ **Your assessment of a client experiencing Cushing's syndrome would reveal a moon face, hirsutism (the growth of hair in unusual places), and ecchymosis (superficial bleeding under the skin or mucous membranes). These symptoms are associated with excessive corticosteroids, especially glucocorticoids.**

1. Clients experiencing Cushing's syndrome have weight gain.
5. Clients experiencing Cushing's syndrome have red cheeks, not facial pallor.

Client Need: Physiological Integrity

2-48

② Consuming foods that are high in bulk and residue will help clients experiencing hypomotility to have a daily soft stool.

④ Physical activity stimulates peristalsis and is highly recommended to avoid or treat constipation.

⑤ Small, frequent meals will not increase gastrointestinal mobility. The type of food and the amount of fluid are more significant than amount of food and time of meals.

1. Consuming 2 to 3 liters of fluid (especially water) daily is recommended for clients who are experiencing hypomotility of the gastrointestinal tract.

3. It is appropriate for clients experiencing gastrointestinal hypomotility to take a laxative or stool softener if needed. These medications will stimulate gastrointestinal motility.

Client Need: Health Promotion and Maintenance

2-49

② Sleeping with the head of the bed raised will help to promote fluid drainage.

③ Exercising extraocular muscles daily can maintain flexibility. Severe exophthalmos can cause paralysis of these muscles.

④ Methylcellulose eyedrops (artificial tears) can help to prevent eye discomfort. When exophthalmos prevents clients from closing their eyes, dryness can occur, along with corneal ulceration.

1. Dietary salt intake should be restricted, since it contributes to periorbital edema.

5. Covering the eyes with a mask or taping the lids closed may be necessary when exophthalmos prevents clients from closing their eyes.

Client Need: Safe, Effective Care Environment

2-50

② Clients with primary adrenal cortical insufficiency (Addison's disease) experience hyperpigmentation of the skin. Skin exposed and unexposed to the sun has a tanned appearance. This is due to elevated adrenocorticotropic hormone (ACTH).

③ The gums and oral mucosa of a client with Addison's disease will be bluish-black in color. This is due to elevated adrenocorticotropic hormone (ACTH).

1. Cyanosis is not associated with Addison's disease. Cyanosis (a blue, gray, slate, or dark purple discoloration of the skin) is usually associated with deoxygenated or reduced hemoglobin in the blood.

4. Pallor (lack of color or paleness of the skin) is not associated with Addison's disease. Pallor is a symptom of conditions such as anemia.

5. Ecchymosis (superficial bleeding under the skin) is not associated with Addison's disease. Ecchymosis is seen in conditions such as disseminated intravascular coagulation (DIC) and hepatitis.

Client Need: Physiological Integrity

2 - 5 1

② Glucocorticoids are administered exogenously usually for their anti-inflammatory effects. Systemic administration of glucocorticoids may be used in allergic reactions or inflammatory disorders. Glucocorticoids such as cortisol are produced by the adrenal cortex and affect metabolism and inflammation.

1, 3, and 4. The glucocorticoids have neither diuretic, analgesic, nor antiarrhythmic properties.

Client Need: Physiological integrity

Practice Test 3

Gastrointestinal System and Nutrition

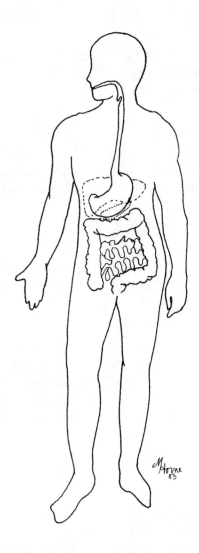

The Gastrointestinal System

OVERVIEW OF THE GASTROINTESTINAL SYSTEM

Digestion is the process of breaking down food mechanically and chemically in the gastrointestinal tract and converting it into forms that can be absorbed and used by the body. The process of digestion takes place in the digestive system (gastrointestinal tract or alimentary canal). Digestion is begun in the mouth, where food enters the body. Digestion is completed at the anus, where the wastes of the digestive process leave the body.

The digestive system is comprised of the oral cavity (mouth), pharynx (throat), esophagus (9- to 10-inch muscular tube), stomach, small intestine (small bowel), and large intestine (large bowel). Three other organs of digestion are the liver, gallbladder, and pancreas.

ORAL CAVITY (MOUTH)

Digestion begins in the mouth, or oral cavity, where food is chewed and also moistened by saliva, which is secreted into the oral cavity from the salivary glands. In addition to moistening food, saliva begins the chemical digestion of carbohydrates.

PHARYNX AND ESOPHAGUS

The pharynx and esophagus serve as passageways. Their muscular walls permit food to progress toward the stomach by peristalsis (progressive, rhythmic contractions).

STOMACH

The stomach receives the swallowed food from the esophagus, where it is mixed with gastric juices. Some absorption of nutrients takes place in the stomach. Protein metabolism starts in the stomach.

SMALL INTESTINE

The small intestine extends from the pyloric sphincter to the beginning of the large intestine. The duodenum (the first portion of the small intestine) receives food from the stomach, where it is mixed with bile from the liver and gallbladder, as well as with pancreatic juices from the pancreas. It is from the small intestine that completely digested nutrients pass via tiny capillaries (vilii) into the bloodstream and lymphatic system.

LARGE INTESTINE

The large intestine receives fluid and waste products from the digestive process that are too large to pass into the bloodstream. Solid waste is formed as water is absorbed for the body's use through the walls of the large intestine. This solid waste passes from the body via the anus in the form of feces.

ADDITIONAL ORGANS OF DIGESTION

The liver, gallbladder, and pancreas are additional organs of digestion. The liver produces and secretes bile, which is stored in the gallbladder. Bile helps to metabolize fats. The pancreas produces pancreatic juices that assist in the digestive process. The pancreas also produces insulin (a hormone needed to release sugars from the blood to be used for energy by all the cells in the body).

THE THREE FUNCTIONS OF DIGESTION

Ingestion

1. Food is taken into the body through the mouth, where it is broken down mechanically and chemically. Digestive enzymes (substances that speed chemical reactions) change sugars by reducing them to simple sugars such as glucose; fats are broken down into fatty acids and triglycerides; and proteins are broken down into amino acids.

Absorption

2. Digested food is absorbed into the bloodstream by passing through the walls of the small intestine. Absorption allows nutrients such as sugars and amino acids to travel to all parts of the body. Nutrients are burned (catabolized) in the presence of oxygen to release energy. The nutrient amino acids are used to build (anabolize) the larger protein molecules needed for growth and the development of cells. Fatty cells and triglycerides are also absorbed through the walls of the small intestine; however, they enter the lymphatic vessels rather than the blood vessels. Fats, which take longer to digest, enter the bloodstream as the lymph vessels join the bloodstream in the upper chest.

Elimination

3. The third function of the digestive system is to eliminate waste materials that cannot be absorbed into the bloodstream. This waste material is referred to as feces. Feces are concentrated in the large intestine and passed out of the body through the anus.

DISEASES/DISORDERS OF THE GASTROINTESTINAL SYSTEM INCLUDE

Anal Fistula

A narrow slot in the anal wall is referred to as an anal fistula.

Colonic Polyposis

Small growths (polyps) that protrude from the mucous membrane of the colon are known as colonic polyposis.

Colorectal Cancer

Cancers of the colon or rectum are known collectively as colorectal cancer.

Crohn's Disease

Crohn's disease is also known as regional enteritis. It is associated with chronic inflammation of the intestinal tract.

Diverticular Disease

Diverticular disease is associated with bulging pouches (diverticula) in the intestinal wall.

Dysentery

Dysentery is a painful disorder characterized by inflamed intestines, usually in the colon. There are two forms of dysentery, amebic and bacillary.

Esophageal Varices

Esophageal varices (varicose veins of the esophagus) are associated with swollen, twisted veins located toward the distal end of the esophagus.

Hiatal Hernia

This disorder is characterized by a protrusion of the upper part of the stomach through the diaphragmatic opening into the chest.

Inguinal Hernia

An inguinal hernia occurs when a small loop of the bowel protrudes through a weak place in the abdominal wall.

Ileus

An ileus is an intestinal obstruction that could be caused by a tumor, peristaltic failure, or twisting of the intestine within the abdomen.

Intussusception

Intussusception is the telescoping or invagination of a portion of the bowel into an adjacent distal portion. This condition appears mostly in children. Surgery may be indicated.

Irritable Bowel Syndrome (IBS) (Mucous Colon) (Spastic Colon)

This is a group of signs and symptoms characterized by diarrhea, constipation, lower abdominal pain, and bloating. It is usually associated with stress and tension.

Peptic Ulcers

Peptic ulcers are also known as gastric or duodenal ulcers. They occur when acid and gastric juices or pepsin cause damage to the epithelial lining of the stomach or duodenum. When an ulcer makes a hole through the intestines, it is a perforating ulcer.

Ulcerative Colitis

This condition is marked by chronic inflammation of the colon in the presence of ulcers.

Volvulus

A volvulus occurs when the intestine twists upon itself. Surgery can be performed to untwist the loop of the bowel.

Cirrhosis

Cirrhosis is a chronic disease of the liver with degeneration of the liver cells. This disorder is associated with alcoholism and malnutrition. Since bilirubin is not eliminated from the body, jaundice occurs.

Gallstones (Cholelithiasis)

Cholelithiasis means gallstones in the gallbladder. Stones (calculi) prevent the bile from leaving the gallbladder. Gallstones are treated by surgery, either open or laparoscopic, or nonsurgically, with a procedure using an endoscope.

Pancreatitis

Pancreatitis, or inflammation of the pancreas, may be acute or chronic. It can develop from alcoholism, gallstones, drugs, or abdominal trauma. It is usually treated with drugs to relieve pain, IV fluids, and adherence to a strict diet. Surgery may be performed to remove affected portions of the gland.

Hepatitis (A, B, C, D, E)

Hepatitis is inflammation of the liver caused by a virus. The virus directly injures liver cells.

HEPATITIS A (HAV) The hepatitis A virus is an RNA virus without envelope that can be contracted through contaminated food or water. A vaccine prevents infection either before or immediately after exposure to the virus. Vaccination is recommended for health-care workers, travelers, day-care center workers, and people with preexisting liver disease.

HEPATITIS B (HBV) HBV is caused by the hepatitis B virus, a double-stranded DNA virus. The virus is transmitted by exposure to blood or body fluids of an infected person. A hepatitis B vaccine is available and provides active immunity.

HEPATITIS C (HCV) Hepatitis C is a chronic blood-borne infection caused by a single-stranded RNA virus that is transmitted from person to person by exposure to blood or body fluids.

HEPATITIS D (HDV) HDV is caused by the hepatitis delta virus. It is considered a defective virus because it can produce an infection only when hepatitis B is present. This disease can be prevented through the hepatitis B vaccine.

HEPATITIS E (HEV) HEV is a form of hepatitis similar to hepatitis A. It is caused by an RNA virus that produces an acute infection. This disease occurs in nations where the water is contaminated and is seen in travelers coming from abroad.

OVERVIEW OF NUTRITION

Nutrition is the study of nutrients and the sources in the environment from which they are obtained and utilized, and also the actions and interactions of nutrients as they are absorbed and transported within the body. Nutrition supplies energy for cellular and metabolic processes and provides building materials for growth, maintenance, and repair of tissues. The body draws six classes of nutritive chemical substances from the environment: Carbohydrates, fats or lipids, proteins, minerals, vitamins, and water.

The energy nutrients are carbohydrates, fats, and proteins. The energy they release is measured in calories.

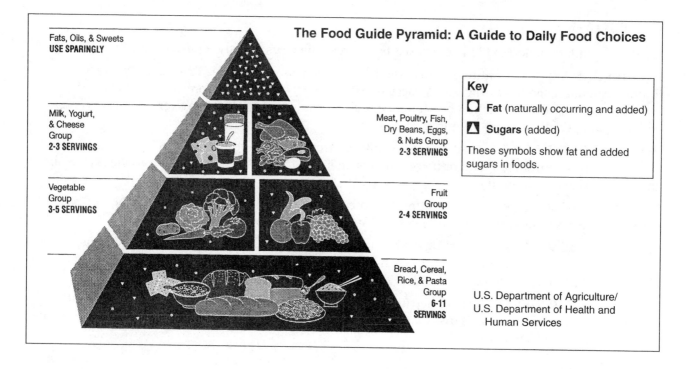

The Food Guide Pyramid: A Guide to Daily Food Choices

Fats, Oils, & Sweets
USE SPARINGLY

Milk, Yogurt, & Cheese Group
2-3 SERVINGS

Meat, Poultry, Fish, Dry Beans, Eggs, & Nuts Group
2-3 SERVINGS

Vegetable Group
3-5 SERVINGS

Fruit Group
2-4 SERVINGS

Bread, Cereal, Rice, & Pasta Group
6-11 SERVINGS

Key

◻ **Fat** (naturally occurring and added)

▲ **Sugars** (added)

These symbols show fat and added sugars in foods.

U.S. Department of Agriculture/
U.S. Department of Health and
Human Services

CARBOHYDRATES (CHO)

Carbohydrates supply sugars, starches, and fiber. Carbohydrate digestion and absorption is completed in the small intestine.

FATS (LIPIDS)

Fats come from both plant and animal sources. Fats have a higher energy value than other nutrients, and they cushion our body parts.

PROTEINS

Proteins can be used for energy. The body stores protein for energy. Proteins build, repair, and maintain tissues. Protein comes from animal and plant foods.

MINERALS

Minerals help to maintain proper body functioning.

Sodium

Sodium maintains water and electrolyte balance.

Potassium

Potassium maintains electrolyte balance, neuromuscular activity, and enzyme reaction.

Chloride

Chloride maintains fluids and electrolyte balance.

Calcium

Calcium functions in the formation of teeth and bones, neuromuscular activity, blood coagulation, and cell-wall permeability.

Phosphorus

Phosphorus functions in the formation of teeth and bones; most of the body's phosphorus is incorporated with the calcium of teeth and bones. The remainder is distributed throughout the body cells. Phosphorus plays an important role in almost all metabolic reactions and is present in nucleic acids, proteins, some enzymes, and some vitamins. It also functions in the regulation of pH.

Iodine

Iodine serves in the regulation of body metabolism and the promotion of normal growth. It is crucial to the proper functioning of the thyroid gland and the secretion of thyroid hormone, which regulates body temperature and metabolic rate.

Iron

Iron is a component of hemoglobin and serves in cellular respiration. All human cells contain iron.

Magnesium

Magnesium is crucial to proper neuromuscular activity, in the activation of enzymes, and in the formation of teeth and bones.

Zinc

Zinc is a constituent of enzymes and insulin. Zinc is active throughout the body and is involved in most metabolic processes.

WATER

Water is a principal constituent of all body fluids and is essential for a healthy body. It is found within intracellular fluid and outside all cells in extracellular fluid. It is crucial for metabolic activities within cells. Water composes approximately 60% of body weight in adults and up to 80% of body weight in infants. Humans can survive only a short time without water.

VITAMINS

Vitamin A (retinol) (fat-soluble)

Functions of vitamin A include: Growth of body cells, promotion of vision, and healthy hair and skin. Vitamin A helps to maintain membrane stability, synthesize the hormone cortisol, and ensure normal output of the hormone thyroxin. Vitamin A assists in maintaining healthy nerve sheaths and in the manufacture of red blood cells. A deficiency of vitamin A causes night blindness. Untreated night blindness can lead to irreversible blindness.

Vitamin B_1 (thiamin) (water-soluble)

Functions of vitamin B_1 include: Carbohydrate metabolism, normal digestion, oxidation of fat, and proper functioning of the thyroid gland. A deficiency of vitamin B_1 is associated with the disease beriberi, characterized by peripheral neurologic and cerebral and cardiovascular abnormalities. Early manifestations of beriberi include: Fatigue, poor memory, sleep disturbances, pericardial pain, abdominal pain, and constipation.

NOTE: Beriberi is endemic in Asia, the Philippines, and other islands of the Pacific.

Vitamin B_2 (riboflavin) (water-soluble and alcohol-soluble)

Functions of vitamin B_2 include: Formation of certain enzymes and normal growth and light adaptation in the eyes. A deficiency of vitamin B_2 causes cheilosis (lips are red and fissures form at the corners of the mouth), glossitis (inflamed tongue), and dermatitis around the nose and mouth.

Vitamin B_3 (niacin) (soluble in hot water and alcohol)

Functions of vitamin B_3 include: Proper functioning in cellular and energy production and proper carbohydrate, fat, and protein functioning. Vitamin B_3 also aids in prevention of appetite loss. Deficiencies of vitamin B_3 include: Pellagra, characterized by cutaneous (skin), gastrointestinal, and neurological and mental symptoms. The skin may become dry and scaly. The cutaneous lesions include erythema (redness). The mucous membranes of the mouth, esophagus, and vagina may atrophy. Anemia is a common manifestation.

Vitamin B_5 (pantothenic acid)

Vitamin B_5 is necessary in the Krebs cycle and for conversion of amino acids and lipids to carbohydrates. A deficiency may cause loss of coordination; however, this is rare.

Vitamin B_6 (pyridoxine) (water-soluble and alcohol-soluble)

Functions of vitamin B_6 include: The promotion of healthy gums, teeth, and red blood cell formation. B_6 deficiency leads to hypochromic anemia, irritability, convulsions, and skin lesions.

Vitamin B_9 (folic acid) (slightly water-soluble)

Functions of vitamin B_9 include: Proper function of protein metabolism, red blood cell formation, and normal intestinal-tract activity. A deficiency of B_9 causes neural deficiency and microcytic anemia (abnormally small red blood cells).

Vitamin B$_{12}$ (cyanocobalamin) (water-soluble and alcohol-soluble)

Functions of B$_{12}$ include: Red blood cell development and proper nerve function. A deficiency of B$_{12}$ leads to pernicious anemia, a condition in which cells do not secrete enough intrinsic factor to ensure intestinal absorption of B$_{12}$.

Vitamin B Complex (biotin)

Biotin is considered to be part of the vitamin B complex. Biotin plays a role in the metabolism of fatty acids. Deficiencies are associated with prolonged administration of total parenteral nutrition that was not supplemented with biotin. A deficiency of biotin is associated with dermatologic, neurologic, and ocular disorders.

Vitamin C (ascorbic acid) (water-soluble)

Functions of vitamin C include: Formation of healthy bones and teeth, iron absorption, formation of collagen, and the formation of blood vessels and capillary walls. A deficiency of vitamin C causes scurvy. This condition is characterized by hemorrhage and abnormal bone and teeth formation. Lack of vitamin C also causes joint tenderness, bleeding gums, and delayed wound healing.

Vitamin D (calciferol) (fat-soluble)

Functions of vitamin D include the accommodation of calcium and phosphorus absorption and the calcification of bones. A deficiency of vitamin D leads to a condition known as rickets in children and osteomalacia in adults. Rickets and osteomalacia are characterized by weak bones, which may result in bowed legs.

Vitamin E (alpha-tocopherol) (fat-soluble)

Functions of vitamin E include: Prevention of oxidative damage of lipids and cell membranes. Vitamin E also helps in promotion of red blood cell stability. A deficiency of vitamin E results in immune system suppression and blood cell hemolysis.

Vitamin K (fat-soluble)

The chief function of vitamin K is in the production of prothrombin. A deficiency of vitamin K can cause hemorrhagic disease.

Practice Test 3

Questions

3 - 1

Your client is receiving continuous nasogastric feedings. You know to change the tube feeding container and line every:

_____.

Fill in the blank

3 - 2

The most accurate assessment for correct placement of a nasogastric tube is to:

1. determine the pH of aspirate.
2. visualize the gastric area by X ray.
3. inject air into the tube and auscultate over the gastric area for the sound of air entering the stomach.
4. palpate the gastric area following the injection of 100 cc of air into the tube.

3 - 3

The nurse is discussing the treatment for gastroesophageal reflux with the parents of a newly diagnosed 4-month-old infant. Which comment by the parents indicates a need for more education?

1. "Our baby may develop pneumonia or breathing problems."
2. "Surgical correction will be needed when our baby is about 1 year of age."
3. "We may need to use formula thickened with rice cereal."
4. "We will try to feed more often and not as much at a time."

3 - 4

A client experiencing upper gastrointestinal bleeding was stabilized in the emergency department and was admitted to the hospital for further evaluation. To determine the cause and specific site of the bleeding, the nurse will anticipate a prescription for which diagnostic test first?

1. gastroscopy
2. gastrointestinal X rays
3. fiberoptic colonoscopy
4. gastric analysis

3 - 5

A client who is to be weighed daily on bed scales is receiving continuous liquid feedings via a percutaneous endoscopic gastrostomy. An important nursing intervention would be to:

1. weigh the day's feeding formula and add it to the client's weight.
2. inform the physician that persons receiving continuous feedings cannot be weighed on the bed scales.
3. defer the daily weights and record this deferment on the chart.
4. turn the feedings off at least 30 minutes prior to the weighing process.

3 - 6

Your client had a resection of a diseased portion of the ileum. Which instruction will you give the client about performing deep breathing and coughing exercises?

1. "Sit in an upright position; take a deep breath, and then cough."
2. "Hold your abdomen firmly, take several deep breaths, and then cough 2 or 3 times as you exhale."
3. "Tighten your stomach muscles as you inhale and then cough forcefully."
4. "Raise your shoulders to expand your chest and then give a deep cough."

3 - 7

Ingestion of which of the following foods has been found to exacerbate gastro-esophageal reflux disease?

1. poultry
2. pastas
3. herbs and spices
4. caffeine and chocolate

3 - 8

A client is experiencing vomiting and gastrointestinal bleeding. You are to prepare an intravenous infusion that contains potassium chloride. The purpose of administering potassium chloride is to:

1. replace the potassium that is lost in the urine.
2. restore lost potassium reserves.
3. provide potassium to promote excretion of sodium.
4. replace the potassium that is being lost through vomiting.

3 - 9

Your client had a subtotal gastrectomy and may experience the dumping syndrome as a direct result of:

1. the removal of a large portion of the stomach.
2. hyperosmolar chyme.
3. consuming large quantities of food.
4. not resting after each meal.

3 - 1 0

How many ounces a day of commercially prepared formula will contain 500 kcal of energy?

_____.

Fill in the blank

3 - 1 1

A 10-lb baby requires how many kilocalories per day for energy?

1. 100 kcal
2. 500 kcal
3. 1000 kcal
4. 1500 kcal

3 - 1 2

A client was admitted to the hospital with Crohn's disease. What do you expect your assessment to reveal?

Select all that apply by placing a ✔ in the square:

❒ 1. diarrhea
❒ 2. jaundice
❒ 3. steatorrhea
❒ 4. ascites

3 - 1 3

Which of the following may result from pro-longed gastroesophageal reflux disease and can quickly become life threatening?

1. pharyngitis
2. colitis
3. esophageal ulceration
4. angina

3 - 1 4

Which of the following diets would be the most appropriate for a client who has hyper-cholesterolemia?

1. hamburger patty, macaroni and cheese, iced tea
2. baked chicken breast, apple, skim milk
3. fish sticks, French fries, cola
4. pizza, tossed salad, beer

3 - 1 5

During a physical assessment your client tells you, "I belch a lot and when I lie down, undigested food comes up into my mouth. I have noticed a gurgling sound after eating, and I have a sour taste in my mouth." You suspect:

1. a diffuse esophageal spasm.
2. gastroesophageal reflux.
4. a hiatal hernia.
5. a pharyngoesophageal diverticulum.

3 - 1 6

Your client has a history of scarring as a result of repeated ulcerations and healings of ulcers distal to the pyloric sphincter. Recent complaints include epigastric fullness, pain, distention, nausea, vomiting, and anorexia. The client states that the pain is worse at night. You suspect:

1. peptic ulcer perforation.
2. acute gastritis.
3. pyloric obstruction.
4. paralytic ileus.

3 - 1 7

Your client is experiencing the acute phase of ulcerative colitis. The client states, "There is blood in my stools. I'm afraid." You will:

1. check the client's stools for the presence of occult blood.
2. recommend that the client keep a record of the number and description of stools.
3. notify the client's physician immediately.
4. explain to the client that blood in the stools is expected in this condition.

3 - 1 8

A client with cirrhosis of the liver has a serum bilirubin level of 50 mg/dl. In order to evaluate these laboratory results, you need to know that the normal serum bilirubin level is:

1. 0.2 to 1.0 mg/dl
2. 3 to 10 mg/dl
3. 10 to 20 mg/dl
4. 20 to 30 mg/dl

3 - 1 9

Your client will have a permanent colostomy following a colon resection. You will teach the client that the colostomy should begin to function postoperatively within:

1. 12 to 24 hours.
2. 2 to 4 days.
3. 4 to 5 days.
4. 5 to 6 days.

3 - 2 0

A child 4 years of age is acutely ill. Which of the following nursing measures will be most helpful in meeting the child's nutritional needs during the acutely ill period?

1. serving foods that are lukewarm
2. giving liquids through a straw
3. offering small, frequent feedings of favorite foods
4. allowing the client to select foods from the regularly scheduled meal trays

3 - 2 1

A client had an abdominoperineal resection with creation of an end colostomy. A sump drain was left in the client's perineal wound. The purpose of the sump drain is to:

1. allow for easy assessment of the character and volume of the drainage.
2. allow for easy passage of flatus until peristalsis returns.
3. prevent contamination of the operative site secondary to frequent dressing changes.
4. allow wound healing from its lowest depth without forming an abscess.

3 - 2 2

Your client has a gastric ulcer and is to receive aluminum hydroxide. The client asks, "Why am I receiving aluminum hydroxide?" You will explain that the expected action of this drug is to:

1. aid in inhibiting the secretion of hydrochloric acid.
2. serve as a catalyst in the breakdown of proteins.
3. absorb air that has been swallowed.
4. neutralize gastric secretions.

3 - 2 3

A 73-year-old client was admitted to the hospital with vomiting and gastrointestinal bleeding. The nurse prepares to administer an intravenous infusion that contains potassium chloride. The nurse will explain to the client that the purpose of the infusion is to:

1. replenish the potassium that is being lost in the urine.
2. replace the potassium that is lost through vomiting.
3. restore the potassium level that elderly clients cannot maintain through normal dietary intake.
4. provide potassium in an amount sufficient to promote excretion of sodium chloride.

3 - 2 4

You are encouraging an elderly client to increase intake of protein. To provide the greatest amount of protein, you will plan to add which of the following to 100 cc of milk?

1. 50 cc of light cream and 2 tablespoons of corn syrup.
2. 30 grams of powdered skim milk and 1 egg.
3. 1 small scoop (90 grams) of vanilla ice cream and 1 tablespoon of chocolate syrup.
4. 2 egg yolks and 1 tablespoon of sugar.

3 - 2 5

You are preparing a client for an upper gastrointestinal series. Which of the following explanations by the nurse would be both accurate and appropriate to share with the client?

1. "In the X-ray department you will be asked to drink a thick liquid, and then several X rays of the upper part of your digestive system will be taken at intervals."
2. "You will be asked to swallow a tube so that your physician can look at the lining of your stomach. X rays will be taken at the same time."
3. "You will be asked to swallow a substance that is radioactive, and then a series of X rays will be taken. This will help to determine what is wrong with your stomach."
4. "This test is carried out in the X-ray department. You will find it a little uncomfortable, but it's not really painful."

3 - 2 6

An adult client is hospitalized with a hiatal hernia. Following a transthoracic hiatal herniorrhaphy, the client returns to the unit with a chest tube attached to a 3-chamber water-seal drain connected to suction. Which of the following actions should the nurse take initially if the client's chest tube is not draining immediately following surgery?

1. Clamp the chest tube near the point of exit from the chest.
2. Increase the suction applied to the drainage system.
3. Ask the client to deep-breathe and cough.
4. Turn the client toward the operative side.

3 - 2 7

The nurse will instruct clients receiving thiaziade drugs to include foods in their diets that are high in:

_____.

Fill in the blank

3 - 2 8

A client complains of nausea. The nurse administers prochlorperazine maleate (Compazine) 25 mg intramuscularly as prescribed. Following prochlorperazine maleate administration, the nurse will assess the client for:

1 hypotension.
2. headaches.
3. confusion.
4. dry mouth.

3 - 2 9

The nurse is caring for a 3-year-old with chronic liver disease and marked ascites. To promote respiratory function and comfort, the child should be placed in which of the following positions?

1. semi-upright
2. semi-prone
3. dorsal recumbent
4. prone

3 - 3 0

The nurse is giving dietary instructions to mothers of infants and toddlers. The nurse will inform the mothers that diets that include milk to the exclusion of other foods may be deficient in:

1. iron.
2. carbohydrates.
3. vitamin D.
4. vitamin K.

3 - 3 1

A client thought to have cholelithiasis has been hospitalized and scheduled for an ultrasonography. Prior to this diagnostic evaluation, the nurse will:

1. administer a sedative approximately 30 minutes before the procedure.
2. question the client about allergies to iodine and seafood.
3. provide a clear liquid diet the evening before evaluation.
4. explain the procedure and its purpose.

3 - 3 2

As a result of a positive guaiac test on the stools of your client, the physician has prescribed a bland diet. The nurse will provide dietary instruction for the client. Which of the following menus, if selected by the client, would indicate the client is able to identify appropriate meals?

1. Hamburger with relish on a roll, ice cream, and coffee.
2. Ham on rye bread, flavored gelatin, and milk.
3. Cream cheese on toasted white bread, canned peaches, and decaffeinated coffee.
4. Bacon, lettuce, and tomato sandwich on whole-wheat bread, applesauce, and tea.

3 - 3 3

To prepare your client for a barium enema, you will:

Select all that apply by placing a ✔ in the square:

❏ 1. administer bowel preparation.
❏ 2. serve a liquid diet 24 hours before the test.
❏ 3. Instruct the client to consume a minimum of 240 ml of clear liquids.
❏ 4. instruct the client that a warm, flushed feeling may be experienced when the dye is infused.
❏ 5. inform the client that the barium preparation has an unpleasant, thick, chalky taste.

3 - 3 4

Which groups of food are highest in iron?

1. milk, pork, and squash
2. steak, spinach, and whole-grain bread
3. oranges, chicken, and green beans
4. tomatoes, strawberries, and liver

3 - 3 5

A client was seen in the emergency department with severe abdominal pain, nausea, vomiting, and diarrhea. Vital signs were: Blood pressure 120/80, heart rate 100 beats per minute, respirations 20 breaths per minute, and temperature of 103°F. The client has a history of angina. What was the client's chief complaint?

1. temperature 103°F
2. angina pectoris
3. severe abdominal pain
4. nausea, vomiting, and diarrhea

3 - 3 6

A client receiving antineoplastic agents asks the nurse why the antigout medication allopurinol has been included in the chemotherapy regimen. The nurse's explanation will include the information that allopurinol:

1. enhances the effects of antineoplastic agents.
2. decreases the side effects of nausea and vomiting.
3. will prevent symptoms of gout that may occur due to rapid cell destruction.
4. will prevent normal cell destruction by promoting folic acid conversion.

3 - 3 7

A client with pancreatitis has an increase in the serum amylase level. This is consistent with a nursing diagnosis of:

1. "altered nutrition, more than body requirements related to excessive intake."
2. "fluid volume excess related to congestive heart failure."
3. "pain related to inflamed pancreas."
4. "altered nutrition, less than body requirements related to inadequate nutrition."

3 - 3 8

A client with a hiatal hernia is receiving the dopamine antagonist metoclopramide hydrochloride. You will explain that the purpose of this medication is to:

1. lower esophageal sphincter pressure.
2. increase gastric emptying.
3. decrease gastric acid production.
4. protect the gastric mucosa.

3 - 3 9

Acid-ash foods for clients with hypercalcemia may be included as part of the treatment for angina. Which of the following will the nurse recognize as foods found on an acid-ash diet?

1. vegetables
2. milk
3. peaches and apples
4. meat

3 - 4 0

Your client has a colostomy. After ambulation, you notice that the client's stoma is a dusky color. You will:

1. have the client lie down and then notify the physician.
2. loosen the drainage pouch and inspect the stoma for ischemia.
3. do nothing, since the stoma should appear dusky in color.
4. prepare the client for a stomal irrigation.

3 - 4 1

Which assessment finding is indicative of a vitamin K deficiency?

1. bruising
2. paresthesia
3. brittle nails
4. loss and thinning of hair

3 - 4 2

A 6-month-old infant with phenylketonuria is brought to the clinic. The client is on a phenylalanine-controlled diet. Which information will the nurse include in the teaching plan that emphasizes the cause of this condition?

1. insufficient fat intake during early infancy
2. deficiency of an enzyme needed to utilize galactose during early infancy
3. inability of the infant to metabolize one of the essential amino acids
4. abnormal accumulation of lipids in the cells of infants

3 - 4 3

A client with cirrhosis of the liver is developing hepatic encephalopathy. You will anticipate laboratory studies that will monitor the client's level of:

1. blood ammonia.
2. serum protein.
3. alpha-fetoprotein.
4. serum amylase.

3 - 4 4

A client with cirrhosis of the liver is concerned about spider angiomas on the nose and cheeks. You teach the client that the angiomas are caused by:

1. splenomegaly.
2. decreased prothrombin levels.
3. increased circulating estrogens.
4. urea crystal deposits on the skin.

3 - 4 5

Your client has achalasia. To decrease esophageal pressure and improve swallowing, the nurse will anticipate a prescription for:

1. antilipemics.
2. bronchodilators.
3. calcium channel blockers.
4. anti-infectives.

3 - 4 6

The results of a diagnostic test reveal that a client has salmonellosis. Which of the following measures, if used by the nurse, would be most effective in preventing the transfer of this organism to others?

1. wearing a protective gown when in proximity to the client
2. discarding any needle used in the treatment of the client
3. washing the hands upon leaving the client's room
4. using disposable dishes for the client's foods

3 - 4 7

After a colonoscopy, which of the following symptoms will suggest that a client has bowel perforation secondary to the procedure?

1. nausea and vomiting
2. abdominal pain and fever
3. abdominal distention and hyperactive bowel sounds
4. hypotension and confusion

3 - 4 8

A client is to have a stool culture for ova and parasites. The accuracy of the results of the client's stool culture would be influenced mostly by which of the following measures taken by the nurse?

1. keeping the specimen warm
2. collecting a large specimen
3. obtaining the specimen before the client has breakfast
4. omitting meat from the client's diet for 3 days

3 - 4 9

A client has liver damage. The nurse will anticipate an abnormally low serum value for:

1. glutaminic-oxaloacetic transaminase.
2. lactic dehydrogenase.
3. albumin.
4. alkaline phosphatase.

3 - 5 0

An adult client is admitted to the hospital with a diagnosis of advanced cirrhosis and ascites. Because the client has advanced cirrhosis of the liver, the nurse would most likely obtain which of the following information during an assessment?

1. clubbing of the fingers
2. an acetone odor of the breath
3. epigastric pain and dysphasia
4. fatigue and muscle wasting

3 - 5 1

A client has been admitted to your unit with a jejunostomy tube. Which nursing action is contraindicated?

1. Administer bolus tube feeding every 4 hours.
2. Flush tube with 30 cc of water every 4 hours.
3. Administer medications in liquid form.
4. Change feeding bag every 24 hours.

3 - 5 2

In planning dietary education for a client on a low-fat diet, the nurse should first:

1. determine a 24-hour recall and a list of foods the client likes best.
2. give the client a list of foods included in a low-fat diet.
3. discuss with the client the important relationship between diet and exercise.
4. tell the client that fruits and vegetables should form the bulk of a low-fat diet.

3 - 5 3

A client is scheduled for a partial glossectomy. The nurse should recognize the primary purpose of oral hygiene preoperatively is to:

1. reduce the bacterial count in the mouth.
2. alter the pH of the salivary secretions.
3. improve the functioning of the taste buds.
4. promote softening of the lesion.

3 - 5 4

A client receives a diagnosis of acute pancreatitis. In assessing the client's condition, the nurse should expect the laboratory test results to show an elevated serum level of which of the following substances?

1. amylase
2. bilirubin
3. cholesterol
4. gastrin

3 - 5 5

A 6-month-old has been vomiting, crying, screaming, and drawing her knees up to her abdomen for 3 hours. The diagnosis is possible intussusception. Which of the following additional signs of intussusception would the nurse observe and record?

1. jaundice
2. hematuria
3. petechia
4. currant jelly-like stools

3 - 5 6

You are to give potassium chloride liquid to a client with a percutaneous endoscopic gastrostomy who is on continual feedings. Prior to administering the medication, you aspirate 30 cc of residual feed. You should:

1. discard the residual feed and withhold the medication.
2. reinstill the residual feed and give the medication.
3. question the administration of potassium chloride via a percutaneous endoscopic gastrostomy.
4. increase the tube feeding rate and give the medication.

3 - 5 7

You are teaching a group of concerned citizens how to minimize risks associated with the ingestion of pesticides. Which comments by the group suggest they understand how to minimize their risks?

Select all that apply by placing a ✔ in the square:

- ❏ 1. "We will trim the fat from meat before we cook it."
- ❏ 2. "We will use a knife to peel oranges and grapefruit."
- ❏ 3. "We will discard the outer leaves of leafy vegetables."
- ❏ 4. "We won't use a scrub brush to wash fresh vegetables."
- ❏ 5. "We will wash and rinse fresh produce in water."

3 - 5 8

Which of the following do you recognize as risk factors associated with cancer?

Select all that apply by placing a ✔ in the square:

- ❏ 1. excessive alcohol intake
- ❏ 2. low-fat diet
- ❏ 3. high fiber intake
- ❏ 4. low vitamin and mineral intake
- ❏ 5. smoking tobacco

3 - 5 9

A client comes to the clinic and tells the nurse, "About an hour or two after I drink milk or eat ice cream, I become bloated and have gas, crampy abdominal pain, and diarrhea." You suspect this client has a deficiency in the enzyme:

_____

Fill in the blank

3 - 6 0

Clients experiencing complications from Crohn's disease may have a deficiency in which of the following vitamins?

Select all that apply by placing a ✔ in the square:

- ❏ 1. A
- ❏ 2. D
- ❏ 3. C
- ❏ 4. E
- ❏ 5. B
- ❏ 6. K

3 - 6 1

Your client has an ileostomy. Which of the following foods is associated with potential obstruction in clients with an ileostomy?

Select all that apply by placing a ✔ in the square:

- ❏ 1. celery
- ❏ 2. nuts
- ❏ 3. onions
- ❏ 4. popcorn
- ❏ 5. beans

Practice Test 3

Answers, Rationales, and Explanations

3 - 1

Fill in the blank correct answer:

24 hours

The tube feeding container and line are normally changed every 24 hours to prevent transmission of bacteria. The feedings themselves should infuse for no longer than 8 hours.

Client Need: Safe, Effective Care Environment.

3 - 2

② **The most accurate assessment for correct placement of a nasogastric tube is an X-ray visualization of the gastric area. With an X ray, one actually sees if the tube is correctly positioned.**

1. Determining the pH of aspirate is one way to check tube placement, but it is not the most accurate way.

3. Auscultation over the gastric area to hear the sound of injected air as it enters the stomach is one method to check the tube placement, but it is not the most accurate.

4. Palpation is not used to determine placement of a nasogastric tube. Injecting enough air to palpate would cause discomfort.

Client Need: Health Promotion and Maintenance

3 - 3

② **The parents should be taught that surgical intervention will not be needed. Medical treatment and allowing time for maturation of the gastrointestinal tract are usually all that is necessary to treat gastroesophageal reflux in the infant. The parents should also be taught to place the infant in an upright position after feedings and also during sleep. Medications may be prescribed to hasten emptying of the stomach and to decrease gastric acidity. If surgery becomes necessary, it is usually beyond infancy. A technique called fundoplication is used to prevent reflux.**

1. Gastric contents are very acidic and irritating to the respiratory tract if aspirated. The upper sphincter of the stomach is somewhat relaxed in infants and allows for regurgitation of gastric contents. Pneumonia and breathing problems could occur.

3. Formula thickened with rice cereal is a common treatment. The heavier, thickened formula is not as likely to reflux and is more likely to empty into the duodenum.

4. Feeding more often and not as much at a time is a common treatment for gastroesophageal reflux. The less full the stomach is, the less likely reflux will occur.

Client Need: Health Promotion and Maintenance

3 - 4

① **A gastroscopy would be the most likely diagnostic procedure, since upper gastrointestinal bleeding is suspected. A gastroscopy allows direct visualization of the mucosal lining of the esophagus, stomach, and duodenum.**

2. Gastrointestinal X rays would be requested only if the gastroscopy was inconclusive and it was thought that additional information would be useful.

3. Fiberoptic colonoscopy would not be requested since the bleeding is occurring in the upper gastrointestinal tract. A fiberoptic colonoscopy allows direct visualization of the colon up to the ileocecal valve. It is used to diagnose conditions such as inflammatory bowel disease, strictures, and bleeding sites. The procedure also allows for removal of polyps.

4. A gastric analysis is usually requested to analyze the pH and volume of the gastric contents. This test could assist in determining the cause of bleeding, such as high acidity of stomach contents. However, gastric analysis cannot locate specific sites of bleeding, since direct visualization is not possible.

Client Need: Health Promotion and Maintenance

3 - 5

④ **The percutaneous endoscopic gastrostomy (PEG) feeding should be turned off at least 30 minutes prior to the weighing process. This will decrease the risk of aspiration.**

1. Weighing the day's feeding formula and adding it to the client's weight is not an appropriate or common practice.

2. Clients receiving continuous PEG feedings can be weighed on bed scales.

3. There is no clinical reason to defer the daily weights.

Client Need: Safe, Effective Care Environment

3 - 6

② **You will instruct clients to hold the abdomen firmly, take several deep breaths, and then cough two or three times as they exhale. Effective splinting of the surgical site will allow the client to breathe deeply and cough more effectively. The client will experience less pain, since stress on the suture line is relieved. The goal of coughing and deep breathing is to fully expand and aerate the lungs, thus allowing secretions to be coughed out. Effective coughing is always preceded by deep breathing.**

1. When possible, the nurse should teach the postoperative client to maintain a sitting (upright) position for coughing and deep-breathing exercises. This position lowers abdominal organs and allows the diaphragm to expand fully. However, a sitting position may not be therapeutic for all surgical clients.

3. The client should not tighten the stomach muscles when coughing and deep-breathing exercises are performed. Also, it is not necessary that coughing be forceful. It would be helpful to have the client slightly flex the knees to take tension off the abdomen.

4. The client should be taught to breathe deeply from the diaphragm. Raising the shoulders tends to facilitate shallow breathing, not deep breathing.

Client Need: Physiological Integrity

3 - 7

④ Ingestion of caffeine and chocolate may exacerbate gastroesophageal reflux. The reflux of stomach contents into the esophagus is due in part to a lowering of esophageal sphincter pressure. Certain foods have been found to lower the sphincter's pressure. These foods include caffeine, chocolate, peppermint, and fatty foods.

1, 2, and 3. Neither poultry, pastas, herbs, or spices have been found to significantly lower esophageal sphincter pressure.

Client Need: Health Promotion and Maintenance

3 - 8

④ Administering potassium chloride will replace the potassium that is being lost through vomiting. Potassium is one of the electrolytes contained in gastric secretions. When excessive vomiting or suctioning of gastric contents occurs, clients lose potassium (K+). If potassium is not replaced, hypokalemia may occur.

1. Potassium is usually lost in urine output during diuretic therapy.

2. Potassium cannot be stored in the body. A minimum of 40 mEq of potassium must be consumed daily. A normal potassium level is 3.5 to 5.5 mEq/l.

3. Potassium does not promote excretion of sodium. When potassium is lost from cells, sodium shifts into the cells to replace lost K+.

Client Need: Physiological Integrity

3 - 9

① The dumping syndrome is a direct result of removing a large portion of the stomach. The dumping syndrome is a set of unpleasant vasomotor and gastrointestinal (GI) symptoms that occur in 10 to 50% of clients who have had gastric surgery. Food passes too rapidly from the stomach remnant into the duodenum and jejunum. Symptoms include weakness, faintness, cramping, and diarrhea.

2. Hyperosmolar chyme occurs as a result of food entering the duodenum and jejunum without proper mixing.

3 and 4. The dumping syndrome occurs as a direct result of gastrointestinal surgery. Eating large quantities of food, not lying down after meals, and drinking liquids with the meal contribute to the problem.

Client Need: Physiological Integrity

3 - 1 0

Fill in the blank correct answer:

<u>25 ounces.</u>

Most commercially prepared formulas contain about 20 kcal/oz, as does breast milk. Some of the formulas made for preterm infants are slightly higher in energy. The following equation may be used to calculate the ounces of formula for a given energy:

$$\frac{20 \text{ kcal}}{1 \text{ oz}} = \frac{500 \text{ kcal}}{X}$$

20X = 500 kcal

X = 25 oz.

Client Need: Health Promotion and Maintenance

3 - 1 1

② Babies require 105 to 110 kcal/kg/day of energy. The following formula may be used to calculate this infant's caloric needs:

$$\frac{105 \text{ to } 110 \text{ kcal/kg}}{\text{day}} \times \frac{1 \text{ kg}}{2.2 \text{ lb}} \times 10 \text{ lb} = \frac{477 \text{ to } 500 \text{ kcal}}{\text{day}}$$

1, 3, and 4. A baby requiring 500 kcal/day would be undernourished, receiving only 100 kcal/day, and overfed receiving either 1,000 or 1,500 kcal/day.

Client Need: Health Promotion and Maintenance

3 - 1 2

① Manifestations of Crohn's disease include diarrhea, fatigue, abdominal pain, and weight loss. Crohn's disease is a chronic, nonspecific inflammatory disorder of unknown origin that can affect any part of the gastrointestinal (GI) tract. It is characterized by inflammation of segments of the GI tract. This condition is also called regional ileitis and regional enteritis.

2. Jaundice and steatorrhea (fatty stools) are symptoms of gallbladder disease.

3. Shortness of breath and tachycardia would be symptoms manifested in a client with chronic obstructive pulmonary disease (COPD).

4. Dependent edema and ascites are seen in right-sided congestive heart failure.

Client Need: Physiological Integrity

3 - 1 3

③ Prolonged gastroesophageal reflux disease can quickly become life threatening, causing esophageal ulceration. A repeated assault on the esophageal mucosa by acid reflux can cause erosion of the esophagus and hemorrhage. This is an uncommon occurrence, but can be morbid if not treated promptly. Symptoms may become very severe and constant with little relief from previously effective treatments. This is a medical emergency.

1 and 2. Neither pharyngitis nor colitis is directly related to gastroesophageal reflux disease (GERD). However, they may occur simultaneously.

4.   The chest pains associated with angina may easily be confused with the "heartburn" associated with GERD, and vice versa. Although one does not cause the other, pain that may be cardiac in origin must always be considered when a client complains of chest pain.

Client Need: Physiological Integrity

3 - 1 4

① A baked chicken breast, an apple, and skim milk would be appropriate foods for a client with hypercholesterolemia. Clients with hypercholesterolemia have elevated serum cholesterol levels, which have been found to contribute to the development of coronary artery disease. The consumption of low-fat foods, such as white meat, fruits, vegetables, grains, and skimmed dairy products, will help lower serum lipid levels.

1, 3, and 4. Beef, cheese, fried foods, and processed meats are all high in fat and contribute to hypercholesterolemia.

Client Need: Health Promotion and Maintenance

3 - 1 5

④ You will suspect a pharyngoesophageal diverticulum. A diverticulum is an outpouching of the mucosa that protrudes through a weak place in the esophageal musculature. Symptoms include dysphagia, belching, regurgitation of undigested food, gurgling sounds after eating (caused by fluid and food filling the diverticulum), coughing caused by trachea irritation, halitosis (bad breath), and a sour taste in the mouth caused by decomposing food lodged in the diverticulum.

1.   A diffuse esophageal spasm is caused by motor excitement of the esophagus that produces alternate periods of contractions and relaxation. Symptoms include dysphagia (difficulty swallowing) and chest pain.

2.   Gastroesophageal reflux is characterized by reflux (backward flow) of the acidic contents of the stomach into the distal portion of the esophagus. Symptoms include pyrosis (heartburn), regurgitation (return of food from the stomach into esophagus and mouth), dysphagia (difficulty swallowing), and painful feeling of a lump in the throat.

3.   Hiatal hernia type 1 is a sliding hernia where the upper stomach and the gastroesophageal junction are pushed upward in and out of the thorax. Type 2 is a herniation of a portion of the stomach through an opening (hiatus) into the esophagus. This condition is also known as esophageal or diaphragmatic hernia. Symptoms of types 1 and 2 include pyrosis (heartburn) and dysphagia (difficulty swallowing).

Client Need: Physiological Integrity

3 - 1 6

③ **Pyloric obstruction is suspected. Scarring at the pylorus is likely to cause pyloric obstruction. As a result of the obstruction, the contents of the stomach are unable to empty properly, which causes gastric fullness, distention, pain, nausea, and vomiting. When clients lie down at night, pain intensifies since the stomach is even less likely to be emptied by peristalsis.**

1. The symptoms of peptic ulcer perforation are different from those of pyloric obstruction. Symptoms of peptic ulcer perforation include sudden onset of severe upper abdominal pain that spreads rapidly throughout the abdomen as the spillage of gastrointestinal contents invade the peritoneal cavity. Clients experience a rigid, board-like abdomen. Respirations become shallow and rapid and bacterial septicemia develops, causing fever and hypovolemic shock.

2. Some of the symptoms of acute gastritis are similar to those of pyloric obstruction. However, the client's history of scarring at the distal end of the pyloric sphincter is highly suggestive of pyloric obstruction.

4. A paralytic ileus is a postoperative complication. Peristalsis stops in a portion of the bowel, which causes diminished or absent bowel sounds. Abdominal distention occurs and the client complains of pain and feelings of fullness. A nasogastric tube is usually required to relieve distention and vomiting until normal bowel peristalsis resumes.

Client Need: Physiological Integrity

3 - 1 7

④ **The nurse should explain to the client that 90 to 100% of clients experiencing ulcerative colitis have blood, pus, and mucus in their stools. Understanding the nature and symptoms of the disease may help to alleviate the client's anxiety.**

1. It is not necessary to check the client's stools for the presence of occult blood since blood in the stools is a typical finding. Ninety to 100% of clients in the acute phase of ulcerative colitis have blood in their stools.

2. The client should participate in maintaining a record of the number and description of stools. However, simply maintaining a record will not give the client the information needed to allay anxiety about blood in the stools.

3. It is not necessary to notify the client's physician since blood in the stools is expected in ulcerative colitis. Nursing care would include a record of the number and a description of stools.

Client Need: Psychosocial Integrity

3 - 1 8

① **The normal serum bilirubin level is 0.2 to 1.0 mg/dl. A serum bilirubin level of 50 mg/dl is associated with late-stage liver disease.**

2, 3, and 4. Serum bilirubin levels higher than 1.0 mg/dl are outside the normal range.

Client Need: Physiological Integrity

3 - 1 9

② **The colostomy should begin to function within 2 to 4 days. It generally takes this long for peristalsis to be restored following abdominal surgery.**

1. It is not usual for a colostomy to function within 12 to 24 hours since peristalsis doesn't return for 48 to 72 hours postoperatively.

3 and 4. A colostomy should begin to function in response to the return of peristalsis. Peristalsis should return within 2 to 4 days postoperatively. If peristalsis has not returned within that time, complications such as a paralytic ileus may be suspected.

Client Need: Psychosocial Integrity

3 - 2 0

③ **Offering frequent small portions of favorite foods following periods of rest will prevent exhaustion in the acutely ill child and will meet nutritional requirements.**

1. The temperature of the food is not the issue. The foods should require little energy to consume and should be foods that the child enjoys.

2. Providing liquids through a straw would conserve energy. However, if the child does not like the liquids, they are not likely to be consumed.

4. If the child does not enjoy any foods from the regularly scheduled meals, they are not likely to be consumed.

Client Need: Health Promotion and Maintenance

3 - 2 1

④ **The sump drain will allow wound healing to take place from its lowest depth without forming an abscess.**

1. The character and volume of drainage can be assessed by using a sump drain. However, this is not the primary purpose for the drain.

2. Flatus will be expelled from the colostomy, not the perineal wound.

3. A sump drain can be as easily contaminated as a dressing.

Client Need: Physiological Integrity

3 - 2 2

④ **Aluminum hydroxide (Amphojel) is an antacid that neutralizes gastric secretions by buffering hydrochloric acid.**

1. Antiulcer (histamine H2 antagonists) such as Tagamet inhibit the secretion of hydrochloride acid. Antacids like Amphojel do not inhibit this secretion.

2 and 3. Aluminum hydroxide does not impact the breakdown of protein, or absorb air that has been swallowed.

Client Need: Physiological Integrity

3 - 2 3

② **The purpose of the infusion is to replace the potassium that is lost through vomiting. Potassium is one of the electrolytes contained in gastric secretions. Excessive vomiting or suctioning of gastric contents results in potassium loss and, if not replaced, can lead to hypokalemia.**

1. There is no indication that potassium is being lost through urinary output. Clients who are treated with diuretics such as furosemide (Lasix) may lose potassium. However, there is no indication that this client is receiving a diuretic.

3. Potassium is not stored in the body. People of all ages need to consume potassium on a daily basis. Foods high in potassium include dried peach halves, lima beans, winter squash, potatoes, bananas, and pinto beans.

4. Potassium does not promote excretion of sodium chloride.

Client Need: Physiological Integrity

3 - 2 4

② **A combination of 30 grams of powdered skim milk and 1 whole egg will provide the highest amount of protein.**

1, 3, and 4. Light cream, corn syrup, ice cream, chocolate syrup, and sugar are high in fat and sugar and would not be encouraged.

Client Need: Health Promotion and Maintenance

3 - 2 5

① An accurate and appropriate explanation would be, "In the X-ray department, you will be asked to drink a thick liquid, and then several X rays of the upper part of your digestive tract will be taken at intervals." This explanation is simple, factual, and understandable to a layperson or a client.

2. A gastrointestinal series (GI series) does not require the client to swallow a tube.

3. The substance used for performing a GI series is radiopaque, not radioactive.

4. A GI series is not uncomfortable.

Client Need: Safe, Effective Care Environment

3 - 2 6

③ If a client's chest tube is not draining immediately following a transthoracic hiatal herniorrhaphy, the nurse should have the client deep breathe and cough. In the immediate postoperative period, bloody drainage is expected. Having the client deep breathe and cough will effect changes in intrapleural pressures and, by observing for oscillation of the fluid in the water-seal chamber of the drainage apparatus, it will be possible to determine if the chest tube and connecting tubing are patent. If plugged, the increased intrapleural pressure manifested during coughing may be sufficient to dislodge any obstruction. A patent system is necessary to prevent a hemo- or pneumothorax.

1. Clamping the chest tube may be done when checking for an air leak. However, clamping of chest tubes is not done when the chest tubes are not draining.

2. Increasing the suction will only draw in air through the vented tubing. It will not affect drainage.

4. The client should be turned toward the operative site after coughing and deep breathing.

Client Need: Safe, Effective Care Environment

3 - 2 7

Fill in the blank correct answer:

Potassium

The nurse should instruct clients on thiazide drugs such as chlorothiazide (Diuril) to include foods in their diet that are high in potassium. Thiazide diuretics are potassium-depleting. Foods high in potassium include peaches, lima beans, winter squash, pears, baked potato with skin, bananas, and oranges.

Client Need: Physiological Integrity

3 - 2 8

① The nurse should assess the client for hypotension following prochlorperazine maleate (Compazine) administration. Hypotension is an adverse reaction to prochlorperazine maleate. Other side effects include drowsiness, dizziness, contact dermatitis, and photo-sensitivity.

2, 3, and 4. Headache, confusion, and dry mouth are not associated with Compazine administration.

Client Need: Safe, Effective Care Environment

3 - 2 9

① The child should be placed in a semi-upright (45-degree) position. A semi-upright position affords maximum lung expansion for the client with ascites.

2. A semi-prone position (client lying on abdomen with head of bed slightly elevated) would not facilitate breathing.

3. A dorsal recumbent position (client lying on back) would restrict diaphragmatic excursion and would not facilitate breathing.

4. A prone position (client lying on the abdomen face down) would be very uncomfortable and would obstruct breathing by pressing the fluid in the abdomen (ascites) up against the diaphragm.

Client Need: Physiological Integrity

3 - 3 0

① The nurse will inform the mothers that diets that include milk to the exclusion of other foods may be deficient in iron. Infants and children between the ages of 6 and 34 months may be vulnerable to iron-deficiency anemia since cow's milk is low in iron. Breast-fed infants or those receiving iron-fortified formula usually receive adequate iron intake.

2, 3, and 4. Cow's milk is not deficient in carbohydrates or vitamins D and K.

Client Need: Health Promotion and Maintenance

3 - 3 1

④ **The nurse will provide the client with an explanation of the ultrasonography and its purpose.**

1. A sedative is not necessary for clients having ultrasonography. There is no pain or discomfort as the transducer glides over the surface of the body.

2. Ultrasonography does not require the client to ingest a contrast media that might cause an allergic reaction.

3. Special dietary preparation is not needed for ultrasonography. However, the client should be instructed not to eat solid food 12 hours before the procedure. The client may have water.

Client Need: Psychological Integrity

3 - 3 2

③ **Cream cheese on toasted white bread, canned peaches, and decaffeinated coffee are foods that are allowed on a bland diet.**

1, 2, and 4. Foods that are not allowed on a bland diet include fried foods, cured meats, high-fiber breads, highly seasoned foods, and foods or drinks that contain caffeine.

Client Need: Health Promotion and Maintenance

3 - 3 3

① **Prior to a barium enema, prescribed bowel preparations should be completed. This includes the administration of laxatives and cleansing enemas.**

② **A liquid diet should be consumed 24 hours before the test. Fecal matter and gas can interfere with test results.**

③ **To ensure adequate hydration, clients should receive a minimum of 240 ml of clear liquids prior to the test.**

4. A warm, flushed sensation occurs when a radiopaque dye is injected intravenously in procedures such as excretory urography (IUP).

5. The preparation for a barium swallow, not a barium enema, has an unpleasant, thick, chalky taste.

Client Need: Physiological Integrity

3 - 3 4

② Steak, spinach, and whole-grain breads are high in iron. Other foods high in iron include muscle meats, eggs, dried fruits, legumes, dark green leafy vegetables, potatoes, enriched bread, and cereals.

1, 3, and 4. Milk, pork, squash, oranges, chicken, green beans, tomatoes, strawberries, and liver are not high in iron.

Client Need: Physiological Integrity

3 - 3 5

③ Severe abdominal pain was the client's chief complaint. The severe abdominal pain is what brought the client to the hospital.

1. The client's temperature is part of the present health status.
2. Angina pectoris is a part of the client's past history.
4. Nausea, vomiting, and diarrhea are a part of the history of the present illness.

Client Need: Physiological Integrity

3 - 3 6

③ Allopurinol (Zyloprim) prevents the symptoms of gout that may occur due to rapid cell destruction by antineoplastic medications.

1. Zyloprim does not enhance the effects of antineoplastic agents.
2. Zyloprim is not an antiemetic and will not decrease nausea and vomiting.
4. Zyloprim does not prevent normal cell destruction.

Client Need: Psychological Integrity

3 - 3 7

③ A client with pancreatitis who has an increase in serum amylase levels will have a nursing diagnosis of pain related to inflamed pancreas. An elevation in serum amylase and lipase is consistent with pancreatitis. A common clinical manifestation of pancreatitis is pain.

1. An increase in the serum cholesterol level may be seen with an increase in food intake.
2. A decrease in the serum sodium level may suggest increased fluid volume seen with congestive heart failure.
4. Hypoalbuminenemia is seen with inadequate intake of nutrients.

Client Need: Physiological Integrity

3 - 3 8

② **Metoclopramide (Reglan) increases the resting tone of the lower esophageal sphincter and facilitates gastric emptying. Persons with hiatal hernia usually receive the dopamine antagonist metoclopramide (Reglan). This medication stimulates motility of the upper gastrointestinal tract without stimulating gastric secretions.**

1. Reglan does not lower esophageal sphincter pressure.
3. Reglan is an antiemetic, gastrointestinal stimulant. It does not decrease gastric acid production.
4. Medications such as sucralfate protect the gastric mucosa, not Reglan.

Client Need: Physiological Integrity

3 - 3 9

④ **Acid-ash foods include protein-rich choices such as meat, fish, poultry, eggs, cheese, grains (breads and cereals), and certain fruits (cranberries, prunes, and plums).**

1 and 3. Vegetables and most fruits are not rich in protein and are therefore not included in an acid-ash diet.
2. Milk is high in calcium and would not be recommended for clients who are experiencing hypercalcemia.

Client Need: Health Promotion and Maintenance

3 - 4 0

② **The drainage pouch should be loosened and the stoma inspected for ischemia. A dusky color indicates stomal ischemia. Blood supply may be promoted by loosening or adjusting the colostomy pouch. If this does not correct the deficiency of blood supply, the physician should be notified.**

1. The nurse would examine the client's stoma to determine the possible cause for the ischemia before notifying the physician.
3. A healthy stoma is pink.
4. Irrigating the colostomy would not affect the color of the stoma.

Client Need: Physiological Integrity

3 - 4 1

① **When there is a deficiency in vitamin K, the client's blood will not clot easily, and therefore, bruising would be evident. Vitamin K plays an important role in blood coagulation.**

2. Paresthesia is indicative of vitamin B_{12} deficiencies, not vitamin K deficiencies.

3 and 4. Brittle nails, hair thinning, and hair loss are consistent with protein deficiency, not vitamin K deficiency.

Client Need: Physiological Integrity

3 - 4 2

③ **In phenylketonuria (PKU), the hepatic enzyme needed to metabolize the amino acid phenylalanine (an essential amino acid formed from protein) is absent, resulting in the accumulation of phenylalanine in the bloodstream and excretion of phenyl acid in the urine.**

1. Phenylketonuria is not associated with fat intake.

2. Galactose is a monosaccharide, not an amino acid. Galactose is readily absorbed in the digestive tract and is converted into glycogen in the liver.

4. The word lipids is a descriptive rather than a chemical term such as protein or carbohydrates. Lipids do not affect the essential amino acid phenylalanine.

Client Need: Health Promotion and Maintenance

3 - 4 3

① **The blood ammonia level will be elevated in clients with hepatic encephalopathy (hepatic coma). The conversion of ammonia to urea normally occurs in the liver; therefore, the ammonia level will be elevated when the liver is affected with cirrhosis.**

2. Serum protein refers to any of the several proteins in the blood serum. Serum protein levels above or below the normal range do not directly affect the conversion of ammonia to urea.

3. Alpha-fetoprotein refers to an antigen present in the human fetus. Elevated levels of alpha-fetoprotein are also found in adults with hepatic carcinomas or chemical injuries. Alpha-fetoprotein does not affect the conversion of ammonia to urea.

4. Serum amylase is a class of enzyme that splits up starches. When the enzyme is found in animals, it is referred to as A-amylase. When found in plants, it is referred to as B-amylase. Serum amylase does not directly affect the conversion of ammonia to urea.

Client Need: Physiological Integrity

3 - 4 4

③ **Spider angiomas are caused by an increase in circulating estrogen as a result of the liver's inability to inactivate it. Spider angiomas are small dilated blood vessels with a bright red center and spidery-looking branches. They appear on the nose, cheeks, upper trunk, neck, and shoulders of clients with cirrhosis of the liver.**

1. Splenomegaly refers to enlargement of the spleen and does not cause spider angiomas. However, splenomegaley may be present in cirrhosis of the liver.

2. Prothrombin is a chemical substance in the circulating blood. Prothrombin is produced by thrombokinase interacting with calcium salts. Prothrombin is not directly associated with spider angiomas.

4. Urea crystal deposits on the skin are associated with renal failure. However, due to early and aggressive treatment of renal failure, this symptom is uncommon today.

Client Need: Physiological Integrity

3 - 4 5

③ **The nurse will anticipate a prescription for calcium channel blockers. Achalasia is the absence of or ineffective peristalsis in the distal portion of the esophagus. It is associated with failure of the esophageal sphincter to relax and permit swallowing. Calcium channel blockers reduce esophageal pressure and thereby improve swallowing by reducing arterial resistance.**

1. Antilipemics are agents that prevent or counteract the buildup of fatty substances in the blood. Antilipemics do not affect esophageal pressure.

2. Bronchodilators dilate the bronchus. They do not affect esophageal pressure.

4. Anti-infectives do not affect esophageal pressure. However, they may be administered for the treatment of aspiration pneumonia that can occur with esophageal spillover.

Client Need: Physiological Integrity

3 - 4 6

③ **The nursing measure that would be most effective in preventing the transfer of the organism salmonella is handwashing.**

1. Gown and gloves must be worn by individuals when in direct contact with infected clients.

2. All used needles should be discarded regardless of a client's diagnosis. However, salmonellosis is not transferred by contaminated needles.

4. Using disposable dishes for the client's food is also effective in preventing the spread of salmonella infection. However, handwashing is the most effective in preventing the transfer of salmonella.

Client Need: Safe, Effective Care Environment

3 - 4 7

② Following a colonoscopy, abdominal pain and fever directly suggest bowel perforation and occurrence of peritonitis secondary to perforation.

1, 3, and 4. Indirect suggestions of perforation include distension, hyperactive bowel sounds, hypotension, confusion, nausea, and vomiting.

Client Need: Physiological Integrity

3 - 4 8

① The accuracy of the results of a stool specimen for ova and parasites is dependent upon the specimen being fresh and warm. Ova and parasites cannot live in temperatures much lower than normal body temperature. Urine will also destroy parasites, so care must be taken not to contaminate specimens with urine.

2. Collecting a large specimen is not necessary. It takes only a small amount of feces to obtain results for ova and parasites.

3. Obtaining the specimen before the client has breakfast is not necessary. However, the specimen does need to be fresh and warm.

4. Omitting meat from the client's diet for 3 days has no impact on a specimen for ova and parasites. It would affect specimens for occult blood, since meat contains hemoglobin, myoglobin, and enzymes that can give false-positive results up to 4 days after meat is eaten.

Client Need: Safe, Effective Care Environment

3 - 4 9

③ The nurse would expect a client with liver damage to have abnormally low serum values of albumin. Liver damage is characterized by decreased ability of the liver to synthesize proteins. Consequently, albumin synthesis is reduced.

1. Serum glutaminic-oxaloacetic transaminase (SGOT) is an enzyme present in serum and body tissue. An elevation of SGOT is associated with myocardial infarction or hepatic cell damage.

2. Lactic dehydrogenase (LDH) is an enzyme found in various tissues and serum. LDH is important in catalyzing the oxidation of lactate. It has no direct impact on liver damage.

4. Alkaline phosphatase (ALP) is an enzyme originating mainly in the bone, liver, and placenta, with some activity in the kidney and intestine. It has no direct effect on clients with liver damage.

Client Need: Physiological Integrity

3-50

④ **When assessing a client with advanced cirrhosis and ascites, the nurse would observe muscle wasting and signs of fatigue. Chronic cirrhosis and malnutrition affect carbohydrate and protein metabolism, leading to generalized weakness, fatigue, and muscle wasting.**

1. Clubbing of the fingers is an indication of a heart condition due to ischemia.
2. An acetone odor in the breath could indicate diabetic ketoacidosis.
3. Epigastric pain and dysphagia could indicate a gastrointestinal problem.

Client Need: Physiological Integrity

3-51

① **Because a jejunostomy tube introduces food directly into the jejunum, a bolus feeding is contraindicated. A bolus feeding would cause a hyperosmolar reaction much like the dumping syndrome. Clients with a jejunostomy tube will need continuous enteral feeding.**

2. The nurse will need to flush the tube with 30 cc of water every 4 hours.
3. The nurse will need to administer medications in a liquid form.
4. The nurse will need to change the feeding bag every 24 hours.

Client Need: Safe, Effective Care Environment

3-52

① **The nurse should first determine a 24-hour recall and a list of foods the client likes best. The client's eating habits and lifestyle should also be considered. This will help the nurse plan an acceptable diet, thus increasing chances of compliance.**

2, 3, and 4. Providing lists of foods, education, and telling the client about fruits and vegetables is less helpful. The nurse should first complete 24-hour recall of the foods the client likes.

Client Need: Health Promotion and Maintenance

3 - 5 3

① The primary purpose of preoperative oral hygiene in clients scheduled for partial glossectomy is to reduce the bacterial count in the mouth. Measures to increase the cleanliness of the oral cavity before surgery will reduce the incidence of postoperative infections such as surgical parotitis.

2. Preoperative oral hygiene will not alter the pH of salivary secretions.

3. Preoperative oral hygiene will not improve the function of the tastebuds.

4. Preoperative oral hygiene is not given to soften lesions.

Client Need: Physiological Integrity

3 - 5 4

① A client with acute pancreatitis will show an elevated serum amylase. Serum amylase levels increase due to activation of this enzyme while it is still in the pancreas. This causes actual tissue damage and autodigestion of the pancreas.

2. Bilirubin is produced from the hemoglobin of red blood cells. It is changed chemically in the liver and excreted in the bile. The accumulation of bilirubin leads to jaundice. Bilirubin does not directly affect the pancreas or cause pancreatitis.

3. Cholesterol is a component in cell membrane and plasma lipoproteins. It is absorbed from the diet and synthesized in the liver and other body tissues. Elevated cholesterol may indicate a risk for pancreatitis and other disorders. However, in acute pancreatitis there will be a marked increase in amylase.

4. Gastrin refers to a group of hormones secreted by the mucosa of the pyloric area of the stomach. Gastrin affects the secretionary activity of the gallbladder, pancreas, and small intestine. However, it does not directly cause an increase in amylase.

Client Need: Physiological Integrity

3 - 5 5

④ The nurse will observe and record currant-jelly-like stools. Currant-jelly-like stools are caused by blood and mucus in the intestinal tract. Other symptoms are absence of stools, increasing abdominal distention and tenderness, sausage-like mass in the upper-right abdomen, dehydration, fever, and a shock-like state.

1, 2, and 3. Jaundice, hematuria, and petechia are not signs commonly associated with intussusception.

Client need: Physiological Integrity

3 - 5 6

② You will reinstall the residual feed into the percutaneous endoscopic gastrostomy (PEG) and give the medication. Reinstallation of the residual volume helps avoid fluid and electrolyte imbalance.

1. Residual volumes are usually reinstalled. There is no reason to withhold the medication.

3. Potassium chloride liquid may be given via the PEG.

4. There is no indication that the tube feeding rate should be increased.

Client Need: Physiological Integrity

3 - 5 7

① The fat in meats, as well as the skin from poultry and fish, should be discarded since pesticide residues concentrate in animal fats.

② Pesticide residues are found in the peels of fruits such as oranges and grapefruit. One should not bite into an unpeeled fruit.

③ The outer leaves of vegetables such as cabbage and lettuce should be discarded since pesticide residues are likely to be found there.

⑤ Fruits and vegetables should be washed in running water and rinsed in running water to take off pesticide residues.

4. It is good to use a scrub brush when washing fresh produce. A scrub brush is very effective in cleaning out crevices and sunken areas around stems.

Client Need: Safe, Effective Care Environment

3 - 5 8

① ④ and ⑤ High risk factors associated with cancer include excessive alcohol intake, low vitamin and mineral intake, and smoking tobacco. Other risk factors include a high-fat diet, contaminated food intake, and low calcium intake.

2. A low-fat diet is not associated with cancer.

3. A high-fiber diet is not associated with cancer.

Client Need: Health Promotion and Maintenance

3 - 5 9

Fill in the blank correct answer:

<u>Lactase</u>

The client's symptoms (bloating, flatulence, crampy abdominal pain, and diarrhea) following the ingestion of milk are associated with lactase deficiency. The enzyme lactase is necessary to break down lactose into two simple sugars, namely, glucose and galatose.

Client Need: Physiological Integrity

3 - 6 0

① ② ④ and ⑥ Complications from Crohn's disease include impaired absorption of fat, which creates a deficiency in the fat-soluble vitamins (A, D, E, and K).

3. Vitamin C is water-soluble and is not affected by Crohn's disease.

5. Vitamin B is water-soluble and is not affected by Crohn's disease.

Client Need: Health Promotion and Maintenance

3 - 6 1

① ② and ④ Foods associated with potential obstruction in clients with an ileostomy include celery, nuts, popcorn, raisins, seeds, raw vegetables, and corn. It should be noted that the effects of food on stoma output are individual.

3. Onions are likely to produce odor and gas, not an obstruction.

4. Beans are likely to produce gas, not an obstruction.

Client Need: Health Promotion and Maintenance

Practice Test 4

Immune and Lymphatic/Hematological Systems and Cancer

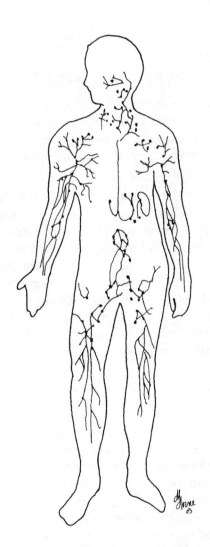

The Immune and Lymphatic Systems

OVERVIEW OF THE IMMUNE SYSTEM

The immune system is the body's physical and chemical defense against infection, whether localized or systemic. The system also responds to protect against allergens, toxins, and malignant cells. Infection occurs when an individual's immune system is not strong or efficient enough to mount a successful defense against microorganisms such as viruses, bacteria, and parasites that our bodies encounter in daily living. Antibiotics, antivirals, and other drugs can be used to help the body eliminate disease-causing organisms.

The immune system includes the lymphoid organs (lymph nodes, thymus, and spleen) as well as their products. It also includes the leukocytes or white blood cells, the chemicals they manufacture, and the organs that create them. The immune system is capable of destroying bacteria, viruses, and poisons. It also assists in healing injured tissue.

THE INFLAMMATORY RESPONSE

The skin and mucous membranes are the body's first-line barriers against foreign organisms. The skin surface is relatively dry, and infectious organisms tend to die without moisture. In addition, glands in our skin secrete fatty acids and other substances that are poisonous to foreign organisms. The membranes that line our nose, sinuses, and air passages are coated with sticky mucus that traps bacteria and viruses carried in the air and moves them into the throat and eventually into the stomach, where they are killed by strong acids and digestive enzymes.

However, when harmful organisms are able to penetrate the skin and mucous membranes, they trigger the body's second line of defense, the inflammatory response. For example, when bacteria enter the body through a cut and initiate an infection, phagocytes (such as neutrophils and macrophages) migrate to the site and begin to ingest the bacteria. The phagocytes also release proteins that attract other immune cells. This activity causes a localized area of heat and inflammation. Once the infection has been contained, macrophages at the site and in the bloodstream converge to clean up the dead cells and debris. This course of action is called the inflammatory response or, sometimes, the inflammatory process. The inflammatory response may be localized or may spread throughout the body in the blood and lymph. Systemic responses include fever, chills, swelling, and malaise, characteristic of infectious diseases like chickenpox, mumps, influenza, pneumonia, and many more.

THE IMMUNE RESPONSE

Not all infections can be stopped at the level of the inflammatory process. When this happens, B- and T-cell lymphocytes (white blood cells responsible for much of the body's immune protection) react in what is known as the immune response. In the immune response, B cells are transformed into plasma cells and secrete antibodies known as immunoglobulins. Immunoglobulins are carried in the bloodstream to the site of the infection, where they act to neutralize antigens. Antigens are substances that cause an immune response. Attached to the surface of bacteria, viruses, molds, and pollens, antigens are recognized by the body as foreign (not body tissue). The body reacts by creating antibodies (immunoglobulins) that are specific to the antigens. Immunoglobulins can also lyse (rupture) bacteria.

Unlike B cells, T cells are able to neutralize antigens directly. T cells are capable of attaching to antigens and destroying them, secreting proteins that assist other cells in destroying antigens, acting as helper cells (T-4 cells) to promote antibody synthesis by the B cells, and suppressing cells in order to inhibit antibody synthesis.

NATURAL, ACQUIRED, AND PASSIVE IMMUNITY

We can become immune (protected from) diseases through the immune response. Immunity can take two forms: natural immunity and acquired immunity. Persons who have natural immunity have an inborn resistance to disease. An example of this is genetically determined resistance to malaria. Acquired immunity, on the other hand, is not inherited. It comes about as a consequence of actually having a disease or by artificial acquisition via vaccines or immune serums. Once a person is exposed to the antigens of a disease, either by having the disease or by having a vaccination that contains live attenuated (weakened) or dead disease organisms, he or she will manufacture her own antibodies to that disease.

If a person needs immediate immunity, an immune serum containing the antibodies for that disease can be given, as for instance the tetanus serum. This kind of immunity is called passive immunity because the body does not build up its own antibodies. Passive immunity also occurs in response to a general "boosting" of the immune system via an injection of gamma globulin, and in the fetus as a result of maternal antibodies crossing the placenta.

Some people are carriers of a disease. This means that they can pass a disease on to others even though they do not show any evidence of having the disease themselves. Typhoid fever and tuberculosis can be transmitted by carriers.

ORGANS OF THE IMMUNE SYSTEM INCLUDE

Lymph Nodes and Nodules

B cells or B lymphocytes are produced in the lymph nodes and other lymphatic tissues. They secrete specialized antibodies that destroy specific invading organisms.

Lymph Vessels

These carry white blood cells and particles from diseased organs to the lymph nodes, where they are trapped and destroyed.

Spleen

This large abdominal organ produces specialized white blood cells that destroy disease-causing organisms in the body.

Bone Marrow

Some leukocytes are produced in the bone marrow.

White Blood Cells (Leukocytes)

Produced in the spleen, bone marrow, and thymus, these cells are the primary destroyers of disease-causing agents in the body.

Thymus

The white blood cells known as T lymphocytes complete their development in the thymus gland.

DISEASES/DISORDERS OF THE IMMUNE SYSTEM INCLUDE

Acquired Immunodeficiency Syndrome (AIDS)

Exposure to the human immunodeficiency virus (HIV) can cause a disease known as acquired immunodeficiency syndrome (AIDS). HIV can cause a loss of immune function by attacking the immune cells themselves. Without cells that recognize invading antigens, the body cannot create antibodies. As a consequence, opportunistic diseases such as tuberculosis, pneumocystis carinii pneumonia, toxoplasmosis, herpes simplex, and histoplasmosis are able to develop.

Leukopenia

This is an abnormal decrease in the total number of white blood cells, caused by radiation therapy, chemotherapy, and steroid drugs as well as by infection, which destroy the bone marrow's ability to produce white blood cells. As the number of circulating white blood cells decreases, the body is increasingly unable to identify and fight infections and diseases.

Allergy

Allergy is an over-response of the immune system to a foreign antigen, causing inflammation and sometimes resulting in organ dysfunction. Allergic disorders include:

ANAPHYLAXIS This potentially life-threatening reaction to a foreign antigen can cause a body-wide (systemic) inflammatory response including respiratory symptoms and fainting.

URTICARIA Swollen, raised, itchy skin caused by an inflammatory reaction to foods, drugs, heat, cold, or agents such as pollens or animal dander.

Autoimmune Disorders

Autoimmunity is the term for the body's tolerance to antigens located on its own cells. Autoimmune disorders result from the absence of this tolerance and are thought to be caused by heredity and environmental influences. Autoimmune disorders include:

RHEUMATOID ARTHRITIS (RA) This is a chronic, systemic, inflammatory disease that affects peripheral joints and connective tissue such as cartilage, bone, and blood vessels. Associated with periods of remission and exacerbation, symptoms include swelling in small and large joints that produce pain, stiffness, and fatigue. Joint fragility may lead to contractures and a decrease in range of motion (ROM).

OVERVIEW OF THE LYMPHATIC SYSTEM

The lymphatic system is closely aligned with the immune system. Lymph is a clear, watery liquid that surrounds cells and circulates around the entire body through its own system of vessels and nodes. The lymphatic system transports proteins and fluids from tissues back to the bloodstream via the veins. Lymphatic vessels in the small intestine absorb lipids (fats) from digested food and transport them to the bloodstream. Lymph is packed with two types of cells, lymphocytes and monocytes, which are formed in the lymph nodes and nodules.

Lymphocytes are responsible for much of the body's immune defense. Approximately 99% of lymphocytes are found in lymph nodes, the spleen, and other lymphoid organs such as the thymus. T cells derived from the thymus make up approximately 75% of all lymphocytes. B cells, derived from bone marrow, make up another 10%.

Monocytes (mononuclear phagocytic white blood cells) and macrophages (mature monocytes) are one of the first lines of defense in the inflammatory process. They surround, engulf, and destroy antigens and cellular debris. Macrophages are found in large quantities in the spleen, lymph nodes, alveoli, and tonsils. They are also found in the liver (Kupffer cells), brain, skin, and bone. Macrophages scavenge the blood to clear it of old cells, cellular debris, and pathogenic organisms such as viruses and bacteria.

ORGANS OF THE LYMPHATIC SYSTEM INCLUDE

All the organs of the immune system, as well as lymphoid tissues found in the small intestine, appendix, tonsils, adenoids, liver, lungs, and brain.

DISEASES/DISORDERS OF THE LYMPHATIC SYSTEM INCLUDE

Lymphoma

Lymphoma is a malignant tumor involving the lymph nodes and lymph tissue. One example of a lymphoma is Hodgkin's disease. This condition is characterized by enlargement of the lymph nodes, splenomegaly (enlargement of the spleen), fever, generalized weakness, weight loss, and anorexia.

Mononucleosis

This is an acute infectious disease associated with enlarged lymph nodes and increased numbers of lymphocytes and monocytes in the blood. It is caused by the Epstein-Barr virus. Symptoms include: Fatigue, generalized weakness, sore throat, and enlarged and tender lymph nodes in the cervical, axillary, and inguinal areas. Hepatomegaly (enlarged liver) and splenomegaly (enlarged spleen) are also present.

Sarcoidosis

This inflammatory disease is associated with small nodules (tubercles) in the lymph nodes as well as in other organs, for instance, the lungs. The cause of this condition is unknown. Symptoms include lymphadenopathy (enlargement of lymph nodes) and symptoms associated with lung involvement, such as: Fatigue, weight loss, anorexia, night sweats, shortness of breath, and a nonproductive cough.

OVERVIEW OF THE HEMATOLOGIC SYSTEM (BLOOD)

One vital function of the blood is to provide a constant environment (temperature and pH) for all the living tissues of the body. This is known as homeostasis. Another vital function is to transport nutrients from the digestive system to all body cells; wastes to the skin, liver, and kidneys for elimination from the body; and chemical messages (hormones and enzymes) to their intended tissues. Blood also transports gases to and from body cells.

The hematologic system aids the immune and lymphatic systems in protecting the body from pathogens such as bacteria, viruses, poisons, and dead or diseased cells. One example of this cooperation involves the production of complement. Antibodies in the blood activate a complex series of proteins, called complement proteins, which in turn assist the antibodies in destroying pathogens. Complement also acts directly, by lysing (rupturing) foreign organisms and by opsonizing organisms (coating them with proteins that make them easier for phagocytes to destroy).

The hematologic system also provides for damage control through a process called hemostasis. When a vessel wall becomes damaged and a tear is produced, red blood cells escape (bleeding), attracting great quantities of platelets. The platelets form a net of fibrin fibers, which begin repairs. Platelets also release chemicals that attract other substances in the blood, called clotting factors. Additionally, they contain protein filaments that are capable of shrinking to bring the edges of a tear together.

The lymphatic and hematologic systems share certain organs, especially the bone marrow, blood vessels, and spleen. Hematopoiesis, or the process of blood formation, occurs primarily in bone marrow, the spongy central core of bones. Here, stem cells (immature blood cells that have not differentiated into particular cell types) develop into red blood cells (RBCs or erythrocytes), white blood cells (WBCs or leukocytes), or platelet-producing cells (thrombocytes). Erythrocytes carry oxygen to tissues and remove carbon dioxide from tissues. Leukocytes act in the inflammatory and immune responses. Thrombocytes play an essential role in blood coagulation, hemostasis, and blood thrombus formation.

The average person has 5 to 6 liters of circulating blood, about 8% of body weight. Blood is 3 to 5 times more viscous than water and has an alkaline pH between 7.35 and 7.45. It is composed of a straw-colored liquid called plasma that transports antibodies and nutrients to the tissues and waste products out of the body, and solid, or "formed," constituents, the red and white blood cells and platelets. Red blood cells give blood its color. The shade of red depends upon the degree of oxygen saturation and hemoglobin levels in the red blood cells. Bright red, oxygenated blood is arterial blood and dark-red, carbon dioxide-filled blood is venous blood.

DISEASES/DISORDERS OF THE HEMATOLOGIC SYSTEM INCLUDE

Anemia

Anemia is generally defined as a deficiency in erythrocytes or hemoglobin.

IRON-DEFICIENCY ANEMIA Iron-deficiency anemia is the most common anemia and is caused by inadequate absorption or excessive loss of iron. The disease is often found in women, young children, and the elderly, especially in underdeveloped countries. In adults, iron-deficiency anemia results from acute or chronic bleeding secondary to trauma; excessive menses; gastrointestinal bleeding associated with peptic or duodenal ulcer, hiatal hernia, diverticulosis, or cancer; or blood donation. Other causes are inadequate dietary intake of foods rich in iron, or malabsorption of iron caused by eating clay (pica), chronic diarrhea, high intake of cereal products with low intake of animal protein, and partial or complete gastrectomy (removal of all or part of the stomach).

In children, iron-deficiency anemia occurs in 25% of lower-income infants and toddlers aged 6 to 24 months, in preterm infants due to reduced fetal iron supply, and in children fed vegetarian diets with limited or no animal sources of iron (meat, eggs, and milk products). Adolescents are also at risk because of their rapid growth rate combined with poor eating habits. The young client can experience iron-deficiency anemia for the same reasons as adults (blood loss, inadequate intake, and impaired absorption), but also are vulnerable because of their bodies' increased demand for the iron required for growth. Pregnancy as a cause of iron-deficiency anemia is related to the fetus's increased demands for iron as it grows, coupled with the mother's own requirements.

Red blood cells (RBCs) in iron-deficiency anemia are microcytic (small in size) and hypochromic (pale in color). Although the total red cell count is usually only moderately low (rarely below 3 million cells/dl), the serum iron level may be as low as 10 mcg/dl. Normal serum iron levels range from 40 to 160 mcg/dl in adult men and women and from 40 to 120 mcg/dl in infants and children.

PERNICIOUS ANEMIA "Pernicious" means ruinous or hurtful. Persons with pernicious anemia are unable to absorb vitamin B_{12} due to a lack of intrinsic factor, found normally in gastric juices. Without intrinsic factor, red blood cells (erythrocytes) cannot mature or function properly. The treatment is taking B_{12} injections for life.

FOLIC ACID DEFICIENCY ANEMIA Without folic acid, red blood cells enlarge (megaloblastic anemia) and are unable to function properly. This condition occurs most commonly in persons experiencing nutritional deficiencies and during hemolysis and pregnancy. A deficiency during pregnancy may result in fetal neural defects.

APLASTIC OR HYPOPLASTIC ANEMIA This condition is caused by deficient red blood cell production due to bone marrow disorders arising from injury to or destruction of stem cells in the bone marrow matrix.

SICKLE-CELL ANEMIA This hereditary condition is characterized by an abnormal crescent or sickle shape of the erythrocytes and hemolysis (destruction of the red blood cells). The abnormal shape of the erythrocytes is caused by abnormal hemoglobin S. The person with sickle-cell anemia experiences acute abdominal pain, arthralgia (joint pain), and ulceration of the extremities. Hemoglobin S is found predominantly in black people. Degrees of severity depend upon the presence of one or two inherited genes for the trait.

THALASSEMIA Thalassemia is an inherited defect in the ability to produce hemoglobin. It is usually seen in persons of Mediterranean ancestry, especially Italian and Greek. However, it also occurs in blacks and in people from southern China, Southeast Asia, and India. This condition takes various forms and degrees of severity; the most severe is Cooley's anemia.

Polycythemia (Excessive Red Blood Cells)

The opposite of anemia, polycythemia is characterized by an excess of red blood cells. It occurs most commonly in people with chronic hypoxemia (decreased oxygen tension concentration in the blood). The body produces increased numbers of red blood cells to provide more places for oxygen to attach to hemoglobin in an attempt to increase blood oxygen levels.

POLYCYTHEMIA VERA This disorder is characterized by a general increase in red blood cells (erythemia) that is not a response to low blood oxygen levels. The blood becomes viscous (sticky) due to the increased number of erythrocytes. The bone marrow shows hyperplasia (excessive proliferation of normal cells in the normal tissue arrangement of an organ), and leukocytosis and thrombocytosis accompany the increase in red blood cells. This condition is most common among males of Jewish ancestry. It seldom affects children or blacks. Treatment includes phlebotomy (removal of red blood cells from the vein) and suppressing production with myelosuppressive drugs. This is a lifetime problem.

Hemorrhagic Disorders

ALLERGIC PURPURAS These are conditions where blood cells leak into the skin or mucous membranes (usually at sites associated with disorders of coagulation or thrombosis). Allergic purpuras may be caused by many agents, including: Foods, drugs, and bacteria.

HEREDITARY HEMORRHAGIC TELANGIECTASIS (RENDUR-OSLER-WEBER SYNDROME) This is a vascular lesion formed by dilation of small blood vessels. It is an inherited vascular disorder where the venules and capillaries dilate to form fragile masses of thin, convoluted vessels. The condition may appear as a birth-mark. Thinning of the walls of blood vessels in the nose, skin, and digestive tract facilitates hemorrhage.

THROMBOCYTOPENIA This condition is characterized by an abnormal decrease in the number of platelets. Since platelets are essential in coagulation, this disorder is a great threat to hemostasis. Thrombocytopenia may be congenital or acquired. Congenital thrombocytopenia may be caused by maternal injections of thiazide, neonatal rubella, or Wiskoff-Aldrich Syndrome (X-linked immune deficiency syndrome). When acquired, there may be a nutritional deficiency in B_{12} and folic acid. Acquired thrombocytopenia is associated with drugs such as: Sulfonamides, antibiotics, and estrogens.

IDIOPATHIC THROMBOCYTOPENIC PURPURA Idiopathic thrombocytopenic purpura (ITP) results from immunologic platelet destruction. This is an autoimmune disorder that may be acute or chronic. Acute ITP usually comes about after a viral infection such as rubella or chickenpox; or may follow immunizations with live virus vaccine. Chronic ITP is linked with immunologic disorders such as systemic lupus erythematosus. The condition is usually linked to drug reactions. ITP occurs frequently in persons who abuse alcohol, heroin, or morphine. It also occurs in persons with AIDS who are exposed to the rubella virus.

HEMOPHILIA This condition is characterized by excessive bleeding caused by a congenital (hereditary) lack of one of the proteins necessary for clotting (factor VIII). The lack of factor VIII results in a prolonged coagulation time. The treatment is the administration of factor VIII by intravenous infusion.

VON WILLEBRAND'S DISEASE This is a hereditary bleeding disorder characterized by a prolonged clotting time. It affects males and females equally. The disease causes bruising, epistaxis (nosebleed), and bleeding from the gums. Persons may bleed excessively after dental treatments, surgery, and minor lacerations. The severity of bleeding seems to decrease with age.

DISSEMINATED INTRAVASCULAR COAGULATION (DIC) DIC is a pathological form of coagulation that leads to generalized bleeding. DIC may occur as a consequence of infection, obstetric complications, neoplastic disease, disorders that produce necrosis, heat stroke, shock, snakebite, and a host of other causes. This condition essentially depletes circulating clotting factors and platelets, which in turn facilitates severe hemorrhage.

Miscellaneous Hematologic Disorders

HYPERSPLENISM (OVERACTIVE SPLEEN) This disorder is associated with increased activity of the spleen resulting in peripheral blood cell deficiency, as the spleen traps and destroys too many blood cells, removing too much blood from circulation. Hypersplenism can be the result of many primary disorders, such as chronic malaria, polycythemia vera, and rheumatoid arthritis.

HYPERBILIRUBINEMIA As the name suggests, hyperbilirubinemia is excessive bilirubin in the blood. This is a hemolytic disease of the newborn, sometimes called neonatal jaundice. Physiologic jaundice (when jaundice is the only symptom) shows mild jaundice and elevated bilirubin levels. Physiologic jaundice is more common and severe in certain ethnic groups, namely: Chinese, Japanese, Koreans, and Native Americans.

HEMOLYTIC DISEASE OF THE NEWBORN (ERYTHROBLASTOSIS FETALIS) Erythroblastosis fetalis is a hemolytic disease of the fetus or newborn arising from incompatibility of fetal and maternal blood, in which maternal blood antibodies attack fetal red blood cells. Treatments include an intrauterine intraperitoneal blood transfusion.

OVERVIEW OF CANCER (ONCOLOGY)

Cancer is the unrestrained multiplication of body cells. These cells penetrate, encompass, and destroy normal tissue. Such unrestrained growth can take place in any part of the body and at any time in the lifespan of its victims. Because cancer may result from the inability of the immune system to perceive certain cells as abnormal, and because cancer cells can detach from a primary tumor site and metastasize (spread) by entering the circulatory systems of the blood and lymph, we have included our overview of cancer in connection with the immune, lymphatic, and hematologic systems.

Cancer cells may develop into neoplasms. A neoplasm is an abnormal formation of cells, such as a growth or tumor that has no function but continues to grow at the expense of healthy tissue. Neoplasms are divided into two broad categories: benign and malignant. Benign tumors usually grow slowly, are typically not life threatening, and remain localized and encapsulated. However, when benign tumors disrupt the normal functions of vital organs, they can threaten life. Malignant tumors always threaten life. The cells of these non-encapsulated tumors travel, via the bloodstream and lymph vessels, away from the original neoplasm and metastasize (spread) to other areas of the body. Malignancy brings about a change in mitosis (a type of cell division). The cells of a malignant tumor become anaplastic (they show loose cellular differentiation and function). The DNA stops making normal cell codes and begins to create new signals that start the production and invasion of cancerous cells into adjacent tissues.

NORMAL CELL REPLICATION (DNA/RNA)

Deoxyribonucleic acid (DNA) is located in the nucleus of all cells and directs cell mitosis (self-replication). DNA, along with RNA (ribonucleic acid), influences protein synthesis (the creation of new cell proteins). Normal cell replication is disrupted by cancer.

Changes in DNA can be brought about by environmental factors and heredity.

Environmental Factors

Environmental carcinogenic factors include: Infection, toxic chemicals, sunlight, drugs, and radiation.

Heredity

The causes of cancer can originate within the body itself and may be passed from parent to offspring through defects in the DNA, the egg, or the sperm cells. Retinoblastoma (a tumor involving the retina of the eye) is an example of a heredity cancer.

NEOPLASTIC DISEASES (CANCER) (NEOPLASMS)

All parts of the body may be affected by cancer. Some regions of the human body that are invaded by cancer cells include:

Head, Neck, and Spinal Cord

Malignant brain tumors, pituitary tumors, laryngeal cancer, thyroid cancer, spinal neoplasms

Thoracic Neoplasms

Lung cancer, mesothelioma, breast cancer

Abdominal and Pelvic Neoplasms

Gastric and colorectal cancer; cancers of the esophagus, pancreas, kidney, liver, bladder, gallbladder, and bile ducts

Neoplasms of the Male and Female Genitalia (sexual organs)

Prostatic, testicular, cervical, uterine, vaginal, and ovarian cancer

Bone, Skin, and Soft Tissue Neoplasms

Primary malignant bone tumors, multiple myeloma, multiple endocrine neoplasia, basal cell epithelioma, squamous cell carcinoma, malignant melanoma

Blood and Lymph Neoplasms

Hodgkin's disease, malignant lymphomas, mycosin fungoides, acute leukemia, chronic granulocytic leukemia, chronic lymphocytic leukemia, Kaposi's sarcoma

---

TREATMENTS FOR CANCER

The primary tools used to treat cancers in the various organs of the body are the antineoplastic drugs, radiation, and surgery. The type of treatment will depend on the type, location, and extent of the neoplasm.

Antineoplastic Drugs

These can be classified as follows:

ALKYLATING AGENTS These agents attach organic side chains to the protein within the cancer cell, therefore poisoning it.

ANTIMETABOLITES These agents interfere with some phase of normal cellular metabolism by taking the place of proteins.

HORMONES These agents may antagonize certain tumors of the reproductive tract along with accessory sex organs. This is carried out by altering normal hormone balance.

ANTIBIOTICS Antibiotics usually act by interfering with DNA and RNA synthesis.

MISCELLANEOUS MEDICATIONS These are a heterogeneous group of drugs with various mechanisms of action. For example, Oncovin is used in the treatment of acute leukemia, and Matulane is used in the treatment of Hodgkin's disease.

Radioisotopes

Radioisotopes destroy certain cellular components by emission of radioactive particles.

Practice Test 4

Questions

4 - 1

A client's wound has eviscerated. Which of the following will you implement first?

1. Stay with the client and notify the physician.
2. Apply a clean, dry dressing to the wound.
3. Cleanse the wound with Betadine and apply bacteriostatic ointment.
4. Place sterile towels soaked in sterile saline over the wound.

4 - 2

A child who is due for an immunization should not receive that immunization if the child:

1. has recently been exposed to an infectious disease.
2. is receiving antimicrobial (antibiotic) therapy.
3. has a moderately severe illness, without fever.
4. had a moderate local reaction to a previous vaccine injection.

4 - 3

The most common early symptom of hepatitis A is:

1. loss of appetite.
2. abdominal distention.
3. ecchymosis.
4. shortness of breath.

4 - 4

Which of the following statements is true regarding chemotherapy-related alopecia?

1. Hair loss is temporary; growth will occur soon after chemotherapy is discontinued.
2. Hair loss is transient and is one of the minor side effects of chemotherapy.
3. Hair loss can be minimized by adjusting the dosage of the causative medication.
4. Hair loss is permanent, so clients need to prepare for alternatives such as wigs.

4 - 5

An infant has hemolytic disease of the newborn. The nurse caring for the infant should teach the parents that the development of jaundice in the newborn in caused by:

1. polycythemia.
2. an abnormal production of melanin.
3. excessive destruction of red blood cells.
4. hypobilirubinemia.

4 - 6

Following a lumpectomy for breast cancer, the cyclophosphamide, methotrexate, fluorouracil protocol was prescribed. Which of the following statements should be included in the teaching plan of the client receiving these medications?

1. Have the client see a cardiologist prior to chemotherapy.
2. Encourage the client to increase fluid intake to approximately 3 liters per day.
3. See that the client protects herself from sun during chemotherapy.
4. Recommend that the client eat only foods she likes because of potential nausea.

4 - 7

A 60-year-old has terminal lung cancer. On admission, a morphine drip was prescribed to treat intractable pain. Which of the following would the nurse recognize as a side effect of this medication?

1. Client awake and alert; requires minimal rescue doses of medication for pain.
2. Requires rescue doses of pain and medication every 4 hours.
3. Client has not had a bowel movement for 5 days.
4. Client's pulse rate is 60 beats per minute.

4 - 8

A 3-year-old with hemophilia (factor VIII deficiency) was admitted to the hospital because of persistent bleeding from a minor laceration. In planning care, the nurse will anticipate which of the following consequences of hospitalization to be most traumatic for the client?

1. inhibition from running about freely
2. separation from family
3. placement in an unfamiliar environment
4. disruption of routines and rituals

4 - 9

A client is admitted to the medical-surgical unit with a diagnosis of anemia. The laboratory results reveal a hemoglobin of 6.8 gm/dl. Which therapy do you anticipate?

1. No therapy is anticipated; this is a normal hemoglobin.
2. albumin intravenously
3. 1 unit of packed red blood cells
4. normal saline intravenously

4 - 1 0

A 41-year-old is admitted to the hospital with chronic granulocytic leukemia. The client also has anemia and thrombocytopenia. Because the client has thrombocytopenia, the nurse should include which of the following measures in the plan of care?

1. placing the client in a semi-upright position
2. limiting the client's intake of fluids
3. protecting the client from injury
4. exercising the client's lower extremities

4 - 11

Which of the following measures should the nurse implement to control bleeding into the joints of a client who is experiencing hemarthrosis?

1. Begin gentle passive exercises.
2. Immobilize the joint in an elastic compression bandage to apply pressure.
3. Wrap the joint in an elastic compression bandage to prevent bleeding.
4. Apply a tourniquet above the joint.

4 - 12

A client who is receiving chemotherapy for treatment of breast cancer tells you that she notices her mouth is extremely dry all the time. You know this is probably a side effect of chemotherapy, and is called:

1. xerostomia.
2. alopecia.
3. xanthoma.
4. anemia.

4 - 13

A client has sickle-cell anemia. The nurse's assessment of the client is least likely to reveal:

1. paleness of hands and soles of feet.
2. height and weight retardation.
3. elevated heart rate with cyanosis.
4. several fresh bruises on the calves of the legs.

4 - 14

A client is to receive a blood transfusion. Prior to administration of the blood, it is important for the nurse to:

1. instruct the client that the transfusion takes less than 30 minutes.
2. administer an antibiotic.
3. infuse dextrose 5% in water with the blood.
4. verify the prescription and check labels carefully with another nurse.

4 - 15

An 8-year-old has rubella. Which of the following recommendations will the nurse stress regarding contact with others?

1. "Do not let the child play with brothers and sisters until there is no longer a rash."
2. "Do not allow friends or relatives who are pregnant to visit for at least 5 days after the rash disappears."
3. "Do not allow your children to sleep with each other until a week after the rash disappears."
4. "Do not allow your children to play with other children in the neighborhood for several days."

4 - 16

A client who has been receiving chemotherapy for liver cancer is making holiday plans. The client's white blood cell count today is 2000/cm^3. Which of the following is the most appropriate advice to give this client regarding holiday plans?

1. "You should avoid being with your family because you may be contagious."
2. "There is little point in celebrating this year, is there?"
3. "Try not to eat foods that are high in carbohydrates over the holidays."
4. "You should try to avoid being in crowded public situations."

4 - 17

Which of the following immunizations should not be given to a 2-month-old infant whose caregiver is currently receiving chemotherapy?

1. oral polio vaccine
2. hepatitis B
3. diphtheria, tetanus, and pertussis
4. Haemophilus influenzae type B

4 - 18

A client who has leukemia has a platelet count of 50 cells x 10⁹/l. Nursing care must include which of the following?

1. scheduled analgesia, since a low platelet count is associated with profound muscle pain
2. measures to prevent bleeding and bruising
3. parenteral medications only, since GI absorption will be poor
4. vigorous range-of-motion exercises

4 - 19

A young child will receive the Haemophilus influenzae type B vaccine. The nurse will teach the child's parents that the vaccine will:

1. protect the child from one cause of serious infections such as epiglottitis or meningitis.
2. protect the child from hepatitis B disease.
3. help prevent human immunodeficiency virus disease in young children.
4. help prevent influenza.

4 - 20

A client experiencing acute hepatitis B should be advised to avoid:

1. citrus juices.
2. sleeping on the right side.
3. antihistamines for pruritus.
4. contact sports.

4 - 21

A client who has been diagnosed with autoimmune chronic hepatitis will have which of the following laboratory results?

1. a positive hepatitis B surface antigen
2. low liver function tests
3. elevated liver function tests
4. low serum bilirubin levels

4 - 22

Which of the following laboratory studies indicates an infectious process?

1. serum potassium level of 4
2. hemoglobin of 13
3. serum cholesterol of 180
4. white blood cell count of 14,000 mm^3

4-23

You are teaching a parent about fever management for a child who has chickenpox. Which of the following treatment modalities is contraindicated?

1. offering plenty of liquids
2. administering aspirin for fever management
3. dressing the child in lightweight clothing
4. teaching the correct technique for using a thermometer

4-24

Who of the following is most likely to experience hepatitis E?

1. an intravenous drug user
2. an immigrant newly arrived from a developing country
3. a toddler in a day-care facility
4. a client receiving hemodialysis

4-25

A client with cancer of the lung is receiving the colony-stimulating factor filgrastim and is complaining of bone pain. What should you administer to relieve the pain?

1. aspirin 10 gr po
2. acetaminophen 650 mg po
3. meperidine hydrochloride 50 mg intramuscularly
4. morphine sulfate 30 mg po

4-26

A client 22 years old has Hodgkin's lymphoma. As a consequence of chemotherapy and radiation therapy, the client is immunocompromised. The nurse's aide reported the client's temperature as 100.3°F. The appropriate nursing action is to:

1. retake the temperature after 2 hours.
2. do nothing; a fever is expected in this condition.
3. give the client aspirin 10 gr.
4. notify the physician and prepare to take cultures.

4-27

A 5-year-old with acute lymphocytic leukemia is to be discharged from the hospital in a state of remission. The nurse will reinforce which of the following understandings about the role of the child's parents?

1. Make few demands on the child and try to make the child as happy as possible, since the condition is terminal.
2. Guide the child through encouragement and setting limits so that the child may develop to full potential.
3. It is not necessary to control the child's behavior since the child's condition will impose limitations.
4. It will be necessary to develop a carefully planned schedule for the child so that energy can be conserved.

4-28

A client has a laceration approximately 2 inches long and 1 inch deep that has been sustained for approximately 2 hours. You will irrigate the wound with a minimum of:

1. 200 ml of saline solution.
2. 150 ml of saline solution.
3. 100 ml of saline solution.
4. 250 ml of saline solution.

4 - 2 9

A 4-month-old infant is brought to the clinic for a well-child checkup. Assuming that immunizations are being given as recommended and were begun at birth, what immunizations should be given at this time?

Select all that apply by placing a ✔ in the square:

- ❏ 1. measles, mumps, and rubella vaccine 4 (MMR #1)
- ❏ 2. diphtheria, tetanus, and pertussis
- ❏ 3. pneumococcal6 (PVC)
- ❏ 4. Haemophilus influenzae type B3 (Hib)
- ❏ 5. inactivated polio (IPV)

4 - 3 0

A 20-year-old college student is seen in the student health clinic because of fatigue, weight loss, and a low-grade fever. Physical examination reveals slight enlargement of the cervical lymph nodes. Which of the following questions pertaining to the client's fever should the nurse ask initially?

1. "When did you first notice your temperature was elevated?"
2. "Has your temperature been over 102°F?"
3. "Have you recently been exposed to anyone who has an infection?"
4. "Have you had a sore throat?"

4 - 3 1

Your client's enzyme-linked immunoabsorbent test was positive. What does this mean?

1. The client is immune to the acquired immunodeficiency syndrome.
2. The client will develop acquired immunodeficiency syndrome in the near future.
3. Antibodies to the human immunodeficiency virus are present in the client's blood.
4. There are no antibodies to the human immunodeficiency virus in the client's blood.

4 - 3 2

A child has acute lymphocytic leukemia. The nurse is planning a room assignment. Which of the following would be the best choice?

1. a private room
2. a room with another child with leukemia
3. a four-bed room with children his age
4. a bed in intensive care

4 - 3 3

Which evidence supports a nursing diagnosis of "high risk for infection related to immunodeficiency?"

1. decreased leukocyte count
2. decreased serum globulin level
3. increased serum hemoglobin level
4. increased number of T-helper cells

4 - 3 4

A client with acquired immunodeficiency syndrome is receiving the antiviral agent zidovudine (AZT). What laboratory studies need to be monitored in the client receiving this medication?

1. serum glutamic-pyruvic transaminase
2. blood urea nitrogen
3. erythrocyte sedimentation rate
4. red blood cell count

4 - 3 5

A client newly diagnosed with hepatitis A should be informed that:

1. this form of hepatitis typically develops into a chronic carrier state.
2. persons who have had hepatitis A have an increased risk for developing liver cancer.
3. hepatitis A is spread only via contaminated serum.
4. the oral-fecal route is the most common cause of the spread of hepatitis A.

4 - 3 6

Your client is at risk for Rh incompatibility. Which client data would support a nursing diagnosis of injury, fetal potential for, related to blood transfusion?

1. a positive indirect Coombs test
2. a negative direct Coombs test
3. an Rh-positive mother and an Rh-negative father
4. Rhogam given at 28 weeks gestation

4 - 3 7

The nurse receives a phone call from a mother of 4 children who completed their primary tetanus immunizations 2 years ago. The nurse would need to advise the mother to have a booster dose of tetanus toxoid for which one of her children?

1. the child who sustained scratches on bare legs while climbing on a backyard fence
2. the child who is hospitalized and having emergency treatment for a perforated appendix
3. the child who is having dental treatment for an abscessed impacted molar
4. the child who walked barefooted in the woods and sustained an injury by stepping on a nail

4 - 3 8

The nurse should recognize which of the following factors in a client's history as most likely to be related to hepatitis A?

1. recently recovered from an upper respiratory infection
2. was bitten by an insect
3. had contact with a person who was jaundiced
4. ate home-canned foods

4 - 3 9

A client presents signs and symptoms of malaise, low-grade fever, and fatigue after being exposed to chickenpox 2 weeks earlier. What stage of illness is the client experiencing?

1. incubation
2. prodromal
3. illness
4. convalescence

4 - 4 0

Infection with the human immunodeficiency virus progresses to acquired immunodeficiency syndrome more quickly in infants. This process is due to:

1. the human immunodeficiency virus attacking the organs of the infant.
2. the infant's immune system being overtaken by the mother's human immunodeficiency virus antibodies.
3. the human immunodeficiency virus attacking the infant's immune system, which has not formed antibodies.
4. the human immunodeficiency virus attacking the infant's organs during their various stages of development.

4 - 4 1

A client with acquired immunodeficiency syndrome has developed Kaposi's sarcoma. The physician has prescribed interferon alpha 2b, 30 million units 3 times a week. The following is a teaching plan related to self-administration of interferon. Which of the following information is incorrect and should not be included in the teaching plan?

1. The client can substitute a less expensive generic interferon in place of the one prescribed.
2. Most clients tend to experience flulike symptoms that should diminish with continued therapy.
3. The drug should be administered at bedtime to minimize daytime drowsiness.
4. The client should avoid contact with persons with viral illness and those who have recently taken vaccines.

4 - 4 2

Which diagnoses would be given the highest priority for a child with varicella?

1. potential sleep pattern disturbance related to pruritus
2. potential nutritional alteration: less than body requirements, related to oral lesions
3. potential for infection related to bacterial invasion of skin lesions
4. impaired social interaction related to isolation during the contagious period

4 - 4 3

To determine if the immune system is functioning adequately, your assessment would reveal:

1. a positive Homans' sign.
2. the absence of fasciculations.
3. a positive Babinski reflex.
4. a positive reaction to skin testing.

4 - 4 4

The nurse is planning care for a client convalescing from the hepatitis A virus. The nurse will expect the client to have the most difficulty:

1. relieving pain.
2. regulating bowel elimination.
3. maintaining a sense of well-being.
4. preventing respiratory complications.

4-45

You have never had chickenpox and learn that you have been exposed to a client with herpes zoster. Within 96 hours, you should receive:

1. the immune globulin.
2. the varicella-zoster immune globulin.
3. a full course of antibiotic therapy.
4. a Tzanck smear to determine herpes.

4-46

Which of the following should be completed before beginning an anti-infective?

1. Allergies should be identified and culture specimens collected.
2. Culture report should be on chart and allergies identified.
3. History should be taken and offending organism identified.
4. Allergy tests, a history, and a physical should be completed.

4-47

A 15-year-old client is admitted to the hospital with sickle-cell anemia. The client states, "My knees are killing me. I guess that's why I can't walk to the bathroom and back to bed without getting short of breath." An appropriate nursing response would be to:

1. agree with the client and assist the client back to bed.
2. explain in understandable terms how sickle-cell anemia can affect mobility.
3. administer an analgesic so that the client will be able to walk back to the bed without getting short of breath.
4. explain that the white blood count is high and the client should be careful walking back and forth to the bathroom.

4-48

A client has been given an antibiotic. Which assessment finding indicates this medication has been effective?

1. passage of a formed stool
2. voiding 500 cc over 2 hours
3. client stating that pain is relieved
4. temperature decreasing to 98.6°F

4-49

The physician has requested peak and trough levels in association with tobramycin therapy. The nurse will know that peak and trough levels are used to:

1. determine efficacy of the drug.
2. determine if the client is allergic to the drug.
3. establish and maintain therapeutic serum levels without excessive toxicity.
4. determine the correct therapeutic loading of the initial dose.

4-50

What changes in laboratory studies are seen as the disease process caused by the human immunodeficiency virus progresses?

1. platelet count increases
2. T-4 lymphocyte count decreases
3. T-8 lymphocyte count decreases
4. erythrocyte sedimentation rate decreases

4 - 5 1

A 7-year-old is diagnosed with typhoid fever. The nurse will:

1. wear gloves due to infectious materials.
2. wear a mask because the client may have a cough.
3. place the client on strict isolation because the client may have a cough.
4. place the client on contact isolation because of wound infection.

4 - 5 2

The nurse will recognize the first sign of testicular cancer as:

1. the ability to transilluminate the testicle using a penlight.
2. urinary frequency and urgency.
3. lumbar pain.
4. painless enlargement of the testicle.

4 - 5 3

The most common pathogen found in the bladder and upper urinary tract is:

1. *Escherichia coli* (*E. coli*).
2. *Streptococcus pyogenes* (group A).
3. *Staphylococcus aureus*.
4. *Salmonella*.

4 - 5 4

Which of the following populations would be most likely to test positive for hepatitis D?

1. children who attend an overcrowded day-care facility
2. health-care workers who have received hepatitis C vaccine
3. persons who are diagnosed with hepatitis B
4. anyone in the population

4 - 5 5

A client diagnosed with hepatitis B should be informed that:

1. hepatitis B is spread only via the oral-fecal route.
2. hepatitis B vaccine may be administered only after a person reaches 18 years of age.
3. there is no hepatitis B immune globulin.
4. standard precautions are indicated for all contacts.

4 - 5 6

The nurse provides a client with information about the most common side effects of mechlorethamine hydrochloride and measures that can be used to counteract these side effects. Which of the following measures, if incorporated in the client's nursing care plan, would diminish the most common side effect of this medication?

1. encouraging high fluid intake
2. providing a diet high in fiber
3. obtaining a prescription for niacin
4. administering a pretreatment antiemetic

4 - 5 7

Typical signs and symptoms affecting the skin that might lead to a tentative diagnosis of systemic lupus erythematosus (SLE) include:

Select all that apply by placing a ✔ in the square:

❑ 1. a butterfly rash across the cheeks.
❑ 2. red, swollen, painful joints.
❑ 3. ulcers in the mouth.
❑ 4. alopecia.
❑ 5. hemolytic anemia.

4 - 5 8

A client with acquired immunodeficiency syndrome has been hospitalized. During your initial assessment of the client, you observe cheesy-looking white patches in the client's mouth. When the patches are rubbed, erythema and bleeding occur. You suspect:

1. herpes simplex.
2. candidiasis.
3. leukoplakia.
4. Kaposi's sarcoma.

4 - 5 9

An appropriate nursing intervention for a client with tetanus is to:

1. decrease environmental stimulation.
2. suction by the nasopharyngeal route.
3. gently massage the large joints.
4. frequently assess level of consciousness.

4 - 6 0

Your client has experienced a bone marrow biopsy and is complaining of tenderness. You would:

1. administer the prescribed analgesic.
2. notify the physician of the client's complaint.
3. tell the client this is a normal reaction to the biopsy.
4. apply direct pressure to the tender area.

4 - 6 1

The binding with, engulfing, and destroying of bacteria and foreign material in the body is known as:

_____

Fill in the blank

4 - 6 2

A 3-year-old has measles. The type of immunity that is developed by having an infection such as measles is known as:

1. passive immunity.
2. natural acquired active immunity.
3. artificially acquired active immunity.
4. immune serum globulin.

4 - 6 3

A client having a kidney treatment is to receive a drug that will suppress the client's immune system. Which of the following drugs do you recognize as immunosuppressants?

Select all that apply by placing a ✔ in the square:

❏ 1. azathioprine (Imuran)
❏ 2. cefdinir (Omnicef)
❏ 3. cyclosporine (Sandimmune)
❏ 4. mycophenolate mofetil (CellCept)
❏ 5. famciclovir (Famvir)

4 - 6 4

It has been determined that your client has a severe allergy to bee venom. You will recommend an emergency kit that contains a premeasured, injectable dose of the drug:

_____

Fill in the blank

4 - 6 5

The human immunodeficiency virus (HIV) is primarily transmitted through:

Select all that apply by placing a ✔ in the square:

❏ 1. Sexual intercourse
❏ 2. intravenous drug use
❏ 3. insect bites
❏ 4. blood transfusions
❏ 5. mother to infant

Practice Test 4

Answers, Rationales, and Explanations

4 - 1

④ The nurse will place sterile towels soaked in sterile saline over the eviscerated wound. An evisceration is the protrusion of visceral organs through a wound opening. The condition is a medical emergency that requires surgical repair. If organs protrude through the wound, the blood supply to the tissues is compromised. When evisceration occurs, the nurse places sterile towels soaked in sterile saline over the extruding tissues to reduce the possibility of bacterial invasion and drying.

1. The physician should be notified, but only after the sterile towels soaked in sterile saline have been placed over the wound.

2. Placing an unsterile dry dressing over an evisceration will expose the wound to infection and dry out the wound.

3. Surgery is required and ointment would have to be removed. Also, Betadine should not be placed on the organs because it is an irritant.

Client Need: Safe, Effective Care Environment

4 - 2

③ A child who has an illness should not receive immunizations, since doing so will compromise the child's health. The child's health is already compromised and immunizations may compromise it further.

1. A child who has been exposed to an infectious disease but has no symptoms of illness could be immunized.

2. Children who are presently receiving antimicrobial (anti-infective) therapy may receive immunizations.

4. The fact that a child had a moderate local reaction to a previous vaccine injection does not mean the child is not a candidate for other vaccinations.

Client Need: Health Promotion and Maintenance

4 - 3

① Anorexia is the most common early symptom of hepatitis A. Chills, nausea, vomiting, dyspepsia, and tenderness of the liver are other early manifestations of type A hepatitis. Type A hepatitis is usually spread by the fecal-oral route as a result of poor hygiene or a breakdown in sanitary conditions. Enteric precautions are recommended.

2, 3, and 4. Abdominal distention, ecchymosis (blue-black hemorrhagic areas of the skin), and shortness of breath are symptoms of advanced liver disease.

Client Need: Physiological Integrity

4 - 4

① The nurse will inform clients receiving chemotherapy that alopecia (hair loss) is temporary and that hair growth will occur soon after chemotherapy is discontinued.

2. Even though alopecia (hair loss) is transient, it is a very traumatic experience for many clients and would be considered more than a minor side effect of chemotherapy.

3. Alopecia (hair loss) cannot be minimized by adjusting the dosage of the causative medication.

4. Alopecia (hair loss) is not permanent. However, the client should be taught that when hair growth returns, the hair could be a different color and texture.

Client Need: Physiological Integrity

4 - 5

③ The nurse will teach the parents that their baby's jaundice is caused by excessive destruction of the red blood cells (RBCs). Hemolytic disease of the newborn (HDN erythroblastosis fetalis) results from excessive destruction of fetal red blood cells caused by maternal antibodies. The end product of red blood cell destruction is excessive bilirubin (hyperbilirubinemia), which the infant's immature liver is unable to metabolize. The result is jaundice.

1. Polycythemia (an abnormal, excessive number of red blood cells) is not associated with HDN.

2. Melanin (the pigment that gives skin and hair its color) is not associated with HDN.

4. An infant who has HDN will have hyperbilirubinemia, not hypobilirubinemia.

Client Need: Physiological Integrity

4 - 6

② The nurse's teaching plan for the client should include the need to increase fluid intake. Hemorrhagic cystitis is a common side effect of cyclophosphamide that may be diminished by increasing fluid intake (approximately 3 liters per day).

1 and 3. None of the prescribed medications require a cardiology workup or cause photosensitivity.

4. Nausea will cause clients to have an aversion to foods they like and defeats the purpose of good nutrition.

Client Need: Physiological Integrity

4 - 7

③   **The nurse will recognize constipation as a common side effect of morphine. Other common side effects of opiates include sedation, nausea, vomiting, and decreased respiratory rate.**

1.   Effective pain relief would require minimal rescue doses of medication.

2.   Frequent rescue doses indicate under-dosage or under-treatment, not a side effect of morphine.

4.   The client's pulse rate would increase, not decrease, to compensate for lack of oxygen.

Client Need: Physiological Integrity

4 - 8

②   **The nurse will anticipate separation from family, especially the mother, as the most traumatic event for a hospitalized toddler.**

1, 3, and 4. Inhibition from running about freely; placement in an unfamiliar environment; and disruption of routines and rituals will all require adjustment by the toddler, but are not considered traumatic.

Client Need: Psychosocial Integrity

4 - 9

③   **The administration of packed red blood cells will be anticipated. Anemia exists when there is a reduction in red blood cells, a decrease in hemoglobin, and a drop in the volume of packed red cells. Therapy is aimed at replacing red blood cells, which carry oxygen to the body.**

1.   6.8 gm/dl is not a normal hemoglobin. The normal hemoglobin count for the female adult is 12 to 16 gm/100 ml. The normal hemoglobin count for the adult male is 14 to 18 gm/100 ml.

2 and 4. The hemoglobin would not be affected by intravenous albumin or normal saline.

Client Need: Health Promotion and Maintenance

4 - 10

③   **The nursing-care plan will include protecting the client from injury. A client with thrombocytopenia (abnormal decrease in number of blood platelets) should be protected from injury because of the low platelet count. Should the client sustain an injury, abnormal bleeding would occur due to an impaired clotting mechanism.**

1.   The immediate concern is to prevent injury and the potential for bleeding. Placing the client in a 45-degree position may facilitate breathing, but positioning is not the major concern.

2.   There is no indication that the client should limit fluids.

4.   Exercising the client's lower extremities is contraindicated. Nothing should be done that would facilitate bleeding. Soft toothbrushes and electric razors should be used. The client should also avoid aspirin.

Client Need: Health Promotion and Maintenance

4 - 11

② Clients who are experiencing hemarthrosis (bleeding into the cavity of a joint) should have the affected joint immobilized. Immobilization of a joint in a position of slight flexion will prevent bleeding from further trauma.

1. Passive exercise should not begin until the active phase of the disease has passed.

3. Wrapping the joint in an elastic bandage to apply pressure would not prevent bleeding, but may be done to assist in immobilizing the joint.

4. A tourniquet would not prevent bleeding in this case but may cause additional trauma due to the restriction of the blood supply.

Client Need: Safe, Effective Care Environment

4 - 12

① Xerostomia is dryness of the mouth due to an alteration in normal secretions. It is a side effect of some chemotherapies and can be very distressing to clients. It places the client at an increased risk for infections of the oral cavity.

2. Alopecia refers to hair loss.

3. Xanthoma is a type of skin lesion.

4. Anemia is a blood disorder whose hallmark is low or abnormal hemoglobin levels.

Client Need: Physiological Integrity

4 - 13

④ The nurse is not likely to observe signs of bleeding such as bruising. Bruising is more likely to indicate bleeding tendencies, especially in fleshy areas. Bleeding tendencies are not common in sickle-cell disease.

1. Paleness is usually present in clients with sickle-cell anemia because of low hemoglobin levels. Palms of hands and soles of feet are good areas to note skin color in persons with dark pigmentation.

2. Growth retardation of both height and weight is commonly found in children with sickle-cell disease.

3. Increased heart rates help compensate for low hemoglobin levels. Cyanosis is usually not present because most, if not all, hemoglobin in arterial circulation is adequately oxygenated.

Client Need: Physiological Integrity

4 - 1 4

④ **Prior to administering blood, the nurse will verify the prescription and check labels carefully with another nurse. Administering incompatible blood by mistake can be a fatal error, causing a hemolytic reaction and shock. The companion check system radically reduces the risk of such an error.**

1. Blood transfusions typically last from 1 to 2 hours. If the blood has been refrigerated, it should be given within 30 minutes of the time it was removed from the refrigerator.

2. Antibiotics are not routinely given prior to blood transfusions.

3. Dextrose may hemolyze the blood. Blood can be administered only with normal saline (physiological saline).

Client Need: Health Promotion and Maintenance

4 - 1 5

② **The nurse should teach the parents of a child with rubella not to allow friends or relatives who are pregnant to visit for at least 5 days after the rubella rash disappears. If a pregnant woman is not immune and contracts rubella in her first trimester, the fetus can develop birth defects such as cataracts, heart murmurs, and deafness.**

1. Trying to prevent the client from playing with brothers and sisters until the client no longer has a rash is unrealistic.

3 and 4. The contagious period for rubella is 7 days before the appearance of the rash and 5 days after the appearance of the rash. Therefore, siblings are already exposed.

Client Need: Safe, Effective Care Environment

4 - 1 6

④ **The nurse will advise the client to avoid crowded public situations. A client with a white blood cell count (WBC) of <2000/cm^3 is at an increased risk for contracting infection because her immune system is compromised. Because of this increased risk, very crowded public situations should be avoided. Clients with a low WBC should also be advised to practice frequent handwashing, as should all persons with whom they have contact.**

1. This client is not contagious. The client is at an increased risk for contracting an infection.

2. It is inappropriate to make judgments regarding a client's desire for celebrations. It is therapeutic for clients to maintain a sense of normality during times of change and crisis.

3. There is no indication that this client should avoid carbohydrates. Many clients who are in the midst of chemotherapy suffer from nutritional deficits, and efforts should be made to encourage them to enjoy their meals.

Client Need: Health Promotion and Maintenance

4-17

① Oral polio vaccine (OPV) is generally considered unsafe to give to an infant whose caregiver may be immunosuppressed, because the virus in the oral vaccine is shed in the stool and the caregiver may be exposed to the virus.

2, 3, and 4. There are no specific contraindications for the intramuscular immunizations for hepatitis B, diphtheria, tetanus, pertussis, or Haemophilus influenzae type B.

Client Need: Safe, Effective Care Environment

4-18

② The nurse should include measures that prevent bleeding and bruising. Platelets are the component of blood that help the blood to clot. Clients with low platelet counts, or those less than 150 cells x 109/l, are at risk for spontaneous hemorrhage. Nursing care must be scrupulous in preventing any bruising or bleeding.

1. A low platelet count is not associated with profound muscle pain.

3 and 4. Both parenteral medication administration and vigorous range-of-motion-exercises should be avoided because of the increased risk for bruising or bleeding.

Client Need: Health Promotion and Maintenance

4-19

① The nurse will teach the child's parents that the Haemophilus influenzae type B (Hib) vaccine is given to protect a child from serious infections such as epiglottitis, bacterial pneumonia, bacterial meningitis, and sepsis.

2 and 3. The Hib vaccine does not prevent hepatitis B or human deficiency virus (HIV).

4. Hib is not associated with the virus that causes influenza.

Client Need: Safe, Effective Care Environment

4-20

④ Clients with acute hepatitis B should be advised to avoid contact sports. Hepatitis is a viral infection in the liver that causes the liver to become friable and enlarged. Sudden jarring motions or potential for blows to the abdomen should be avoided in persons experiencing such an infection.

1. An increase in carbohydrates is accepted therapy for persons experiencing viral hepatitis.

2. Clients may sleep in any position of comfort during an illness with hepatitis B.

3. Antihistamines in moderation are appropriate for the pruritus that may occur with jaundice.

Client Need: Health Promotion and Maintenance

4 - 2 1

③ Clients with autoimmune chronic hepatitis will have elevated liver function tests. Autoimmune chronic hepatitis is characterized by chronic inflammation of the liver that is not caused by viruses or toxin ingestion. As implied by the name, it is thought to be autoimmune in its etiology. Liver function tests are typically markedly elevated, as is typical of all the hepatitis variations. Serum bilirubin levels are usually elevated, too. There are also specific titers for some of the antibodies associated with this disorder.

1. Autoimmune chronic hepatitis is not associated with hepatitis B. Unless the two disorders occurred coincidentally, there would be no concurrent elevation of hepatitis B surface antigen in the presence of autoimmune chronic hepatitis.

2 and 4. Liver function and bilirubin levels both tend to be elevated in clients with autoimmune chronic hepatitis.

Client Need: Physiological Integrity

4 - 2 2

④ A white blood cell count (WBC) of 14,000 mm³ indicates an infectious process. A normal WBC is 4,000 to 10,000 mm³.

1. A normal potassium level is 3.5 to 5.5. Potassium levels are not associated with infection.

2. A normal hemoglobin level is 14 to 18 for men and 12 to 16 for women. Hemoglobin levels are not associated with infection.

3. Cholesterol levels should be less than 200. Therefore, a cholesterol level of 180 is within normal limits. Cholesterol levels are not associated with infection.

Client Need: Physiological Integrity

4 - 2 3

② Aspirin should not be given to children with a viral illness such as chickenpox due to the association between the use of aspirin and Reye's syndrome.

1. Adequate hydration is essential in fever management. Otherwise, a client can easily become dehydrated.

3. Dressing the child in lightweight clothing and exposing the skin to air is an effective means of fever reduction after an antipyretic is administered.

4. Proper temperature assessment is vital when initiating therapeutic interventions.

Client Need: Health Promotion and Maintenance

4 - 2 4

② An immigrant newly arrived from a developing country is most likely to experience hepatitis E. Hepatitis E is virtually unknown in North America. It is one of the viral liver infections spread via the fecal-oral route and is typically found only in developing countries. Hepatitis E should be considered as a possible cause of illness in those persons who have recently traveled to a developing country.

1. An intravenous drug user is more likely to contract hepatitis B, C, and perhaps D.
3. A toddler in a day-care facility is more likely to contract hepatitis A.
4. Clients receiving hemodialysis are more likely to contract hepatitis B, C, and perhaps D.

Client Need: Health Promotion and Maintenance

4 - 2 5

② The nurse will administer acetaminophen (Tylenol) 650 mg po. The most common side effect of Neupogen (filgrastim) is bone pain. The pain is readily relieved by nonnarcotic analgesics such as acetaminophen (Tylenol).

1. Clients with bone marrow suppression should avoid aspirin to prevent potential bleeding.
3. Meperidine hydrochloride (Demerol) is an opioid analgesic. However, it is not necessary to administer an opioid when the pain can be relieved by acetaminophen (Tylenol). Also, it is better to give the medication po to prevent bleeding.
4. Morphine sulfate (Astramorph) is an opioid analgesic. However, it is not necessary to administer an opioid when the pain can be relieved by acetaminophen (Tylenol).

Client Need: Physiological Integrity

4 - 2 6

④ The appropriate nursing action is to notify the physician and prepare to take cultures.

1. A client with a body temperature of 100.3°F should be monitored more frequently than every 2 hours. Also, there is no reason to think that the temperature will subside with the passing of time unless treatment is begun.
2. A body temperature of 100.3°F is not normal. It may be expected, since the client's immune system is compromised. However, treatment should be begun to prevent further compromise of the client's health.
3. Giving aspirin is contraindicated because immunosuppression lowers the platelet count and aspirin would increase the risk of gastrointestinal bleeding. Acetaminophen (Tylenol) is the drug of choice. Aspirin would only mask the symptoms. Since the client's immune system is compromised, there is a need to identify the causative organism.

Client Need: Physiological Integrity

4 - 2 7

② **The nurse will support the parents as they guide, set limits, and encourage their child.**

1. A child with acute lymphocytic leukemia has a greater than 90% chance of achieving an initial remission and approximately one-third may be cured if treated for 30 months.

3. The child is in remission and will need discipline from parents. During remission, the child will not be limited by the condition.

4. During remission, the child will not need a carefully planned schedule that focuses on conservation of energy.

Client Need: Psychosocial Integrity

4 - 2 8

④ **The nurse will irrigate the wound with a minimum of 250 ml of saline solution. Generally, wounds are irrigated with 50 ml of solution per 1 inch of the depth and length for each hour sustained.**

1, 2, and 3. The amounts of solution are not enough.

Client Need: Health Promotion and Maintenance

4 - 2 9

②③④ and ⑤ **It is recommended that an infant 4 months old should receive the third dose, in a series of 5 doses, of diphtheria, tetanus, and pertussis vaccine (DTP); the Haemophilus influenzae type b3 vaccine (Hib), the inactivated polio vaccine (IPV); and the pneumococcal 6 vaccine (PCV).**

1. The measles, mumps, and rubella 4 vaccine (MMR #1) should be started when an infant is between 12 and 15 months of age.

Client Need: Health Promotion and Maintenance

4 - 3 0

① **The nurse should determine when the client first noticed an elevation in temperature. In an attempt to clarify the etiology of the fever, determining when the fever first occurred would be the most appropriate initial question.**

2. The elevation of the fever is not as important in determining the etiology of the fever, as knowing when the fever was first noted.

3. Infection is only one cause for a fever. Knowing when the fever first occurred would be the best initial question. Also, a question about exposure to infection does not directly relate to fever.

4. Asking about a sore throat may or may not be directly related to the fever experienced by the client.

Client Need: Physiological Integrity

4 - 3 1

③ The enzyme-linked immunoabsorbent assay (ELISA) test determines the presence of antibodies directed specifically against the human immunodeficiency virus. The ELISA test does not establish a diagnosis of acquired immunodeficiency syndrome, but does indicate that an individual has been exposed to or infected with the human immunodeficiency virus.

1. There is no known immunity to the human immunodeficiency virus (HIV) that causes acquired immunodeficiency virus (AIDS).

2. Determining that a client is infected with or has been exposed to the human immunodeficiency virus should not be interpreted to mean that the client will develop acquired immunodeficiency syndrome (AIDS) in the near future.

4. Having a positive enzyme-linked immunoabsorbent assay (ELISA) test confirms the presence of the antibody associated with the human immunodeficiency virus (HIV).

Client Need: Physiological Integrity

4 - 3 2

① In planning a room assignment for a child with acute lymphocytic leukemia, the nurse's best choice would be a private room.

2 and 3. Neutropenia (an abnormally small number of neutrophils) predisposes clients with acute lymphocytic leukemia to infection; therefore, placing them in a room with other sick children could be potentially life threatening.

4. Unless the child is critically ill, the intensive care unit would be inappropriate. Until the degree of involvement is determined, a private room is the safest.

Client Need: Safe, Effective Care Environment

4 - 3 3

① The data that supports a nursing diagnosis of "high risk for infection related to immunodeficiency" is a decreased leukocyte count.

2, 3, and 4. Clients with immunodeficiency will have an increased serum globulin level, a decreased serum hemoglobin level, and a decreased number of T-helper cells.

Client Need: Physiological Integrity

4 - 3 4

④ **Persons experiencing acquired immunodeficiency syndrome (AIDS) who receive zidovudine (AZT) should have their red blood count monitored. AZT can be very toxic to bone marrow, producing dose-limiting anemia and neutropenia.**

1. Serum glutamic-pyruvic transaminase (SGPT) tests would be appropriate in diagnosing liver disease and the presence of myocardial infarction.

2. The test for blood urea and nitrogen (BUN) gives an indication of glomerular function and the production and excretion of urea.

3. The erythrocyte sedimentation rate (ESR) test provides information about the inflammatory process in conditions such as rheumatic fever and rheumatic arthritis.

Client Need: Health Promotion and Maintenance

4 - 3 5

④ **A client newly diagnosed with hepatitis A should be informed that the hepatitis A virus is spread via the oral-fecal route and parenterally. It is found in food and water. Hepatitis A is a viral infection of the liver most commonly found in crowded areas and where food is handled, such as restaurants, schools, day-care centers, and homeless shelters.**

1. Hepatitis A is not associated with a chronic carrier state.

2. Hepatitis A is not associated with an increased risk for developing liver cancer.

3. Hepatitis A may be spread via contaminated serum, but is more commonly spread via the oral-fecal route.

Client Need: Health Promotion and Maintenance

4 - 3 6

① **A positive indirect Coombs test would support a nursing diagnosis of injury, fetal potential for, related to blood transfusion, for a client at risk for Rh incompatibility. A positive Coombs test indicates fetal antigens on maternal cells.**

2. A negative direct Coombs test indicates absence of maternal antibodies on fetal cells.

3. Rh-negative incompatibility requires an Rh-negative mother who is carrying an Rh-positive fetus.

4. Rhogam given at 28 weeks gestation will not cause injury.

Client Need: Health Promotion and Maintenance

4 - 3 7

④ **The nurse would advise the mother to have a booster dose of tetanus toxoid for the child who stepped on a nail when walking barefooted in the woods. Even though all the children's immunizations are up-to-date, the child who walked barefooted in the woods and sustained an injury by stepping on a nail would have a need for a booster dose of tetanus toxoid. This child sustained an injury in an environment (dirt) where the causative organism (*Clostridium tetani*) is found. *Clostridium tetani* is able to grow in an anaerobic state at the site of the wound.**

1. Sustaining scratches on the legs when climbing a backyard fence is unlikely to expose a child to the *Clostridium tetani* organism.

2. A perforated appendix would not expose a child to the *Clostridium tetani* organism.

3. Dental treatments would not expose a child to the *Clostridium tetani* organism.

Client Need: Health Promotion and Maintenance

4 - 3 8

③ **The nurse will associate contact with a jaundiced person as a likely factor in acquiring hepatitis A. The hepatitis A virus (HAV) may appear sporadically and can be transmitted by close contact with infected persons. The disease is usually spread by the fecal-oral route. It is often associated with overcrowding, poor hygiene, or breakdown of normal sanitary conditions, and may occur in small or large epidemics.**

1. Recent recovery from an upper respiratory infection is not associated with hepatitis A. Hepatitis A is usually spread from person to person via the fecal-oral route and from consuming water contaminated with the hepatitis A virus (HAV).

2. Hepatitis A is not spread via the bite of insects.

4. Consuming home-canned foods would not expose a person to hepatitis A. However, improperly processed foods would expose people to *Clostridium botulinum*.

Client Need: Physiological Integrity

4 - 3 9

② **A client who has been exposed to chickenpox and has a low-grade fever and fatigue is experiencing the prodromal stage of that condition. The prodromal stage is the interval from onset of nonspecific signs and symptoms to the more specific symptoms associated with a condition.**

1. The incubation period is the period of time between exposure to an infection and the appearance of the first symptom of the condition.

3. An illness is the experience of the specific symptoms of a condition such as those associated with tuberculosis, measles, or hepatitis.

4. Convalescence is a period of time following an illness or an injury during which a client recovers.

Client Need: Physiological Integrity

4 - 4 0

③ The human immunodeficiency virus (HIV) progresses to acquired immunodeficiency syndrome (AIDS) more quickly in infants because the infant's immune system has not yet formed antibodies. Within a short period of time (as soon as 2 months) the infant develops symptoms of acquired immunodeficiency syndrome (AIDS).

1. The HIV virus doesn't attack the organs of the infant.

2. The infant's immune system does not receive the mother's HIV antibodies.

4. The HIV virus that causes AIDS does not attack the infant's organs during their various stages of development.

Client Need: Physiological Integrity

4 - 4 1

① The care plan should not include the recommendation that the client substitute a less expensive generic interferon. Different brands of interferon (Intron-A) cannot be interchanged due to equivalency and dosage differences.

2. Clients taking interferon alfa-2b (Intron-A) will initially experience flulike symptoms. These symptoms usually diminish with continued use.

3. Since interferon alfa-2b does cause drowsiness, it is helpful to have the client take the medication at hour of sleep (hs).

4. Since the client's immune system is compromised, it is not recommended that the client be in contact with persons with viral illnesses.

Client Need: Health Promotion and Maintenance

4 - 4 2

③ The diagnosis with the highest priority for a child with varicella (chickenpox) is potential for infection related to bacterial invasion of skin lesions. Secondary bacterial infections are a common complication, since children are likely to scratch the lesions.

1, 3, and 4. Sleep pattern disturbances related to pruritus; nutrition alteration related to oral lesions; and impaired social interaction related to isolation are discomforts of short-term consequences and would not be the nursing diagnosis with the highest priority.

Client Need: Health Promotion and Maintenance

4 - 4 3

④ **The nurse can determine if a client's immune system is functioning properly if the client has a positive reaction to a skin test after exposure to a disease such as tuberculosis. For example: If a client has been exposed to the tubercular bacillus or has an active case of tuberculosis, the client should have a positive reaction to the purified protein derivation (PPD) skin test.**

1. A positive Homans' sign may be an indication of phlebitis.
2. Absence of fasciculations does not relate to the immune system. (Fasciculation refers to involuntary contractions or twitching of muscle fibers).
3. A positive Babinski reflex is indicative of an upper motor neuron disorder and is not associated with the proper functioning of the immune system.

Client Need: Physiological Integrity

4 - 4 4

③ **The nurse will expect clients recovering from hepatitis A to have difficulty maintaining a sense of well-being. The recovery is slow and clients may continue to have anorexia, malaise, and irritability. It is important for the nurse to work with these clients and their families during the course of the recovery.**

1. Clients experiencing hepatitis A virus (HAV) may experience vague epigastric distress, nausea, heartburn, and flatulence. During the icteric phase (jaundice) the client may experience tenderness of the liver. However, relieving pain is not expected to be a problem.
2. Bowel elimination is not a concern during the convalescent period.
3. Mild flulike upper respiratory tract infection is seen when symptoms first appear. However, respiratory complications are not a concern during convalescence.

Client Need: Health Promotion and Maintenance

4 - 4 5

② **For persons who are susceptible, the varicella-zoster immune globulin should be given within 96 hours of exposure. The infection of herpes zoster is contagious until the crusts have dried and fallen off the skin.**

1. Immune globulin is used for prophylaxis of measles, hepatitis A, and the treatment of hypogammaglobulinemia in immunodeficient clients.
3. Herpes zoster is an acute infectious disease caused by the varicella-zoster virus. Therefore, antibiotics are not effective in treating this condition.
4. A Tzanck test consists of examining tissue from the lower surface of a lesion in a vesicular condition to determine the cell type. The Tzanck test is not associated with immunity from the varicella-zoster virus.

Client Need: Safe, Effective Care Environment

4 - 4 6

---

① **Before administering anti-infective therapy, a client's allergies should be identified and culture specimens should be collected. It is important to know a client's allergies so that allergic reactions such as anaphylaxis can be avoided.**

2. You do not need to wait until the culture report is actually in the client's chart to begin anti-infective therapy.

3. The organism does not need to be identified before an anti-infective therapy can be started. A physical and history can provide enough information to administer anti-infective therapy.

4. Allergy tests are not usually necessary prior to administering anti-infective therapy. A client's history is usually sufficient.

Client Need: Safe, Effective Care Environment

4 - 4 7

---

② **An appropriate nursing response would include in understandable terms how sickle-cell anemia can affect mobility. The client should understand that activity intolerance due to discrepancy between oxygen supply and demand is associated with shortness of breath, not the pain the client is experiencing in the knees.**

1. One of the primary responsibilities of a nurse is client education. A client with sickle-cell anemia should be taught that pain is caused by a lack of oxygen to the tissues due to low hemoglobin.

3. An analgesic will not prevent the client from becoming short of breath.

4. An abnormally high white blood cell count does not cause shortness of breath. An abnormally low red blood cell count would cause shortness of breath.

Client Need: Physiological Integrity

4 - 4 8

---

④ **If the antibiotic is effective against infection, the temperature should return to normal. Antibiotics inhibit the growth or destroy microorganisms. A person's temperature becomes elevated in response to infection.**

1. A laxative or stool softener would facilitate the passage of a formed stool.

2. A diuretic would decrease fluid volume by increasing urine output.

3. An analgesic would relieve pain.

Client Need: Physiological Integrity

4 - 4 9

③ **The nurse will know that establishing a peak and trough level for a medication means to establish and maintain therapeutic serum levels without excessive toxicity.**

1. The efficacy of medications such as the anti-infectant tobramycin (Tobrex) is determined by relief of symptoms. Tobramycin's bactericidal action against susceptible bacteria relieves symptoms of infections including bone infections, central nervous system infections (CNS), respiratory infections, septicemia, and endocarditis.

2. Allergies are not associated with peak and trough levels. Allergies should be determined before medications are administered.

4. The initial loading dose of tobramycin is determined by factors including client body weight. All doses after the initial loading dose are determined by renal function and blood levels, since tobramycin is nephrotoxic.

Client Need: Physiological Integrity

4 - 5 0

② **As the effects of the human immunodeficiency virus (HIV) progress, the T-4 lymphocyte count decreases. Other laboratory changes include anemia, increased sedimentation rate, thrombocytopenia, and increased levels of B$_2$ macroglobulin.**

1. Decreases in platelet counts occur after HIV has progressed to the point of attacking the bone marrow. This does not occur in all clients who have HIV.

3. The T-8 lymphocyte count remains unchanged, but the ratio of T-4 cells to T-8 cells gradually reverses.

4. The erythrocyte sedimentation rate (ESR) increases as HIV disease progresses.

Client Need: Health Promotion and Maintenance

4 - 5 1

① **The nurse caring for a client with typhoid fever should wear gloves due to infectious materials. The causative organism for typhoid fever is *Salmonella typhis*. The source of *Salmonella typhis* is contaminated water, food, infected urine, and feces (the fecal carrier is the most common source). Control is through vaccinations, establishment of sanitary conditions, good handwashing, treatment and control of carriers, pasteurized milk and dairy products, and sanitary disposition of human feces.**

2. A mask is not required, since typhoid fever is not transmitted via the respiratory tract.

3. Typhoid fever does not require strict or contact isolation.

4. The client is not placed on contact isolation because of wound infection. Clients with typhoid fever require enteric precautions. The nurse should observe standard precautions. Contact isolation is instituted for conditions such as acute respiratory infections, herpes, and wound infections.

Client Need: Safe, Effective Care Environment

4 - 5 2

---

④ **The nurse will recognize the first sign of testicular cancer as painless enlargement of the testicle. Another early sign includes heaviness of the scrotum.**

1. If blood or tissue is present in the testicle, transillumination cannot be accomplished.
2. Urgency and urinary frequency are seen in more advanced stages of testicular cancer.
3. Lumbar pain is a sign seen in more advanced stages of testicular cancer and is usually due to metastasis.

Client Need: Health Promotion and Maintenance

4 - 5 3

---

① *Escherichia coli* **(E. coli) is the most common pathogenic organism found in the bladder and upper urinary tract.**

2. *Streptococcus pyogenes* (group A) is found in the nasopharynx (upper respiratory tract), and on the skin, hair, and perianal area.
3. *Staphylococcus aureus* is found on the skin, hair, and perianal area along with *Streptococcus pyogenes* (group A).
4. *Salmonella* is found in the small bowel and colon.

Client Need: Safe, Effective Care Environment

4 - 5 4

---

③ **The most likely persons to test positive for hepatitis D are those diagnosed with hepatitis B. Hepatitis D is a viral superinfection that occurs only in the presence of hepatitis B. It is thought to be spread in the same manner as hepatitis B but requires the helper function of hepatitis B for its expression. Only persons with hepatitis B may contract hepatitis D.**

1. Children attending an overcrowded day-care facility are at risk for developing hepatitis A, which is spread via the oral-fecal route and is found in food and water.
2. There is no vaccine for hepatitis C.
4. Hepatitis D can be found only in persons who experience hepatitis B.

Client Need: Safe, Effective Care Environment

4 - 5 5

④   A client diagnosed with hepatitis B should be informed that standard precautions are indicated for all contacts. Hepatitis B is spread via body fluids. The antigen (virus) is found in serum, saliva, stool, semen, and urine. All body fluids are to be treated as contaminated and universal or standard precautions must be taken at home.

1.   Hepatitis B is spread via body fluids such as serum, saliva, stool, semen, and urine.

2 and 3. Hepatitis B vaccine may be administered to individuals as young as 24 hours old. There is a hepatitis B immune globulin that should be administered as soon as possible after exposure to the virus.

Client Need: Safe, Effective Care Environment

4 - 5 6

④   Administration of a pretreatment antiemetic would diminish the most common side effect of mechlorethamine hydrochloride (Mustargen). Mechlorethamine hydrochloride (Mustargen) is an antineoplastic (alkylating agent). One of the most common side effects of Mustargen is nausea and vomiting. Administration of pretreatment antiemetics should be completed 30 minutes before Mustargen is administered. Acute toxic signs include nausea and vomiting lasting 12 to 24 hours.

1 and 2. A high-fluid and high-fiber diet is not recommended. However, the diet should be adjusted so that it is tolerated by the client. This will help to maintain fluid and electrolyte balance as well as good nutrition.

3.   Niacin is a lipid-lowering agent administered to treat clients with pellagra and hyperlipemia.

Client Need: Physiological Integrity

4 - 5 7

① ③ and ④   Signs and symptoms affecting the skin that are associated with systemic lupus erythematosus (SLE) include a butterfly rash, ulcers in the mouth, and alopecia. (hair loss).

2.   Red, swollen, painful joints are associated with SLE but have nothing to do with the skin.

5.   Hemolytic anemia is associated with SLE but has nothing to do with the skin.

Client Need: Health Promotion and Maintenance

4 - 5 8

② You will suspect candidiasis. Candidiasis (thrush) appears as cheesy white patches that, when rubbed, cause erythema (redness of mucosa) and bleeding. Predisposing factors include immunosuppression.

1. Herpes simplex appears as a singular vesicle or clustered vesicles that usually occur where the mucous membrane joins the skin. It is an opportunistic viral infection (an infection or disease caused by an organism that does not normally cause disease except under certain circumstances, such as in immunosuppressed clients).

3. Leukoplakia is a disease affecting the mucous membranes of the cheeks, gums, and tongue. It appears as white thick patches that have a tendency to fissure (cleft or furrow). Leukoplakia is associated with use of tobacco and poorly fitted dentures.

4. Kaposi's sarcoma appears first on the oral mucosa as a reddish, purple, or blue malignant lesion. Lesions may be singular or multiple in number. Kaposi's sarcoma is an opportunistic neoplasm affecting clients with acquired immune deficiency syndrome (AIDS).

Client Need: Physiological Integrity

4 - 5 9

① An appropriate nursing intervention for a client with tetanus (lockjaw) would be to decrease environmental stimuli. Stimulation of these clients causes severe muscle spasms, without loss of consciousness. Although strong sedation and muscle relaxants are usually administered, care should be exercised to avoid unnecessary stimulation.

2. Suctioning by the nasopharyngeal route would be too stimulating and is not necessary, since there are no excess secretions.

3. Gentle massage to the large joints may be too stimulating. The discomfort of tetanus is felt more in the muscles than in the joints.

4. Frequent assessment is not necessary, since the level of consciousness (LOC) is not affected by tetanus.

Client Need: Safe, Effective Care Environment

4 - 6 0

① A client experiencing tenderness following a bone marrow biopsy would receive the prescribed analgesic. Tenderness is expected following a bone marrow biopsy. Administering the prescribed analgesics will usually resolve the problem.

2. If tenderness is accompanied by other signs of infection, it would be appropriate to notify the physician.

3. Because tenderness is a normal expectation, an analgesic is anticipated.

4. Applying direct pressure will probably increase the tenderness and is not recommended.

Client Need: Safe, Effective Care Environment

4 - 6 1

Fill in the blank correct answer:

<u>Phagocytosis</u>

Phagocytosis is the process of binding with, engulfing, and digesting (destroying) bacteria, viruses, and other foreign material. Phagocytosis is a part of the immune response that protects the body from infection.

Client Need: Health Promotion and Maintenance

4 - 6 2

② Any time clients have infections such as measles, chickenpox, pertussis, hepatitis, or polio, they will develop natural acquired active immunity. It should be noted that even though a client has a specific disease, such as measles, it may not produce a response that will provide lifelong immunity.

1. Passive immunity occurs when ready-made antibodies are given to a susceptible person. This only provides short-lived protection from the antigen. Newborns receive passive immunity as the mother's antibodies can cross the placenta barrier.

3. Artificially acquired active immunity develops through immunization, not actually having a disease. Examples of immunization that provide protection include diphtheria, tetanus, pertussis (DTP); inactivated polio (IVP); and varicella (chickenpox).

4. Immune serum globulin, also known as gamma globulin or immunoglobulin, is not a type of immunity. Immune globulin is a drug created from serum containing antibodies. It may be used to bolster the immune system of those with deficiencies.

Client Need: Health Promotion and Maintenance

4 - 6 3

① ③ and ④ Azathioprine (Imuran), cyclosporine (Sandimmune), and mycophenolate mofetil (CellCept) are immunosuppressant drugs. Mycophenolate mofetil is specifically administered to prevent kidney transplant rejections. Immunosuppressants help to minimize organ rejection by preventing activation of the immune response.

2. Cefdinir (Omnicef) is an anti-infective, not an immunosuppressant.

5. Famciclorin (Famvir) is an antiviral, not an immunosuppressant.

Client Need: Health Promotion and Maintenance

4 - 6 4

Fill in the blank correct answer:

<u>epinephrine (adrenaline)</u>

Epinephrine is recommended for clients who are known to have severe allergic reactions to the venom of insects such as bees, wasps, and hornets as well as to anthropods (spiders) such as the black widow.

4 - 6 5

①②and ⑤ HIV is transmitted primarily by sexual intercourse, intravenous drug use, and mother-to-infant during pregnancy and through breast milk. When infected blood, milk, semen, or vaginal secretions from one person are deposited onto the mucous membranes or into the bloodstream of another person, infection can occur.

3. HIV is not transmitted through the bites of insects.

4. Transmission of HIV used to occur through blood transfusions as well as through other blood products; however, blood donations are now screened for HIV and are therefore not a primary source of infection today.

Practice Test 5

Integumentary System and Burns

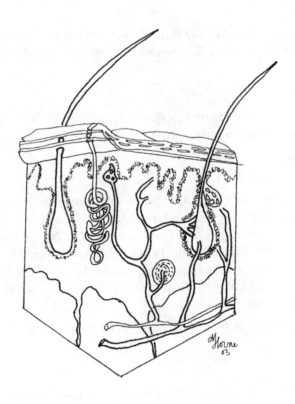

The Structure of the Skin

OVERVIEW

The integumentary system includes the skin (the outer covering of the body), sebaceous glands, and sweat glands, as well as hair and nails.

The skin is the largest organ of the body. It serves as a protective membrane over the entire body and guards the deeper tissues. It also prevents excessive loss of water, salts, and heat. As a physical barrier, the skin is the body's first line of defense. It guards against invasion of pathogens and their toxins and also protects the body against microorganisms by its slightly acidic secretions.

The skin also contains nerve endings or fibers that act as receptors for sensations such as pain, temperature, pressure, and touch and relay these sensory messages to the brain and spinal cord. We rely on these messages for critical information about our environment.

STRUCTURE OF THE SKIN

The skin consists of three layers: The epidermis, a thin, cellular membrane-like layer; the dermis or corium, a dense, fibrous layer of connective tissue; and the subcutaneous tissue, a thick, fat-containing layer.

Epidermis

The epidermis is the outermost layer of the skin. It does not contain blood vessels, lymphatic vessels, or connective tissue. It is dependent upon the corium to supply nourishment from its capillaries.

Dermis

The dermis (corium) lies below the epidermis. It is rich in blood vessels, lymph vessels, and nerve fibers. The dermis contains the accessory organs; namely, hair follicles, sebaceous glands, and sweat glands.

Subcutaneous Tissues

The subcutaneous tissues consist of connective tissue with a special formation of fat. This layer protects the deeper tissues in the body and serves as a heat insulator. The body's temperature is maintained by thermoregulation involving several different tissues in the skin. Nerve fibers coordinate thermoregulation by carrying messages to the skin from the heat centers in the brain that are sensitive to increases and decreases in body temperature. The impulses generated from these fibers cause the blood vessels to dilate, bringing blood to the surface of the skin, thus causing the sweat glands to produce sweat. Sweat regulates heat through its evaporation.

The skin contains two types of glands that produce needed secretions:

Sebaceous Glands

The sebaceous glands produce an oily secretion called sebum that helps to lubricate the surface of the skin. Ducts bring sebum to the skin's surface, where it is excreted through tiny openings called pores.

Sweat Glands

Like the sebaceous glands, the sweat glands produce a substance that is brought to the skin's surface by ducts. Through these ducts a watery substance known as sweat is excreted. Sweat helps to cool the body as it evaporates from the skin's surface.

DISEASES/DISORDERS OF THE SKIN INCLUDE

Impetigo

A contagious bacterial infection of the skin caused by either staphylococcus or streptococcus or a combination of the two.

Folliculitis/Furunculosis

A bacterial infection resulting from boils.

Carbunculosis

Carbunculosis is a bacterial infection of the hair follicle caused by *Staphylococcus aureus*. Predisposing factors include: Infected wounds, poor hygiene, diabetes, alcoholism, and debilitation. This condition usually affects males between 20 and 40 years of age.

Staphylococcal Scalded Skin Syndrome

Another name for staphylococcal scalded skin syndrome is Ritter's disease or Ritter-Lyell syndrome. This is a severe skin disorder most prevalent in infants. It can develop in children and is uncommon in adults. Most people recover fully. However, there is 2% to 3% mortality. Death usually results from complications such as loss of fluids and electrolytes, sepsis, and other systemic involvement.

Tinea Versicolor (Fungal Infestation)

Tinea versicolor (pityriasis versicolor) is a chronic superficial fungal infection. It usually affects adolescents and may produce a multicolored, scaly rash. The cause is uncertain.

Dermatophytosis (Fungal Infection)

Another name for dermatophytosis is tinea. Tinea infections result from dermatophytes (fungi) and usually affect males more than females. With effective treatment, the cure rate is high; however, some people will develop chronic infections.

The six types of dermatophytosis are:

- tinea capitis — affecting the scalp
- tinea corporis — affecting the body
- tinea unguium — affecting the nails
- tinea pedis — affecting the feet (athlete's foot)
- tinea cruris — affecting the groin (jock itch)
- tinea barbae — refers to bearded skin (infection of the bearded area)

Scabies (Itch) (Parasitic Infestation)

Scabies are caused by the itch mite. Scabies are associated with overcrowded conditions and poor hygiene. Mites can live their life cycle in the skin of humans. The female burrows into the skin and lays her eggs. Scabies can be transmitted by sexual contact as well as through the skin.

Cutaneous Larva Migrans (Parasitic Infestation)

Cutaneous larva migrans is a skin reaction to infestation by nematodes (hookworms or roundworms) that usually infest dogs and cats. Humans are usually affected by coming in contact with infected soil or sand. The ova are present in the feces of dogs and cats. When the ova hatch, they can burrow into human skin.

Pediculosis (Head Lice)

These lice infest humans and feed off their blood. The lice lay eggs (nits) in body hair and clothing. When the nits hatch and become mature lice, they bite and inject a toxin into the skin that causes irritation and purpuric spots (little hemorrhages on the skin). With proper treatment, this condition responds well.

Acne Vulgaris (Follicular and Glandular Disorder)

Acne vulgaris is an inflammatory disease of the sebaceous follicles. It affects mostly adolescents between 15 to 18 years of age; however, lesions can appear as early as 8 years of age. Acne vulgaris affects boys more often than girls. The cause is unknown. Experimental investigations are ongoing.

Hirsutism (Excessive Growth of Body Hair)

Hirsutism is usually seen in women and children. When seen in the adult male, it is associated with excessive hair growth. The causes of this condition are thought to be endocrine abnormalities and also genetic predisposition.

Alopecia (Hair Loss) (Follicular and Glandular Disorder)

Alopecia usually occurs on the scalp, but it can occur on bearded areas, eyebrows, and eyelids. People with the nonscarring types of alopecia are usually able to re-grow hair. This condition may be related to androgen levels and aging. It also has a genetic component. Radiation, drug therapies, and drug reactions also cause alopecia.

Rosacea (Follicular and Glandular Disorder)

Rosacea is a chronic skin eruption manifested by flushing and dilation in small blood vessels in the face, in particular, the nose and checks. The cause of this condition is unknown; however, the symptoms are made worse by stress, infection, vitamin deficiency, menopause, and endocrine disturbance.

Albinism (Disorder of Pigmentation)

Albinism is a genetic nonpathological condition characterized by partial or total absence of pigment in the skin, hair, and eyes. It may be accompanied by astigmatism (defective divesture of the cornea or lens of the eye), photophobia (intolerance to light), and nystagmus (involuntary back-and-forth or cyclical movement of the eye) because the choroid is not completely protected from light due to lack of pigmentation.

Melasma (Chloasma or Mask of Pregnancy) (Disorder of Skin Pigmentation)

Melasma is best described as a hypermelanotic skin condition (caused by increased melanin production). This disorder may be related to hormonal changes during pregnancy, menopause, ovarian cancer, and the use of contraceptives. Certain medications may contribute to this disorder. Persons with acquired immunodeficiency syndrome (AIDS) have a similar hyperpigmentation.

Vitiligo (Disorder of Skin Pigmentation)

Vitiligo (obvious white patches of skin) results from loss of pigment cells, or melanocytes. Vitiligo has no racial preference but is more visible in dark complexions. It does not favor one sex over the other.

Photosensitivity Reactions (Disorders of Skin Pigmentation)

A photosensitivity reaction causes skin eruptions due to a toxic or allergic response to light or chemicals such as dyes, coal, and tar. Also, oil of bergamot, a component found in perfume, colognes, and pomades, may cause a reaction. These sensitivity reactions are manifested by erythema (redness).

Dermatitis (Inflammatory Reaction) (Inflammatory Disorder)

Dermatitis is an inflammation of the skin occurring in several forms: Atopic, seborrheic, nummular, contact, chronic, localized neurodermatitis, exfolicitive, and stasis.

MISCELLANEOUS DISORDERS OF THE SKIN

Toxic Epidermal Necrolysis (Scalded Skin Syndrome)

Toxic epidermal necrolysis is a life-threatening disorder that primarily affects adults. It is a rare skin disorder that causes epidermal erythema, superficial necrosis, and skin erosions. The mortality rate is high among debilitated and elderly persons. The cause of this disorder is obscure; however, it is thought that 30% of the cases are caused as a result of reactions to drugs such as: Sulfonamides, penicillin, barbiturates, and isoniazid.

Warts (Verrucae)

Warts are common benign viral infections of the skin. Warts may occur at any age; however, the incidence is highest in children. Some warts disappear gradually after treatment, while others may require extensive and prolonged treatment. There are different types of warts: Common (verrucal vulgaris), filiform, periungual, flat (referred to as juvenile), plantar, digitate, and condyloma acuminatum (moist warts).

Psoriasis

Psoriasis is a chronic skin disorder affecting approximately 2% of the population. It is denoted by red scaly patches with defined borders. Psoriasis may be genetically determined; however, the onset may be influenced by environmental factors. Also, pregnancy, endocrine changes, climate, and emotional stress may cause flare-ups.

Corns and Calluses

Corns and calluses are usually located on areas exposed to repeated trauma, such as the feet. They may be caused by the excessive pressure of ill-fitting shoes and sometimes by internal pressure from arthritic bones. A callus is an area of thickened skin found on the feet or hands and produced by external pressure or friction. Persons who play the guitar or do manual labor will develop calluses. The severity of corns and calluses depends upon the degree and duration of the trauma.

Pityriasis Rosea

Pityriasis rosea, an acute, self-limiting, and noncontagious inflammatory disorder, may develop at any age but typically develops in adolescents and young adult women. The incidence of pityriasis rosea rises in the spring and fall. The cause is unknown; however, the virtual absence of recurrence suggests a viral agent or an autoimmune disorder.

Hyperhidrosis (Bromidrosis) (Fetid Sweat)

Hyperhidrosis is an excessive secretion of sweat from the exocrine glands, especially sweat that occurs in the axillae (mostly after puberty) and on the palms and soles (often occurring during infancy and/or childhood). The cause is unknown. Genetic factors may contribute to the development of hyperhidrosis; however, emotional stress appears to be the most prominent cause. It is thought that increased central nervous system (CNS) impulses may cause the release of excessive amounts of acetylcholine, which produces a heightened sweat response. Exercise and a hot climate can cause profuse sweating in persons with hyperhidrosis. In addition, certain foods such as tomato sauce, chocolate, coffee, and spices, as well as some drugs (antipyretics, emetics, meperidine, and anticholinesteroses) can cause excessive sweating.

Pressure Ulcers (Pressure Sores or Bedsores)

Pressure ulcers are localized areas of cellular necrosis. The ulcers occur most often in the skin, subcutaneous tissue, and over bony prominences. Pressure exerted over these areas causes tissue ischemia and increased capillary pressure. Repositioning people with pressure ulcers can alleviate the ulcers.

Lichen Planus

Lichen planus is a relatively rare disease, manifesting benign but pruritic (itching) skin. Eruptions occur most often in middle age and are uncommon in the young and elderly. Lichen planus is found in all geographic areas and is equally distributed among races. The cause of this condition is unknown.

Practice Test 5

Questions

5 - 1

A child sustains deep partial-thickness burns to the arms and anterior chest. It has been 8 hours since admission. All of the following are assessment findings at this time. Which one of the following should have the highest priority for intervention?

1. decreased urine output
2. increased restlessness and irritability
3. radial pulses less palpable
4. hoarseness and stridor

5 - 2

A 5-year-old was hospitalized promptly after sustaining third-degree burns on the anterior chest, upper arms, forearms, and hands. Intravenous infusion was begun, an indwelling urethral catheter inserted, and pressure dressings applied to burned areas. While performing a nursing assessment, which of the following would suggests a need to implement nursing measures to counteract the initial effects of shock?

1. restlessness and bradycardia
2. air hunger and hyperreflexia
3. intense pain and convulsions
4. pale, clammy skin and thirst

5 - 3

A child 6 years old has sustained third-degree burns. To plan for the need for fluid replacement, the nurse will consider which of the following?

1. The younger the child, the greater the fluid needs in proportion to body weight.
2. The proportion of body weight contributed by water is smaller during early childhood than it is during adulthood.
3. The fluid needs per kilogram of body weight are variable until the kidneys become functionally more mature at adolescence.
4. The total volume of extracellular fluid per kilogram of body weight increases gradually from birth to adolescence and then stabilizes at the adult level.

5 - 4

You are irrigating a draining wound with sterile saline solution. Which of the following would be the most appropriate procedure to follow?

1. wash hands, don clean gloves, remove soiled dressing, remove gloves, wash hands, prepare sterile field, don sterile gloves
2. prepare sterile field, put on sterile gloves, and remove soiled dressing
3. pour solution, wash hands, and remove soiled dressing
4. remove soiled dressing, flush wound, and wash hands

5 - 5

An infant has localized scaling and red areas on the cheeks, neck, and elbows that have been diagnosed as atopic dermatitis. Which of the following instructions regarding the infant's care is most important for the nurse to reinforce for the mother?

1. Bathe the infant daily with a mild soap.
2. Keep the infant's nails cut short.
3. Use only short-sleeved clothing for the infant.
4. Have the other children in the family avoid contact with the infant.

5 - 6

A client experiencing acne vulgaris may benefit from a prescription for:

1. amphotericin B cream.
2. butoconazole nitrate cream.
3. ciclopirox olamine cream.
4. benzoyl peroxide cream.

5 - 7

A client involved in an industrial accident was exposed to a gasoline fire. The client is complaining of painful burns to the feet, but denies pain on the burned legs. The nurse will:

1. remove the footwear to assess the feet only, leaving the rest of the clothing intact.
2. keep the client fully clothed to avoid chilling.
3. remove all the clothing, then cover the client in a clean sheet.
4. remove the footwear and immediately cover the client's feet in antibiotic ointment.

5 - 8

A client who has experienced 25% body surface second-degree burns may require analgesia with:

1. acetaminophen.
2. morphine sulfate.
3. ibuprofen.
4. a transcutaneous electrical nerve stimulator unit.

5 - 9

A client who has experienced deep partial-thickness burns to the left forearm will require which of the following interventions?

1. casting of the left arm to immobilize the elbow and wrist joints
2. antifungal cream bid to the affected area for 10 days
3. immediate surgical intervention to the left arm to restore the skin's integrity
4. a tetanus prophylaxis injection if the client's last injection is 10 years old

5 - 1 0

Your client has experienced extensive burns and is scheduled for daily hydrotherapy. The chief purpose of hydrotherapy is to:

1. prevent infection.
2. restore fluid balance.
3. maintain wound sterility.
4. remove loose tissue and debris.

5 - 1 1

Two weeks after a skin graft, a client is concerned about the possibility of scarring at the donor site. Which of the following responses by the nurse concerning the care of the donor site would be most appropriate?

1. "Clean the area with soap and water every day and leave it alone."
2. "Apply hydrogen peroxide to the area several times a day."
3. "Use an antibacterial soap and keep the area covered."
4. "Keep the area soft with lanolin cream or lotion."

5 - 1 2

You are to administer a tepid sponge bath to a client with an elevated temperature. To achieve the desired outcome of this procedure, which of the following measures should be used?

1. Stroke the client's skin to cause friction.
2. Give fluids to drink.
3. Allow moisture on the skin to evaporate.
4. Lower the temperature of the room.

5 - 1 3

A client has been diagnosed with Hansen's disease. The nurse will recognize the pharmacologic treatment for this condition as:

1. rifampin and dapsone.
2. amphotericin B and nystatin.
3. ciclopirox and haloprogin.
4. miconazole and clotrimazole.

5 - 1 4

Which of the following medications would be appropriate to administer one-half hour prior to the debridement of a full-thickness burn?

1. acetaminophen
2. fluoxetine
3. meperidine
4. captopril

5 - 1 5

Which intravenous fluid and rate would be most appropriate to administer immediately to an adult with a full-thickness burn on 18% of the body?

1. keep the vein open with normal saline
2. lidocaine (20 to 50 mcg/kg/min) infusion up to 200 to 300 mg in 1 hour
3. keep the vein open with dextrose 5% in water
4. lactated Ringer's at 250 cc/hour

5 - 1 6

A client who had abdominal surgery has a wound drain in place. On the evening following surgery, the dressing covering the incision is saturated with a large amount of blood-tinged drainage. Which of the following interpretations and actions is most accurate?

1. Hemorrhage is occurring and the physician should be notified.
2. Wound dehiscence is imminent and a firm binder should be applied.
3. This drainage is expected and the dressing should be reinforced.
4. The drain is obstructed and it should be irrigated before the dressing is changed.

5 - 17

Your client is extremely edematous. Which of the following nursing interventions is most appropriate?

1. Cough and deep breathe every 2 hours.
2. Massage extremities with lotion every 4 hours.
3. Turn and reposition every 1 to 2 hours.
4. Place lamb's wool the full length of the bed.

5 - 18

A client is admitted to the emergency department with partial- and full-thickness burns on the chest, arms, and hands. On arrival to the emergency facility, which of the following will the nurse anticipate as an immediate action?

1. arterial blood gasses
2. morphine sulfate to be given intramuscularly
3. assessment of the client's home environment
4. body weight assessment

5 - 19

A client who has experienced "sunburn" after 2 hours of unprotected exposure to the summer's sun most likely has:

1. a superficial partial-thickness burn.
2. a deep partial-thickness burn.
3. a full-thickness burn.
4. no real thermal burn. "Sunburn" is merely a lay term.

5 - 20

A client experienced extensive burns. What is the first consequence of capillary permeability in the surrounding tissues?

1. fluid loss
2. pain
3. edema
4. nausea

5 - 21

A child was admitted with burns over 30% of the body due to clothes catching fire. It is now 24 hours later. The lowest-priority information to collect at this time is:

1. body weight.
2. bowel sounds.
3. breath sounds.
4. vital signs.

5 - 22

According to the "rule of nines," burn victims experiencing burns to their anterior chest and abdomen have an injury that approximates:

1. 8% of their body's surface.
2. 18% of their body's surface.
3. 29% of their body's surface.
4. above 29% of their body's surface.

5 - 23

Which of the following will you remove in order to reduce sources of heat in a thermally burned client?

1. jewelry
2. dentures
3. makeup
4. hairpieces

5 - 2 4

Clients experiencing fungal skin infections should be advised to avoid using:

1. detergents.
2. cornstarch.
3. cotton clothing.
4. topical creams.

5 - 2 5

A client was recently placed on a regimen of prednisone for severe poison oak. Which of the following instructions should be given to the client?

1. "Take a tablet only when the itch gets really bad."
2. "Make sure you drink a big glass of orange juice with each dose."
3. "Save any leftover pills and take them next time you get poison oak."
4. "Don't stop taking this medicine abruptly; the dosage must be tapered."

5 - 2 6

An adolescent is experiencing severe acne caused by the microorganism *P. acnes*. Which pharmacological agent is administered to treat this condition?

1. tetracycline
2. pyrimethamine
3. miconazole
4. famciclovir

5 - 2 7

A client has anemia and is experiencing the following integumentary changes: pallor, jaundice, and pruritus. The nurse knows that pruritus occurs as a result of:

1. reduced hemoglobin and decreased blood flow to the skin.
2. increased serum and skin bile salt concentration.
3. increased concentration of serum bilirubin that increases red blood cell hemolysis.
4. low viscosity of blood.

5 - 2 8

Parents of pediatric clients with chickenpox should be advised to avoid administering:

1. calamine lotion over or around lesions.
2. acetaminophen po for pain.
3. diphenhydramine po for itch.
4. diphenhydramine ointment liberally over the entire body.

5 - 2 9

Your client received a partial-thickness (first-degree) burn. You know this degree of burn affects the:

1. epidermis.
2. epidermis and dermis.
3. epidermis, dermis, and subcutaneous tissue.
4. skin and nerve endings.

5 - 3 0

A 4-year-old is experiencing cellulitis of the right forearm. There is swelling above the wrist and beyond the elbow. You will teach the caregiver how to apply:

1. elastic bandages to reduce swelling.
2. elbow restraints for immobilization.
3. warm, moist compresses.
4. range-of-motion exercises to prevent contracture.

5 - 3 1

A client with condylomata acuminata has been treating the growths with a self-application of the topical medication podofilox. The client tells the nurse, "I just learned that I am pregnant. Will this interfere with my medication?" The nurse's best response is:

1. "The medication is contraindicated during pregnancy."
2. "It will be necessary to change the route of administration."
3. "There is no reason the medication can't be continued as usual."
4. "Treating the growths now will prevent complications for the baby during delivery."

5 - 3 2

You are teaching the parents of a child with impetigo how to treat the child's lesions. Which statement made by the parents indicates a need for further teaching?

1. "We will wash and soak the lesions with warm, soapy water 3 times a day."
2. "We will gently remove the crusts after soaking."
3. "We will apply the prescribed topical antibiotic ointment to the affected areas."
4. "We will cover the affected areas with sterile gauze pads."

5 - 3 3

A 7-year-old child has pediculosis capitis. The medication permethrin 1% has been prescribed. The nurse will teach the parents how to administer this topical liquid medication. Which comment by the parents indicates a need for further teaching?

1. "We will apply the medication after our child's hair has been washed with shampoo, rinsed, and towel-dried."
2. "We will apply about 35 ml of the liquid medication to saturate our child's hair and scalp."
3. "We will allow the medication to remain on our child's hair and scalp for 10 minutes before rinsing it off with water."
4. "We will administer a second application of the medication 7 to 10 days after the first application."

5 - 3 4

Your client is experiencing vitiligo. This condition is best described as:

1. raised, firm, thickened scabs that form at the site of a wound.
2. ingrown hairs producing papules, pustules, and occasional keloids.
3. unpigmented skin patches.
4. a fungal infection producing yellow or fawn-colored patches on the skin.

5 - 3 5

A 4-year-old has recently had an autograft following a burn on the anterior chest. Your plan of care is least likely to include:

1. maintaining the client in a supine position.
2. hydrotherapy to stimulate circulation.
3. use of elbow restraints.
4. aspiration of fluid accumulated under the graft.

5-36

What would you expect your assessment to reveal in a postburn client during the early stages of shock?

1. restlessness
2. marked decrease in blood pressure
3. shallow respirations
4. oliguria

5-37

A preterm neonate weighing 1,430 grams is under a radiant warmer for phototherapy. The most appropriate nursing diagnosis for this neonate is:

1. skin integrity impaired.
2. gas exchange impaired.
3. fluid volume deficit, potential for.
4. infection, potential for.

5-38

Warm, moist packs have been prescribed qid to treat ulceration on a client's foot. Aseptic technique will be used to:

1. destroy bacteria on the skin.
2. inhibit the growth of pathogens.
3. prevent the introduction of additional microorganisms.
4. minimize the risk of spreading the infection to others.

5-39

Which of the following is not associated with congenital anomaly?

1. Mongolian spotting over the buttocks
2. short stature, low posterior hairline, webbing of the neck, broad chest, and widely spaced nipples
3. a simian crease across the palms of both hands
4. the top of the pinna falling below an imaginary line from the outer orbit of the eye to the occiput

5-40

A dark-skinned client is experiencing erythema. You will expect the skin to appear:

1. pale.
2. dusky red or violet.
3. black.
4. yellow.

5-41

You are teaching a group of parents about initial first aid at the scene of a fire involving a child whose clothes are on fire. Which comments by the group suggest a correct understanding of your teaching?

Select all that apply by placing a ✔ in the square:

❏ 1. "I will throw water on the child to put out the fire."
❏ 2. "I will throw a blanket over the head and body of the child."
❏ 3. "I will lay the child flat and roll him in a blanket."
❏ 4. "I will call the Fire Department."
❏ 5. "I will call 911."

5 - 4 2

Signs of heat or smoke inhalation injury include:

Select all that apply by placing a ✔ in the square:

- ❑ 1. singed nasal hairs, eyebrows, and eyelashes.
- ❑ 2. stridor.
- ❑ 3. shortness of breath.
- ❑ 4. burns around the face and neck.
- ❑ 5. soot around the mouth and nose.

Practice Test 5

Answers, Rationales, and Explanations

5 - 1

④ **Hoarseness and stridor are assessment findings that have the highest priority for intervention at this time. These findings are likely indications of airway edema, which is potentially life threatening.**

1, 2, and 3. A decrease in urine output, increased restlessness and irritability, and less palpable radial pulses would not take precedence over potential airway obstruction.

Client Need: Physiological Integrity

5 - 2

④ **Pale, clammy skin and thirst indicate a need to implement nursing measures to counteract the effects of shock. Burns result in an initial fluid loss due to diuresis and increased capillary permeability.**

1. Initial signs of shock include tachycardia, not bradycardia.
2. Air hunger is associated with a decrease in hemoglobin, not dehydration. Also, the burned client is most likely to experience hyponatremia (sodium depletion), not hypernatremia, which would cause increased muscle tone and deep tendon reflexes.
3. Intense pain and convulsions would be associated with the actual burn, especially painful deep second-degree burns.

Client Need: Physiological Integrity

5 - 3

① **The younger the child, the greater the amount of fluids needed in proportion to body weight. At 6 years of age, the client's body surface in proportion to body weight leads to increased insensible fluid loss through the skin.**

2. The proportion of body weight contributed by water is greater, not smaller, during early childhood compared to adulthood.
3. The kidneys are functionally mature at birth.
4. The total volume of extracellular fluid per kilogram of body weight does not increase gradually from birth to adolescence. As a person matures, body fluid will decrease due to body growth.

Client Need: Health Promotion and Maintenance

5 - 4

① **In this situation, the nurse should wash hands, don clean gloves, remove soiled dressing, remove gloves, wash hands, prepare sterile field, and don sterile gloves. Nurses should wash their hands first before beginning any procedure.**

2, 3, and 4. None of these options follow the sequence necessary to maintain sterile technique.

Client Need: Safe, Effective Care Environment

5 - 5

② **Keeping an infant's fingernails cut short will lessen the chance of secondary infection and the "itch-scratch-itch" cycle. Infants with atopic dermatitis (eczema) may try to scratch themselves because of intense itching.**

1. Soaps should be avoided because of the drying effects they have on the skin. Dry skin triggers and exacerbates atopic dermatitis.

3. Long-sleeved clothing is recommended because it discourages scratching. Also, it is advisable to wear soft cotton fabrics directly next to the skin.

4. Atopic dermatitis is not contagious. There is no need for family members to avoid a child with this condition.

Client Need: Health Promotion and Maintenance

5 - 6

④ **Benzoyl peroxide is an anti-acne medication whose action is due to its bacteriostatic properties and its penetration. Acne vulgaris is a common skin disorder of adolescents caused by the microorganism *P. acnes*.**

1, 2, and 3. Amphotericin B, ciclopirox olamine (Loprox), and butoconazole nitrate (Femstat) are all antifungal agents and do not impact on acne vulgaris.

Client Need: Health Promotion and Maintenance

5 - 7

③ The nurse will remove all the clothing and cover the client in a clean sheet. The initial treatment of a burn victim includes removing clothing and covering the victim. Clothing may still be smoldering and may increase the extent of the burn. A complete assessment must be done. In this instance, it is very probable that the burns on the legs involved all layers of the skin, as well as the nerves, and are therefore painless. Burns that are painless are often the most serious because nerve endings have been damaged.

1 and 2. In order to allow a thorough survey and assessment and to avoid further injury due to smoldering garments, clothing of the burn victim should be removed.

4. Oil-based ointments are contraindicated in the initial treatment of burns. The initial application to burned skin is usually a cooling liquid such as chilled saline or water.

Client Need: Safe, Effective Care Environment

5 - 8

② Morphine sulfate (morphine) is an opioid analgesic whose impact on the central nervous system makes it a very potent pain reliever. Because of the very painful nature of second-degree burns, adequate pain management is a challenge and is likely to necessitate an opioid.

1 and 3. Acetaminophen (Tylenol) and ibuprofen (Motrin) are used to treat mild to moderate pain.

4. A transcutaneous electrical nerve stimulation (TENS) unit is for localized pain and is attached to the skin, making it unsuitable for burn analgesia.

Client Need: Physiological Integrity

5 - 9

④ Tetanus prophylaxis is indicated for any client who has a nonsurgical wound or injury and has not received a tetanus immunization within 10 years. Unlike some other diseases that are considered eradicated, such as smallpox, tetanus remains a threat to any person who is not immunized and has a break in the skin's integrity. Only those allergic to the injection are exempt.

1. Casting is not an accepted treatment for deep partial-thickness burns. These injuries require dressings.

2. Fungal infections are much less common in the burn injury than bacterial infections, so bacteriostatic ointments are used to prevent infection.

3. Surgical intervention is usually not required in deep partial-thickness burns. All full-thickness burns require surgical consultation at least.

Client Need: Physiological Integrity

5-10

④ **The chief purpose of hydrotherapy for clients with extensive burns is to cleanse the wounds by removing loose tissue and debris. Hydrotherapy also allows for active range-of-motion exercises.**

1. The prevention of infection is accomplished by use of topical silver sulfadiazine (Silvadene).
2. Fluid replacement is essential and is achieved through intravenous infusion (IV). Burn shock requires IV administration of fluid to maintain circulating volume.
3. Wounds are not sterile; therefore, using an antibacterial soap is not necessary.

Client Need: Physiological Integrity

5-11

④ **To keep the donor site soft and scarring at a minimum, lotion or lanolin cream should be applied several times a day.**

1, 2, and 3. Soaps and hydrogen peroxide are irritants and should be avoided.

Client Need: Health Promotion and Maintenance

5-12

③ **Temperature reduction is promoted by the evaporation of moisture from the skin. This is the desired outcome of the procedure.**

1. Friction produces heat and would be counterproductive.
2. Offering fluids would affect hydration but would not directly affect body temperature.
4. Lowering room temperature could cause chilling and sudden fluctuations in the client's body temperature.

Client Need: Safe, Effective Care Environment

5-13

① **Rifampin (Rifadin) and dapsone (Avlosulfon) are antitubercular antileprotics that are used as first-line pharmacologic treatment on skin and mucosal lesions such as those associated with Hansen's disease (leprosy).**

2. Amphotericin B (Fungizone) and nystatin (Mycostatin) are antifungal agents administered to treat fungal infections. They do not have an impact on bacteria.
3. Ciclopirox (Loprox) and haloprogin (Halotex) are antifungal agents and do not have an impact on bacteria.
4. Miconazole (Monistat) and clotrimazole (Mycelex-G) are antifungal agents and do not have an impact on bacteria.

Client Need: Physiological Integrity

5 - 1 4

③ **Meperidine (Demerol) would be appropriate to administer one-half hour prior to the debridement of a full-thickness burn. Demerol is an opioid whose effect on pain perception makes it a very effective analgesic. Because of the painful nature of many burn debridements, analgesia is often given beforehand.**

1. Acetaminophen (Tylenol) is an antipyretic analgesic indicated for mild or moderate pain only.

2. Fluoxetine (Prozac) is an antidepressant medication.

4. Captopril (Capoten) is an antihypertensive medication.

Client Need: Health Promotion and Maintenance

5 - 1 5

④ **The nurse would prepare lactated Ringer's (LR) solution. There are numerous formulas used to calculate intravenous replacement for burn victims. The consensus formula is simply:**

$$\frac{2 \text{ to } 4 \text{ ml} \times \text{ kg body weight} \times \% \text{ body surface area burned}}{2}$$

If the average adult weighs approximately 75 kg, one might quickly estimate:

$$\frac{3\text{ml} \times 75 \text{ kg} \times 18 \%}{2} = 2{,}025 \text{ in 8 hours or 250 cc LR/hr.}$$

1. Normal saline at a keep-vein-open (KVO) rate is too slow to rehydrate a burned client.

2. Lidocaine (20 to 50mg/kg/min) infusion is administered to treat ventricular arrhythmias, not to rehydrate clients who have been burned.

3. Dextrose 5% in water (D5W) administered at a keep-vein-open (KVO) rate is too slow to rehydrate a burned client.

Client Need: Physiological Integrity

5 - 1 6

③ **A large amount of blood-tinged drainage is expected and the dressing should be reinforced. It is the purpose of a wound drain to prevent the accumulation of blood in the wound.**

1. Since the drainage is blood-tinged, it cannot be hemorrhage. Venous blood is dark and arterial blood is bright red.

2. There is no indication that a dehiscence (bursting open of a wound) is imminent.

4. There is no indication that the wound is obstructed. In fact, the dressing is saturated with blood-tinged drainage.

Client Need: Health Promotion and Maintenance

5 - 1 7

③ **The nurse should turn and reposition the client. Turning and repositioning the client every 1 to 2 hours will relieve pressure and aid in the prevention of skin breakdown.**

1. Coughing and deep breathing will help to prevent pneumonia and atelectasis, not pressure ulcers.

2. Massaging the extremities is not recommended, since edema interferes with circulation and the development of thrombi is possible.

4. Lamb's wool would be helpful but not as effective as repositioning the client every 1 to 2 hours.

Client Need: Health Promotion and Maintenance

5 - 1 8

① **Arterial blood gasses (ABGs) should be drawn. Arterial blood gases are usually the first laboratory evaluation performed on clients who have been burned in order to establish pulmonary function levels.**

2. Although pain relief is an important consideration, intramuscular medications are not indicated. Intravenous medications are administered until fluid resuscitation is completed.

3. Assessment of the client's home environment is a lower-level priority in the immediate care of clients who are burned.

4. Body weight assessments are useful to determine fluid resuscitation requirements, but this does not take priority over pulmonary function levels, which may indicate airway obstruction.

Client Need: Physiological Integrity

5 - 1 9

① **The client has probably sustained a superficial partial-thickness burn. Superficial partial-thickness burns are usually very painful, have hair follicles present, are intact, and will usually heal on their own if they are not complicated by infection. A prolonged exposure to the sun's rays can cause a superficial partial-thickness burn, which is typically called a "sunburn." All clients should be advised to wear protective clothing or sunscreen to protect against such an injury.**

2. Deep partial-thickness burns are less common in the sun-exposed client who is conscious and able to retreat from the sun's rays.

3. Full-thickness burns, which involve all layers of the skin, are usually caused by hot liquids or fire.

4. Sunburn is a very real injury and should be treated as such.

Client Need: Physiological Integrity

5-20

③ Edema is the first consequence of capillary permeability in the surrounding tissue of clients who are burned. Increased capillary permeability is a direct cause of edema. As the capillary walls become more permeable, water, sodium, and other proteins such as albumin move into the interstitial spaces surrounding the affected tissue.

1. Body fluid loss occurs as a consequence of edema.

2. Pain is not the first consequence of increased capillary permeability. Pain develops as a consequence of edema pressing against the nerve endings.

4. Nausea is often associated with intense feelings of pain and is not the first consequence of increased capillary permeability.

Client Need: Physiological Integrity

5-21

① The lowest priority data to collect at this time would be body weight. Body weight is obtained initially to help calculate drug dosage and fluid requirements. There will be little change of body weight in 24 hours.

2. A partial paralytic ileus may occur in children with 20% or greater burns, most often in the first 2 to 3 days. Therefore, bowel sounds should be assessed.

3. Breath sounds should be assessed, since common pulmonary problems include infections, aspiration, inhalation, and pulmonary edema.

4. Vital signs can give data about fluid status and infection and should be assessed often.

Client Need: Physiological Integrity

5-22

② Eighteen percent of a client's body is affected if the anterior chest and abdomen are burned. The "rule of nines" is a quick assessment chart used to evaluate the extent of a victim's burn injury based on body surface. It does not address the thickness of the injury. Using the "rule of nines," an adult's head and neck are assigned 9% of the body surface, the upper right extremity 9%, the upper left extremity 9%, the anterior chest and abdomen 18%, the posterior chest and abdomen 18%, each leg 18%, and the perineal area 1%. Treatment is based on the extent and depth of injuries.

1, 3, and 4. All are incorrect calculations using the "rule of nines".

Client Need: Physiological Integrity

5 - 2 3

① The nurse can reduce sources of heat from a client's body by removing metals such as jewelry, coins, eyeglasses, and watches. Metals retain heat once exposed to fire.

2, 3, and 4. Dentures, makeup, and hairpieces should be removed to facilitate assessment of the client. However, these articles do not retain heat like metals.

Client Need: Physiological Integrity

5 - 2 4

② Clients with fungal skin infections should avoid the use of cornstarch. Fungal, or mycotic, skin infections may be due to numerous microorganisms. These infections are nourished by nonhuman nutrients. The carbohydrates in cornstarch may provide nutrition to fungal infection and should be avoided.

1 and 3. There is no evidence that detergents or cotton clothing will worsen a fungal infection.

4.   There are many effective antifungal creams available, such as nystatin (Mycostatin) and oxiconazole nitrate (Oxistat).

Client Need: Safe, Effective Care Environment

5 - 2 5

④ The client should be taught to taper the dosage of prednisone. Prednisone, like all glucocorticoids, is normally produced by the adrenal glands. Exogenous replacement of this hormone will interrupt the adrenal's normal hormone production. Abrupt cessation may cause adrenal crisis.

1.   Prednisone should be taken on schedule, not as needed (prn).

2.   There is no indication that prednisone must be taken with orange juice.

3.   The physician should prescribe any medication needed for future illness.

Client Need: Health Promotion and Maintenance

5 - 2 6

① Tetracycline (Tetracap) is an antibacterial agent that may be taken orally to treat severe cases of acne, or it may be applied topically as a cream. Acne is a common skin disorder of adolescence and is caused by the bacterium *P. acnes.*

2.   Pyrimethamine (Daraprim) is an antimalarial agent and does not have an impact on bacterial infections.

3.   Micanazole (Monistat) is an antifungal agent and does not have an impact on bacterial infections.

4.   Famciclovir (Famvir) is an antiviral agent and does not have an impact on bacterial infections.

Client Need: Health Promotion and Maintenance

5 - 2 7

② **You will teach clients with anemia that pruritus occurs as a result of increased serum and skin bile salt concentrations.**

1. The pallor seen in clients with anemia is a result of reduced amount of hemoglobin and decreased blood flow to the skin.

3. The jaundice seen in clients with anemia is a result of increased concentration of serum bilirubin that increases red blood cell hemolysis.

4. Low viscosity of blood occurs in clients with severe anemia. It does not affect the integumentary system, but it may contribute to systolic murmurs.

Client Need: Physiological Integrity

5 - 2 8

④ **The nurse should advise parents to avoid applying diphenhydramine (Benadryl) liberally over the entire body of their child. Diphenhydramine affects the inflammatory response. It is an antihistamine that is very useful in relieving local skin irritation when applied topically. It is, however, absorbed systemically, especially if open lesions are present. Dosing may be excessive if ointment is applied too liberally.**

1. Calamine lotion is a drying agent and would be an appropriate treatment.

2. Acetaminophen (Tylenol) is an analgesic antipyretic and would be an appropriate treatment.

3. Diphenhydramine is an antihistamine that can provide relief from the discomfort of chickenpox when taken po as directed.

Client Need: Physiological Integrity

5 - 2 9

① **A partial-thickness (first-degree) burn affects only the epidermis. With a first-degree burn, pain and mild edema occur. However, there are no blisters. An example of a first-degree burn would be a superficial sunburn.**

2. Deep (second-degree) burns involve the epidermis and dermis. Vesicles develop and clients experience severe pain caused by nerve injury.

3 and 4. Full-thickness burns involve the epidermis, dermis, subcutaneous tissue, and destruction of nerve endings. Coagulation necrosis is also present.

Client Need: Physiological Integrity

5 - 3 0

③ You will teach the caregiver of a child with cellulitis how to apply warm, moist compresses to the affected area. Cellulitis is a bacterial infection caused by streptococcus. Treatment includes oral antibiotics such as penicillin and erythromycin. Warm, moist soaks are applied every 4 hours to increase circulation and relieve pain.

1 and 2. Elastic pressure bandages and elbow restraints will compromise circulation and are contraindicated.

4. Movement is not encouraged. The child should rest in bed with the affected arm elevated and immobilized.

Client Need: Physiological integrity

5 - 3 1

① The nurse will inform the client that the medication podofilox (Condylox) is contraindicated during pregnancy because of its abortifacient properties (causes or induces abortion). Podofilox places the developing fetus at risk because of its potentially myelotoxic (destructive to bone marrow) and neurotoxic (destructive to nerve cells) properties. Condylomata acuminata (genital warts) are caused by a virus and cannot be cured because there is no specific antiviral therapy.

2. Podofilox is available only in a 0.5% topical solution.

3. Podofilox is contraindicated during pregnancy because of its abortifacient properties.

4. The client should not continue to treat the condition with this medication. Other treatments include cryotherapy using liquid oxygen, cryoprobe, carbon dioxide lasers, electrocautery, and surgical excision.

Client Need: Health Promotion and Maintenance

5 - 3 2

④ The nurse will teach parents not to cover areas of their child's skin affected by impetigo. Areas of the skin affected by impetigo should be left open to the air. Impetigo is the most common childhood infection of the skin. It is caused by staphylococcus aureus. The lesions can be spread simply by touching an unaffected part of the skin after scratching an infected area. The importance of thorough and frequent handwashing on the part of the child and parents cannot be overemphasized.

1. Treatment of impetigo includes washing and soaking the lesion 3 times a day in warm, soapy water.

2. Crusts should be removed after soaking.

3. Applying topical antibiotic ointment and leaving the areas open to the air are appropriate interventions.

Client Need: Physiological Integrity

5 - 3 3

④ **The nurse will teach the parents that only one application of permethrin 1% (Nix) is necessary since it kills both lice and eggs (pediculosis capitis).**

1. Applying the medication after the hair is shampooed, rinsed, and dried is the correct procedure.

2. Between 25 and 50 ml of the liquid medication is recommended to saturate the hair and scalp.

3. It is recommended that the medication remain on the hair and scalp for 10 minutes before rinsing off with water.

Client Need: Health Promotion and Maintenance

5 - 3 4

③ **Vitiligo is best described as unpigmented skin patches associated with lack of melanin formation. The condition is more common among black clients.**

1. Keloids are raised, firm, thickened, red scars that form at the site of a wound. The abnormal increase in scar size is due to unusually high amounts of collagen deposits in the tissue.

2. Pseudofolliculitis ("razor bumps") are so-called ingrown hairs that produce symptoms that include papules, pustules, and keloids.

4. Tinea versicolor is a fungal infection that produces yellow or fawn-colored patches on the skin.

Client Need: Physiological Integrity

5 - 3 5

② **The least likely plan of care would include the use of hydrotherapy to stimulate circulation. Clients with autografts should not be immersed or showered until the graft has taken and the wound is closed.**

1. The supine position (lying on the back with face upward) will allow the graft to remain in place.

3. Elbow restraints are required to keep the child's hands away from the affected area.

4. Aspiration of fluid accumulation under the graft will help the graft to remain flat and in full contact with the tissue bed below.

Client Need: Physiological Integrity

5 - 3 6

① Nursing assessment will reveal restlessness in the early stages of shock. Other assessment findings include an increase in blood pressure, deeper respirations, and a slight decrease in urinary output. These findings, however, are within normal limits. Shock is circulatory failure resulting in impaired tissue perfusion that leads to cellular dysfunction.

2. There will be a marked increase in blood pressure, not a decrease.

3. The respirations will not be shallow but progressively deeper.

4. The client's urinary output will decrease slightly, but not to the extent of oliguria.

Client Need: Physiological Integrity

5 - 3 7

③ The most appropriate nursing diagnosis for a neonate under a radiant warmer receiving phototherapy is fluid volume deficit, potential for.

1. There should be no problems with the neonate's skin integrity if the neonate is turned every 2 hours.

2. There is no association between gas exchange and the use of a radiant warmer.

4. There is no association between infection and the use of a radiant warmer.

Client Need: Physiological Integrity

5 - 3 8

③ The use of sterile technique reduces the risk of introducing additional microorganisms into the wound.

1 and 2. Warm, moist packs are not bactericidal. An anti-infective might be prescribed to kill or inhibit the growth of pathogenic bacteria.

4. To minimize the risk of spreading infection to others, the nurse would dispose of all contaminated materials properly.

Client Need: Safe, Effective Care Environment

5-39

① **Mongolian spotting (blue-gray pigmentation) over the buttocks and sacrum is not associated with congenital anomalies. The spotting occurs most often in dark-skinned clients and disappears on its own during early childhood.**

2. Short stature, low posterior hairline, webbing of neck, broad chest, and widely spaced nipples are physical characteristics of an infant born with Turner's syndrome (45, XO).

3. A simian crease across the palms of both hands is associated with trisomy 21 (Down syndrome).

4. Low ears are associated with a number of congenital anomalies such as Down syndrome (trisomy 21) and Edward's syndrome (trisomy 18).

Client Need: Physiological Integrity

5-40

② **A dark-skinned client's skin will appear dusky red or violet with erythema (a form of macula). A light-skinned client's skin will appear diffusely red.**

1. Paleness is loss of skin color. For example, clients with anemia may experience paleness.

3. Dark-skinned clients experiencing cyanosis will appear black, while light-skinned clients experiencing cyanosis appear blue or dark purple.

4. A temporary yellow discoloration of the skin of light-skinned clients may indicate jaundice. A dark-skinned client with jaundice would manifest the condition by a yellow appearance in the sclera of the eyes, mucous membranes, and body fluids.

Client Need: Physiological Integrity

5-41

③ **A person whose clothes are on fire should be placed flat on the ground or floor and rolled in a blanket. This will prevent the fire, hot air, and smoke from rising up toward the face and being inhaled.**

1. Throwing water on the client, especially near the face, can be dangerous.

2. Throwing a blanket over the head of the client can trap fumes and smoke and facilitate smoke inhalation.

4. Calling the Fire Department takes time. When a client's clothes are on fire, time is of the essence.

5. The personnel responding at the 911 number would advise you to lay the child flat and roll him in a blanket.

Client Need: Safe, Effective Care Environment

5 - 4 2

① ② ③ and ⑤ Signs of heat and smoke inhalation injury include singed nasal hairs, eyebrows, and eyelashes; stridor, shortness of breath, soot around the mouth and nose, sore throat, hoarseness, carbon in the sputum, and excessive secretion of mucus.

4. Burns around the face and neck are not a sign of heat or smoke inhalation. However, people who have burns around the head and neck should be assessed for signs of heat and smoke inhalation.

Client Need: Safe, Effective Care Environment

Practice Test 6

Musculoskeletal System

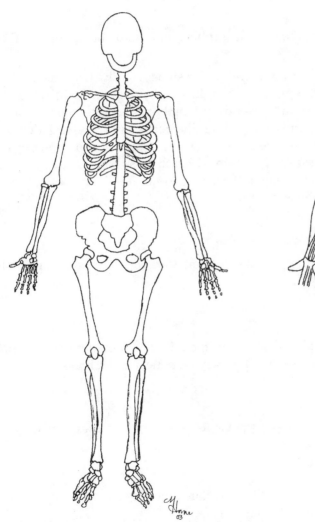

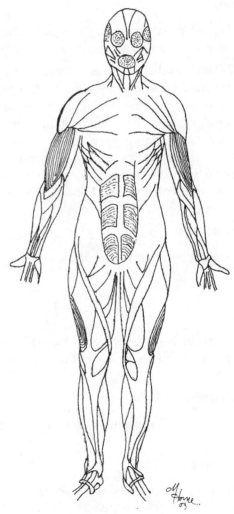

The Skeletal System

The Muscular System

OVERVIEW

The musculoskeletal system is comprised of bones, muscles, and joints. The musculoskeletal system gives shape and form to the body. It protects vital organs and makes movement possible. The bones store calcium, as well as other minerals, and offer sites for hematopoiesis (the production and development of blood cells).

SKELETAL SYSTEM/BONES

There are 206 bones in the human skeleton. These bones are composed of inorganic salts, such as calcium and phosphate, which are embedded in a framework of collagen fibers. Bones are classified by shape, such as long, short, flat, or irregular.

Long Bones

Long bones are located in the thigh (femur), the lower leg (tibia and fibula), the upper arm (humerus), and the lower arm (radius and ulna).

Long bones, such as the femur, are identified by anatomical divisions: The shaft, known as the diaphysis; the two ends of the bone, known as the epiphysis; and the epiphyseal plate, which is an area of cartilage tissue associated with bone growth. All but the ends of long bones are overlaid with a strong, fibrous, vascular membrane known as the periosteum. Under the periosteum is a hard, dense, compact layer that covers the shaft of long bones. Within the compact layer is a system containing blood vessels that bring oxygen and nutrients to the bones. The canals in which these substances travel are known as haversian canals and haversian systems. In the center of the long bones lies the medullary cavity containing the soft organic material known as bone marrow.

Short Bones

Short bones have small, irregular shapes. Examples of short bones are those found in the wrists and ankles.

Flat Bones

Flat bones surround soft body parts. Examples of flat bones include: The shoulder bone (scapula), the ribs, and the pelvic bones. Bones of the skull, such as the parietal bone, are flat bones.

Sesamoid Bones

Sesamoid bones are oval nodules found near joints. The kneecap (patella) is a sesamoid bone.

Irregular Bones

Irregular bones have a variety of shapes and generally articulate (join together as a joint) with several other bones. Irregular bones include: The vertebrae and facial bones.

DISEASES/DISORDERS OF THE SKELETAL SYSTEM INCLUDE

Ewing's Tumor

Ewing's tumor is a myeloma (a tumor originating in cells of the hematopoietic portion of the bone marrow).

Fractures

A fracture is a broken bone. There are four types of fractures characterized according to the cause of the break, namely: Pathological, direct violence, indirect violence, and muscular contraction.

Paget's Disease

Another name for Paget's disease is osteitis deformans. This is a chronic bone inflammation that affects the elderly. The disorder is associated with thickening and hypertrophy of long bones as well as deformity of the flat bones.

Osteogenic Sarcoma

A sarcoma is a cancer arising from connective tissue such as bone or muscle. An osteogenic sarcoma is made up of osseous tissue (bone and cartilage).

Osteomyelitis

Osteomyelitis is an inflammation of the bone and bone marrow caused by bacterial infection.

Osteomalacia

Osteomalacia is characterized by a softening of the bone due to an inadequate amount of calcium in the bone. When seen during infancy and early childhood, this condition is known as rickets.

Kyphosis

This condition is commonly called round back or humpback. It is associated with an abnormal exaggeration of the normal posterior curve of the spine.

Scoliosis

This is a lateral curvature of the spine. In most cases, two curves are seen; the original abnormal curve, and a second curve that develops as a compensatory curve to "balance" the affected person in the opposite direction.

Osteoporosis

This condition is associated with a decrease in bone mass (density) and is commonly seen in post-menopausal women with estrogen deficiency. Bones become thin, weak, and subject to fracture. Osteoporosis can also occur as a consequence of atrophy or disuse of a limb, such as casting.

Talipes

Talipes, also known as clubfoot, is a congenital deformity involving the bones of the feet.

JOINTS

A joint is an articulating juncture between two bones. Joints permit motion and provide stability. Joints are classified according to movement.

1. Fibrous joints (synarthroses) allow for very little movement. They provide stability where a tight union is necessary. Examples of fibrous joints are those that join the cranial bones.
2. Cartilaginous joints (amphiarthroses) allow for limited motion. Examples of cartilaginous joints include the vertebrae.

3. Synovial joints (diarthroses) allow for the greatest degree of motion. Examples of synovial joints include the knee.

DISEASES/DISORDERS OF THE JOINTS INCLUDE

Arthritis

Arthritis is the inflammation of joints. Common forms of this condition are:

- Ankylosing spondylitis (arthritis mainly of the spine)
- Gouty arthritis (inflammation of the joint due to uric acid buildup)
- Osteoarthritis (a degenerative joint disorder due to loss of articular cartilage and hypertrophy of bone)
- Rheumatoid arthritis (a painful inflammation of the joints that produces crippling deformities)

Carpal Tunnel Syndrome (CTS)

This condition occurs when the medial nerve is compressed between bones, tendons, and the carpal ligament.

Dislocation

A dislocation is the temporary disconnection of a bone from a joint.

Ganglion

A ganglion is a cystic mass (tumor) that has developed on a tendon. The wrist is a common location for a ganglion.

Herniated Disk

This condition is characterized by an abnormal protrusion (out-pouching) of a cartilaginous vertebral pad into the neural canal or spinal nerves. A herniated disk is commonly referred to as a slipped disk.

Sprain

A sprain typically occurs as a result of trauma to a joint. A sprain is associated with pain, swelling, and injury to ligaments.

Systemic Lupus Erythematosus (SLE)

SLE is a chronic inflammatory disease affecting the joints, skin, kidneys, heart, lungs, and nervous system. It is thought to be an autoimmune disorder.

MUSCLES

Muscles move the bones of the body, resist movement, help maintain body alignment, and participate in the movement of fluids such as blood, lymph, and urine. The contracting and relaxing of muscles produces heat, which aids in the equilibrium of body temperature.

There are three types of muscles:

1. Striated muscles, also known as skeletal or voluntary muscles. Striated muscles move the head, trunk, and limbs. They produce facial expression and allow us to write, talk, chew, swallow, and breathe. These muscles can be controlled by conscious effort.

2. Smooth muscles, also called involuntary muscles. They are characteristically found in layers within the walls of organs, such as those in the gastrointestinal system. These muscles are also located in blood vessels and secretory ducts.

3. Cardiac muscle is found only in the heart. Cardiac muscle provides the force necessary to circulate blood through the heart and blood vessels. Cardiac muscle is involuntary.

DISEASES/DISORDERS OF THE MUSCLES INCLUDE

Muscular Dystrophy

Muscular dystrophy is a group of inherited diseases associated with chronic and progressive weakness and degeneration of muscle fibers. The most common form of muscular dystrophy is known as Duchenne's dystrophy. In this disease, fat replaces functional muscle cells that have atrophied (wasted).

Polymyositis

Polymyositis is a rare inflammatory disease of skeletal muscle associated with symmetric weakness of proximal muscles of the limbs, neck, and pharynx.

Practice Test 6

Questions

6 - 1

A child is in a hip spica cast. Discharge instruction should include teaching the parents to move the child from room to room and to change diversions frequently. This is most important for a child in which age group?

1. toddlers
2. preschoolers
3. school-age children
4. adolescents

6 - 2

Your client has been scheduled for an arthroscopy following an injury to the left knee. After the arthroscopy, the joint will be wrapped with a compress dressing and the affected leg will be:

1. placed in a flexed position by placing a pillow under the knee.
2. kept in an extended position and elevated.
3. placed in a slightly flexed position and elevated.
4. placed flat on the bed with a trochanter roll on either side of the knee.

6 - 3

Your client is scheduled for an electromyography today. What do you need to do to prepare your client for this procedure?

1. Maintain nothing by mouth for 6 hours prior to the procedure.
2. Omit any scheduled diazepam for 24 hours prior to the procedure.
3. Inform the client that he will not feel any pain during the procedure.
4. Inform the client that he will have to lie still during the procedure.

6 - 4

An infant is being treated for congenital hip dysplasia with a Pavlik harness. Teaching about care of the infant has been effective if the caregiver:

1. maintains the infant's leg position with a smaller pillow or foam wedge during diaper changes.
2. carefully inspects and cleans the inguinal area during diaper changes.
3. places an undershirt over the harness to minimize soiling.
4. releases the straps 4 times a day, one at a time, and inspects the skin underneath.

6 - 5

An infant is being treated for bilateral club-foot with long leg casts. Treatment was begun at 2 weeks of age and will continue for 3 months. Education about home care should include:

1. keeping the child's hands diverted so that objects won't be inserted under the cast.
2. outlining areas of blood on the cast and noting the time.
3. handling the casts with fingertips, not palms of hands.
4. checking circulation in the toes frequently, at least with each diaper change.

6 - 6

An 84-year-old client asks the nurse, "Why am I 5′ 4″ now, but was 5′ 7″ when I graduated from high school?" The nurse's best response would be to say:

1. "I will be glad to measure your height now and see how tall you really are."
2. "Who ever measured your height last must have made a mistake since you know you were 5′ 7″ tall in high school."
3. "It's possible you weren't standing as straight as you could have when your height was measured."
4. "The disks in your backbone have become thinner as you have gotten older."

6 - 7

An athlete fell and broke the radius in the right arm. Following the application of a cast, the athlete says to the nurse, "I'm afraid I'm going to lose muscle strength in my arm because I can't exercise it." Your best response would be:

1. "It must be difficult for an athlete to be unable to maintain an exercise program because of injuries."
2. "You can minimize the effects of immobility by performing isometric exercises of the immobilized muscles."
3. "Would you like for me to speak with the physician about participating in a physical therapy program?"
4. "There will be some atrophy of the muscle. However, you should be able to regain full muscle strength once the cast is removed."

6 - 8

A client is suspected of metastatic bone disease. To aid in the confirmation of this condition, you anticipate which of the following?

1. a venogram
2. a discography
3. an electromyography
4. a bone scan

6 - 9

A fracture of your client's acetabulum is suspected. Which of the following diagnostic tools is most likely to be used to identify the specific location and extent of the suspected injury?

1. an angiography
2. a magnetic resonance imaging
3. a computed tomography
4. an arthroscopy

6 - 1 0

During the assessment of a 76-year-old client, you notice an increased roundness of the thoracic spinal curve. You will document this observation as:

1. scoliosis.
2. osteoporosis.
3. kyphosis.
4. lordosis.

6 - 1 1

Your client experienced a fractured ulna. You observe swelling at the site of injury and the client is complaining of pain. The client is in which stage of bone healing?

1. inflammatory
2. cellular proliferation
3. callus formation
4. ossification

6 - 1 2

A client was admitted to your unit with carpal tunnel syndrome. What will you expect your assessment to reveal?

1. weakened grasp
2. shoulder pain in the deltoid area
3. flexion of the fourth and fifth fingers
4. numbness of the thumb and first and second fingers

6 - 1 3

The nurse in the newborn nursery has completed an initial physical assessment. Observations reveal asymmetry of gluteal folds with a positive Ortolani's sign. The most likely implication of this finding would be:

1. congenital hip dysplasia.
2. normal examination of the hip.
3. cerebral palsy.
4. rickets.

6 - 1 4

Your client, a 76-year-old, has developed contractures. In order to prevent the contractures from becoming worse, you will:

1. place the client in a warm whirlpool bath daily.
2. perform range-of-motion exercises qid.
3. turn the client from side to side every 2 hours.
4. support contracted joints on pillows at all times.

6 - 1 5

A client has sustained a closed fracture of the humerus. After application of the cast, the nurse teaches the client about cast care. Which of the following measures would be contraindicated?

1. Avoiding the use of powder around the cast edges.
2. Placing a plastic bag over the cast while bathing.
3. Calling the physician if drainage or odors are observed around the cast.
4. Using a coat hanger to relieve itching under the cast.

6-16

A client was admitted to the nursing unit with a soft-tissue injury following a snake-bite on the right index finger. The client's fingers are cold and pale on the affected hand. What should the nurse do first?

1. Elevate the extremity.
2. Administer pain medication.
3. Call the physician.
4. Provide passive range-of-motion exercises to the client's fingers.

6-17

A 12-year-old in a spica cast complains of discomfort after eating. Which of the following measures should the nurse take to prevent this problem?

1. Give the client smaller but more frequent meals.
2. Continue to give the client three meals a day, but give smaller portions.
3. Restrict the fluid intake.
4. Encourage the client to eat slowly and to alternate liquids with solids.

6-18

Your client had a bilateral total knee replacement to treat degenerative joint disease. During the first 24 to 72 hours after surgery, you will assess the client for which of the following?

1. bowel impaction and abdominal pain
2. confusion, dyspnea, and petechiae
3. redness and edema at the incision site
4. pedal pulses

6-19

What type of gait would be utilized by a client with a broken leg who is walking up stairs with the assistance of crutches?

Fill in the blank

6-20

A client is experiencing weakness in the left leg and is learning to use a walker. Which observation made by the nurse would indicate that the client understands the instructions given?

1. The client advances the walker and steps forward, alternating the feet with each advancement.
2. The client advances both feet, moves the walker forward, then moves both feet again.
3. The client advances the walker and steps forward with the left foot at the same time.
4. The client advances the right foot and then moves the walker forward, dragging the left foot.

6-21

Which statement is correct concerning the best method of performing passive range-of-motion exercises?

1. A joint should never be forced beyond its capacity.
2. Range-of-motion exercises will cause some discomfort if they are to be beneficial.
3. Support should be maintained above the joint being exercised.
4. Range-of-motion movements should be repeated a minimum of 10 times.

6 - 2 2

A client is to have a modified radical mastectomy. While the nurse is giving instructions on arm exercises prior to surgery, the client asks, "Why will I have to exercise my arm after surgery, when it will hurt?" Which of the following responses would be best for the nurse to make?

1. "These exercises prevent stiffness of the shoulder and will help you regain use of your arm."
2. "Exercising the arm will actually decrease the amount of postoperative pain."
3. "Exercises will eliminate the postoperative swelling that occurs at the incision."
4. "You are practicing now so that it won't be so uncomfortable for you later."

6 - 2 3

Which of the following assessment observations indicates scoliosis?

1. head in alignment with gluteal fold
2. symmetrical thoracic area
3. equal leg length
4. asymmetry in the flank area

6 - 2 4

An adult client has experienced a bone marrow aspiration. Immediately following this procedure, the nurse will:

1. apply firm pressure to the site of the aspiration for at least 5 minutes.
2. place a plain adhesive bandage over the aspiration site.
3. apply a topical antibiotic on the aspiration site and leave open.
4. apply an ice pack to the aspiration site for at least 10 minutes.

6 - 2 5

An 11-month-old infant has been placed in Bryant's traction for treatment of a fractured femur. The plan of care will include:

1. turning the child from side to side at least every 2 hours.
2. elevating the head of bed 15 to 30 degrees when meals are served.
3. keeping pin insertion sites clean and free from exudate.
4. keeping toys within easy reach of the child.

6 - 2 6

Your client is in traction to treat a fractured femur. The physician has prescribed a 2-view X ray of the femur. Which of the following is contraindicated as a nursing action?

1. Release the weight of the traction to move the client to the radiology department.
2. Maintain the correct body alignment while positioning for the X ray.
3. Administer pain medication 30 minutes following the procedure.
4. Explain the procedure to the client.

6 - 2 7

When assisting clients with walkers, it would be best for the nurse to walk:

1. directly behind the client.
2. in front of the client, guiding the walker.
3. closely behind and slightly to the side of the client.
4. beside the client.

6 - 2 8

Following a simple mandibular fracture, your client is scheduled for an intermaxillary fixation. Immediately after surgery, you will place the client in which position?

1. a side-lying position with the head slightly elevated
2. an upright position with the neck flexed
3. a horizontal recumbent position
4. a prone position

6 - 2 9

Which of the following self-care behaviors should the nurse include when teaching a client about a continuous passive motion machine?

1. how to operate the on/off switch
2. how to increase/decrease flexion and extension movements
3. how to adjust speed controls
4. how to adjust internal and external rotation movements

6 - 3 0

A child 7 years old has juvenile rheumatoid arthritis. During a period of exacerbation, the plan of care will include:

1. clustering of care to allow uninterrupted periods of rest.
2. short-term use of narcotics administered by client-controlled analgesia.
3. a high-protein, high-vitamin diet.
4. cool packs to the inflamed joints bid and hs.

6 - 3 1

A client fractured his left femur during a soccer game. During your initial assessment in the emergency department, the client says, "My leg feels numb." The nurse understands that the probable cause of the numbness is:

1. blood loss.
2. nerve damage.
3. paralysis.
4. muscle spasms.

6 - 3 2

Your client has had a total hip replacement and you are changing the client's position. Which action should you take to prevent hip dislocation?

1. Cross the client's legs at the knees.
2. Place a pillow along the client's back.
3. Use a drawsheet to facilitate turning the client.
4. Support the client's legs with an abductor pillow between the legs.

6 - 3 3

Which of the following medications might contribute to the further development of osteoporosis?

1. methylprednisolone 8 mg po, qid
2. calcium carbonate 500 mg po, qid
3. ranitidine 150 mg po, bid
4. ramipril 10 mg po, qd

6 - 3 4

A 67-year-old client comes to the local clinic with acute gouty arthritis. An immediate nursing intervention would be to:

1. relieve pain.
2. administer anti-inflammatory agents.
3. relieve pressure on the tender joints.
4. apply cold packs to reduce inflammation.

6 - 3 5

A client complains of feeling faint following a traumatic fracture. The nurse's assessment reveals dyspnea, restlessness, tachycardia, progressive cyanosis, and mental confusion. Which of the following complications will the nurse suspect?

1. nerve damage
2. fat embolism
3. hypostatic pneumonia
4. progressing paralysis

6 - 3 6

A client is experiencing left-sided weakness. You are to get the client into a wheelchair. The intravenous pole and nasogastric suction equipment are on the left side of the bed. Where should you position the wheelchair prior to transfer?

1. On the left side of the bed with the wheelchair facing the head of the bed.
2. On the right side of the bed with the wheelchair facing the head of the bed.
3. On the left side of the bed with the wheelchair facing the foot of the bed.
4. On the right side of the bed with the wheelchair facing the foot of the bed.

6 - 3 7

A 9-year-old has a fractured left femur and a long leg cast has been applied. Which of the following behaviors by the client indicates acceptance of the cast?

1. The client whittles at the cast with a table knife.
2. The client asks for help to replace the waterproof petal around the edges of the cast.
3. The client stuffs paper inside the cast.
4. The client refuses to go to the playroom.

6 - 3 8

Which of the following crutch gaits would be appropriate for clients who have paralysis of the legs and hips?

Fill in the blank

6 - 3 9

An 8-year-old client fractured the right femur and is in 90-90 traction. Three of the following options describe purposes of traction. Which of the following is not a purpose of traction?

1. to reduce dislocation
2. to immobilize the leg
3. to lessen muscle spasm
4. to provide comfort

6 - 4 0

What is the appropriate site for an intramuscular injection for an infant 6 months of age?

Fill in the blank

6 - 4 1

In addition to local joint symptoms, which of the following manifestations are common in clients who have rheumatoid arthritis?

1. pedal edema
2. generalized erythema
3. fever and complaints of fatigue
4. bradycardia and slow respirations

6 - 4 2

A client who has sustained a musculoskeletal injury due to dislocation will require immediate intervention. The need for immediate intervention is based on the possible development of:

1. shock.
2. inadequate blood supply.
3. fat emboli.
4. contractures.

6 - 4 3

A client had the right leg amputated above the knee as the result of an automobile accident. Immediately following the surgery, the nurse will know to place the client's affected limb in a position of:

1. extension.
2. flexion.
3. internal rotation.
4. external rotation.

6 - 4 4

A 45-year-old is suspected of having myasthenia gravis. To confirm this tentative diagnosis, the nurse will anticipate a prescription for which of the following diagnostic tests?

1. tensilon test
2. cold stimulation test
3. magnetic resonance imaging
4. electroencephalography

6 - 4 5

Calcium gives firmness and rigidity to bones and teeth and is also necessary for proper functioning of muscles, including the heart muscle. Good dietary sources of calcium include:

Select all that apply by placing a ✔ in the square:

☐ 1. milk.
☐ 2. cottage-cheese.
☐ 3. canned salmon.
☐ 4. sardines.
☐ 5. turnip greens.

6 - 4 6

After menopause, the leading cause of osteoporosis among aging women is a deficiency in:

Fill in the blank

6 - 4 7

Your client requires a hip spica cast. To prevent constipation due to inactivity and a change in toileting routines, you will encourage foods that are high in fiber, such as:

Select all that apply by placing a ✔ in the square:

❑ 1. bran and whole grains.

❑ 2. dairy products, such as milk and yogurt.

❑ 3. legumes, such as dried peas and beans.

❑ 4. vegetables, such as cabbage and carrots.

❑ 5. meat and meat substitutes.

6 - 4 8

Your client sustained extensive trauma to his right leg as a result of an automobile accident. The client has returned to his room following the amputation of the affected leg. To prevent edema, you will elevate the stump for the first:

1. 8 to 12 hours.

2. 12 to 24 hours.

3. 24 to 48 hours.

4. 48 to 72 hours.

Practice Test 6

Answers, Rationales, and Explanations

---

6 - 1

① Toddlers are involved in environmental exploration, especially through use of large muscles. Confinement can hinder autonomy and speech development. Toddlers also have a short attention span.

2, 3, and 4. Preschoolers, school-age children, and adolescents have a longer attention span and greater capacity for self-direction.

Client Need: Psychosocial Integrity

---

6 - 2

② Immediately following an arthroscopy of the knee, the nurse will elevate the leg with the knee in an extended position. This will reduce swelling and pain. An arthroscopy is an endoscopic procedure that allows for direct visualization of joints.

1 and 3. The affected joint should be extended, not flexed, following an arthroscopy. Extension will prevent edema and take pressure off the joint.

4. The leg should be elevated to help prevent edema.

Client Need: Health Promotion and Maintenance

---

6 - 3

② Persons scheduled for electromyography (EMG) should omit diazepam (Valium), since it causes loss of muscle tone. Electromyography aids in the diagnosis of muscular dystrophy, amyotrophic lateral sclerosis, and myasthenia gravis by evaluating electrical potential associated with skeletal muscle contraction. Clients may have to move their muscles voluntarily during the procedure, and they may experience some discomfort from needle insertion.

1. There is no special client preparation required prior to an electromyography.

3. The client should be told that a sensation similar to receiving an intramuscular injection will be experienced and that the muscle may ache for a short period of time afterward.

4. Because clients may need to move muscles voluntarily, it is not necessary that they lie still during the procedure.

Client Need: Psychosocial Integrity

6 - 4

② **The nurse will know that teaching has been effective if the caregiver carefully inspects and cleans the inguinal area during a diaper change. The skin surfaces of the inguinal area are especially prone to breakdown because of thigh flexion.**

1. The caregiver should be taught that the harness will maintain positioning during diaper changes.

3. To help prevent skin irritation, the infant's undershirt should be placed under the harness.

4. The harness should be removed only for bathing or not at all, according to the prescription.

Client Need: Health Promotion and Maintenance

6 - 5

④ **An infant being treated for bilateral clubfoot with long leg casts should have circulation checks of the toes with each diaper change. Even though casts are changed often (every few days for 1 to 2 weeks, then at 1-to-2-week intervals), the child will be growing rapidly and could develop circulatory impairment.**

1. An infant is not likely to be capable of stuffing objects under the cast.

2. Casting does not require surgery. Therefore, bleeding is not a concern.

3. Hardening casts should be handled with the palms of hands, not the fingertips. Fingertips tend to press into the cast and create pressure areas that could compromise skin integrity.

Client Need: Physiological Integrity

6 - 6

④ **The client should be taught that thinning of the intervertebral disks occurs with age. Other gerontologic changes may include weakened muscles, osteoporotic bones, enlarged joints, and decreased range of motion. The nurse will also teach the client how to minimize the effects of aging.**

1. Offering to measure the client's height suggests some error has been made. It is likely that no error was made and that the client has lost 3 inches of height due to intervertebral thinning.

2. No error was made. The client has lost 3 inches of height due to thinning of the intervertebral disks.

3. The nurse should not attempt to pacify the client by suggesting that the client was not standing erect at the time of the last height measurement. The client should be told about various changes that occur during the aging process and how to minimize their effects.

Client Need: Health Promotion and Maintenance

6 - 7

② Clients who are concerned about loss of muscle strength due to casting should be taught that they can minimize the loss by performing isometric exercises. Isometric exercises may be defined as contraction of a muscle that is not accompanied by motion of the joints that would ordinarily be moved by that contraction.

1. Telling the client that it must be difficult to be unable to exercise because of an injury leaves the client with the impression there is nothing that can be done to minimize muscle loss until the cast is removed. The client could perform isometric exercises on the affected arm.

3. The physical therapy department may be contacted. However, the nurse should encourage the client by teaching the client about the therapeutic benefits of isometric exercises.

4. The client needs to know that isometric exercises can be performed while the affected arm is in a cast.

Client Need: Physiological Integrity

6 - 8

4 A bone scan (bone scintigraphy) would be anticipated to aid in the confirmation of suspected metastatic bone disease. Radioactive isotopes search out bone. The degree of isotope uptake by the bone indicates the presence of conditions such as osteosarcoma, metastatic bone disease, and osteomyelitis.

1. Venograms are used to study the venous system and help to identify conditions such as venous thrombosis. A venogram would not detect bony metastasis.

2. Discography is a test to study intervertebral discs, requiring a contrast medium that is injected into the discs. A discography would not detect bony metastasis.

3. Electromyography is a diagnostic tool that provides information about the electrical condition of the muscles and the nerves leading to muscles. An electromyography would not detect bony metastasis.

Client Need: Physiological Integrity

6 - 9

---

③ **The nurse will anticipate a prescription for a computed tomography (CT) scan. The CT scan is very useful in identifying soft-tissue injuries to ligaments and tendons. Also, the presence of tumors can be identified and the extent and location of fractures in areas that are hard to evaluate, such as the acetabulum (the rounded cavity that holds the head of the femur).**

1. An angiography would not be anticipated, since it is a diagnostic tool used to study the vascular system. X rays are taken of suspected areas following the administration of a radiopaque contrast agent.

2. Magnetic resonance imaging (MRI) would not be anticipated, since it is not likely to identify more difficult areas of suspected injuries such as the acetabulum. Also, clients with pacemakers, metal implants, and braces are unable to use MRI because of its use of magnetic fields.

4. Arthroscopy would not be anticipated, since it requires an invasive operative procedure. It allows for direct visualization of a joint.

Client Need: Physiological Integrity

6 - 1 0

---

③ **You will document your observation as kyphosis (an increased roundness or convexity of the thoracic spinal curve). Kyphosis is often noted in the elderly who are experiencing osteoporosis (loss of bone mass).**

1. Scoliosis (a lateral curving of the thoracic spine) may be congenital, idiopathic (no known cause), or the consequence of injury or disease.

2. Osteoporosis (loss of bone mass) is associated with the aging process. Osteoporosis may contribute to kyphosis.

4. Lordosis (exaggeration of the concave portion of the thoracic spine—swayback) is normal for the toddler and is also seen in pregnant women, whose center of gravity has changed during pregnancy. Lordosis is considered abnormal when noted in other populations, such as adolescents.

Client Need: Health Promotion and Maintenance

6 - 1 1

① The client is experiencing the inflammatory stage of the bone healing process. During this stage (stage 1), there is bleeding into the injured tissue and the formation of a hematoma, white blood cells begin debridement of dead cells, and the client experiences pain.

2. The cellular proliferation stage occurs within the first 5 days. Fibrin strands begin to form and the interrupted blood supply is recreated. Cartilage and fibrous connective tissue develop.

3. The callus formation stage occurs within the continued growth of the cartilage from each bone fragment. The gap created by the fracture begins to bridge the distance. After approximately 3 to 4 weeks, the fractured bone fragments will be united.

4. The ossification stage is identified by the formation of bone substance (ossification) and the continued unification of the fracture. This process may take as long as 3 to 4 months. The final remodeling (stage V) of the affected bone may take additional months to years depending on the injury, the bone, and the healing process generally.

Client Need: Physiological Integrity

6 - 1 2

④ You would expect your assessment to reveal numbness of the thumb and first and second fingers. Carpal tunnel syndrome is a neuropathy caused by entrapment of the median nerve at the wrist. Compression occurs due to a thickened flexor tendon sheath, skeletal encroachment, or soft-tissue mass on the median nerve at the wrist. Symptoms include pain, numbness, paresthesia, and possibly weakness along the median nerve (thumb and first and second fingers).

1. A weakened grasp is associated with epicondylitis (tennis elbow).

2. Pain in the shoulder is not associated with carpal tunnel syndrome. Carpal tunnel syndrome affects the wrist.

3. Flexion of the little and ring fingers is seen with Dupuytren's contracture (the ring and little fingers bend into the palm so they cannot be extended).

Client Need: Physiological Integrity

6 - 1 3

① Asymmetry of the hip with a positive Ortolani's maneuver is indicative of congenital hip dysplasia. Ortolani's maneuver refers to an audible click when reducing a dislocated hip.

2. Asymmetry of the gluteal folds with a positive Ortolani's maneuver is not a normal finding. Ortolani's maneuver indicates an inability of the hip to fully abduct. The hip is unstable and the femur head actually slides out of the socket.

3. Cerebral palsy may be ruled out by assessing for tight abductor muscles at 4 to 6 weeks old.

4. Deficiency of vitamin D leads to poor bone formation or rickets, not congenital hip dysplasia.

Client Need: Physiological Integrity

6 - 1 4

② **You will perform range-of-motion exercises. Exercise is the only preventive measure for contractions. Exercise keeps tendons, ligaments, and muscles flexible. For clients with existing contracture, the exercising is done to the limit of their contractures.**

1. Range-of-motion may be easier to accomplish after relaxation of the joint in a warm bath, but daily bathing is contraindicated because of the fragile, dry skin of geriatric clients.

3. Turning clients from side to side will not exercise the client's joints.

4. Supporting contracted joints on pillows will provide comfort, but it will worsen the contractures.

Client Need: Physiological Integrity

6 - 1 5

④ **Placing sharp objects, such as coat hangers, down a cast can cause skin irritation or breakdown and create a site for infection, and is contraindicated.**

1. Clients should avoid the use of powder around the cast because it can predispose the skin to irritation, breakdown, and infection.

2. Plastic bags should be used during bathing to protect the cast from moisture.

3. The physician should be notified of any signs of infection, such as odor or drainage, under the cast.

Client Need: Health Promotion and Maintenance

6 - 1 6

③ **The physician must be notified immediately. Cold, pale fingers are classical symptoms of compartment syndrome, which is a progressive degeneration of muscles and nerves resulting from severe interruption of blood flow.**

1. Elevation of the extremity is not the primary intervention.

2. Pain relief is important but not the first priority.

4. Range-of-motion exercises are contraindicated for this condition since they will cause the venom to enter the bloodstream more rapidly.

Client Need: Physiological Integrity

6 - 1 7

(1) Small, frequent feedings will prevent discomfort by limiting the amount of food in the stomach at any given time. The nurse should instruct the client about smaller but frequent portions to ensure understanding and cooperation. The nurse will also recommend that the client in a spica cast be placed in a prone position while eating to prevent aspiration.

2. A 12-year-old would resent smaller portions of food if given only three meals a day. Also, the client needs the proper nourishment.

3. Fluids should not be restricted because constipation is a potential problem for clients in a spica cast.

4. Alternating liquids with solids is not realistic. Persons in a spica cast should be served small bite-size pieces of food. Fluids should be taken through a straw.

Client Need: Physiological Integrity

6 - 1 8

(2) Clients who have bilateral total knee replacements are at high risk for fat embolus during the first 24 to 72 hours postoperatively. Symptoms of fat emboli include confusion, dyspnea, anxiety, and petechiae.

1. Bowel impaction is common with decreased activity, but assessment for bowel impaction would not take priority at this time.

3. Infection is not usually present during the first three postoperative days.

4. Assessment for pedal pulses is important but does not take priority over the assessment for a fat embolus. A fat embolus is life threatening.

Client Need: Health Promotion and Maintenance

6 - 1 9

Fill in the blank correct answer:

Modified Three-Point

To walk up stairs with crutches, clients with a broken leg would utilize a modified three-point gait. Clients would start at the bottom of the stairs, transferring their body weight to the crutches. The unaffected leg will be advanced between the crutches to the stairs, the weight will be shifted from the crutches to the unaffected leg, and then the client will align both crutches on the stairs. Three points are on the stairs at all times. With a two-point gait, each crutch is moved at the same time as the opposing leg. This requires partial weight-bearing on each foot, which would not be possible for a client with a broken leg. A four-point gait requires weight bearing on both legs. With this gait, each leg is moved alternately with each crutch. The swing-through gait is utilized primarily by paraplegics. The paralyzed legs are supported by braces, and with a client's weight being supported on the braced legs, the client places the crutches one stride in front and then swings to or through the crutches while the crutches support the body's weight.

Client Need: Safe, Effective Care Environment

6-20

③ The walker and the weaker left leg are moved first. The body weight should be borne by the stronger right leg. The stronger leg is moved into the walker while weight is borne by the arms on the walker and the weak leg.

1, 2, and 4. The walker and the weak left leg should be moved first. Body weight should be borne by the stronger leg. The weaker left leg should not be left dragging due to the probability of further injury.

Client Need: Safe, Effective Care Environment

6-21

① A joint should never be forced beyond its capacity. The nurse should not move the joint past the position where the client might experience discomfort.

2. Exercise should be stopped before the pain occurs. "No pain, no gain" does not apply to range-of-motion exercises.

3. The nurse should support the joint being exercised by holding areas proximal and distal to the joint.

4. Each movement should be repeated only 5 times.

Client Need: Health Promotion and Maintenance

6-22

① Rehabilitation is necessary after a modified radical mastectomy because underlying tissues are removed. The aim of rehabilitation is to restore use of the affected arm as soon as possible to prevent contractures and muscle shortening, maintain muscle tone, and improve circulation in the arm.

2. Exercising the arm after a modified radical mastectomy will not decrease postoperative pain. Pain will decrease as the incision site heals.

3. Exercise will not eliminate postoperative swelling that occurs at the incision site. Swelling will diminish after the injured cells have healed and normal blood flow returns.

4. Preoperative exercises are performed to teach clients what is expected of them postoperatively when they will be experiencing pain.

Client Need: Health Promotion and Maintenance

6-23

④ **Asymmetry in the flank area is indicative of scoliosis. Scoliosis is lateral curvature of the spine.**

1, 2, and 3. Scoliosis can be ruled out if the client's head is in alignment with the gluteal fold, there is symmetry of the thoracic area, and both legs are equal in length.

Client Need: Physiological Integrity

6-24

① **The nurse will apply firm pressure to the site of the aspiration for at least 5 minutes. Bone marrow aspiration on adult clients is usually done from the sternum or iliac crest. Because there is a slight risk of hemorrhage, firm pressure is applied over the site of aspiration for approximately 5 minutes. If a bone marrow biopsy is performed from the iliac crest (the sternum is too thin for a biopsy), pressure should be applied for approximately 60 minutes. This is accomplished by having the client lie in a recumbent position on the affected side with a pressure dressing in place.**

2, 3, and 4. Applying an adhesive bandage, topical ointments, and ice packs are not procedures that need to be implemented immediately.

Client Need: Physiological Integrity

6-25

④ **Keeping toys within reach of the child will facilitate maintenance of proper body alignment. Also, the buttocks should be kept slightly off the bed to provide countertraction. The sheets need to be kept clean, dry, and wrinkle-free to prevent skin breakdown.**

1. Turning the child in Bryant's traction from side to side should be discouraged, since the body should be kept in good alignment.
2. The upper body needs to be kept flat to provide sufficient countertraction.
3. Bryant's traction does not utilize pins. It is a type of skin traction.

Client Need: Health Promotion and Maintenance

6-26

① **Traction weight may not be removed without a physician's prescription.**
2. Body alignment should always be maintained.
3. Pain medication should be administered for the client's comfort approximately 30 minutes prior to the procedure.
4. All procedures should be explained to the client.

Client Need: Safe, Effective Care Environment

6-27

③ **The nurse should walk closely behind and slightly to the side of the client. The greatest degree of safety is provided when the nurse walks behind and slightly to the side of the client. Vulnerability for the client with a walker is at the back, where the walker is open. The nurse must be able to see ahead of the client.**

1. Walking directly behind the client will not give the nurse the visibility needed to help the client move forward.

2. Walking in front of the client is contraindicated because the greatest degree of vulnerability for the client is behind the open walker.

4. Walking beside the client does not give the client the support that is needed, since the walker is open in the back.

Client Need: Safe, Effective Care Environment

6-28

① **Immediately following intermaxillary fixation, the client should be placed in a side-lying position with the head slightly elevated. The side-lying position is the safest position following surgery due to the potential for vomiting. Also, a slight elevation of the head will facilitate breathing. The ultimate goal is to prevent the aspiration of vomitus. Vomiting may occur following surgery due to inadequate ventilation during anesthesia. Also, vomiting may occur when a client emerges from anesthesia to relieve the stomach of mucus and saliva swallowed during anesthesia.**

2. An upright position (90-degree angle) would be unsafe should the client vomit. Flexing the neck (tilting the chin toward the chest) would interfere with breathing and potentiate aspiration should vomiting occur.

3. A horizontal recumbent position (lying on the back) is dangerous. Aspiration is likely if the client vomits.

4. A prone position (lying on the stomach) would interfere with breathing and potentiate aspiration should vomiting occur.

Client Need: Safe, Effective Care Environment

6-29

① **Clients should know how to operate the on/off switch of a continuous passive motion machine in case of emergencies.**

2 and 3. The physician prescribes the flexion and extension movements as well as the speed of the machine. The client should not make any adjustments.

4. External and internal rotation movements are not available options.

Client Need: Safe, Effective Care Environment

6 - 3 0

(1) **Rest is very important for the child with juvenile rheumatoid arthritis and would be facilitated by clustering of care. Clustering of care will provide uninterrupted periods of rest.**

2. Anti-inflammatory medication is more effective than narcotics for control of pain.

3. High protein and high vitamins are not recommended. The diet needs to be well balanced.

4. Heat is more soothing than cool packs to the inflamed joints.

Client Need: Health Promotion and Maintenance

6 - 3 1

(2) **The most likely cause for the client's complaint of numbness is nerve damage or nerve entrapment due to edema, bleeding, or bony fragments.**

1. Blood loss and other injuries may cause hypovolemic shock.

3. Paralysis may be caused by nerve damage. However, the client would be more likely to complain of lack of sensation as opposed to numbness. Untreated nerve damage could cause paralysis.

4. Involuntary muscle contractions (muscle spasms) may occur near the fracture. Pain is experienced as a result of muscle spasms, not numbness.

Client Need: Physiological Integrity

6 - 3 2

(4) **To prevent hip dislocation after a total hip replacement, the hip should be kept in abduction and in a neutral rotation. This can be accomplished by placing abductor splints or pillows between the client's legs.**

1, 2, and 3. Crossing the client's legs, placing pillows along the client's back, and using a drawsheet to facilitate turning could cause a dislocation of the affected hip.

Client Need: Physiological Integrity

6 - 3 3

(1) **Methylprednisolone (Meprolone) is a glucocorticoid medication. These medications are thought to contribute to the development of osteoporosis because they tend to impair calcium transport, which affects bone density.**

2. Calcium carbonate (Tums) is used in the treatment or prevention of osteoporosis.

3. Ranitidine (Zantac) is an antiulcer drug and does not affect osteoporosis.

4. Ramipril (Altace) is an angiotensin converting enzyme (ACE) inhibitor and does not affect bone density.

Client Need: Health Promotion and Maintenance

6 - 3 4

① An immediate nursing intervention would be to relieve pain. A gouty attack is sudden. The joint is intensely painful, swollen, and extremely tender. Relief of pain is the immediate goal. Narcotics may be used until definitive treatment is established. Colchicine is the drug of choice to prevent gout attacks, but it may take 2 to 24 hours to relieve pain.

2. Anti-inflammatory agents are administered. These would be given after relief of pain is accomplished.

3. Relieving pressure on the affected joints would be considered after relief of pain.

4. Application of cold packs may be done to reduce inflammation after the relief of pain.

Client Need: Physiological Integrity

6 - 3 5

② The nurse will suspect a fat embolus. A fat embolus is caused by a globule of fat entering a torn or lacerated blood vessel and causing an obstruction. A fat embolus is a complication that may occur following a fracture of the pelvis or a long bone. Onset is within 72 hours of trauma or other insult.

1. Symptoms of nerve damage would include persistent localized pain, numbness, tingling, and motor weakness not previously present.

3. Symptoms of hypostatic pneumonia would include chest pain, fever, productive cough, dyspnea, headache, and fatigue.

4. Dyspnea, restlessness, tachycardia, progressive cyanosis, and mental confusion are not related to paralysis.

Client Need: Physiological Integrity

6 - 3 6

① The wheelchair should be placed on the left side of the bed where the equipment is located. The wheelchair needs to be facing the head of the bed so the client can reach for the chair arm with the uninvolved strong arm and help with the transfer.

2 and 4. The wheelchair needs to be on the left side of the bed. If the wheelchair could be placed on the right side of the bed, then it would need to be placed facing the foot of the bed to facilitate transfer from the bed to the chair.

3. With the wheelchair facing the foot of the bed, the client would not be able to reach with the uninvolved arm to grasp the wheelchair.

Client Need: Safe, Effective Care Environment

6 - 3 7

② The client's request for assistance in placing a waterproof petal around the edges of the case demonstrates interest in keeping the cast in good condition.

1. Whittling at the cast is a way of defacing the cast. Damaging a cast indicates the child has not accepted the cast.

3. Stuffing paper in the cast is viewed by the child as a possible reason to remove the cast.

4. Refusing to go to the playroom may indicate that the client may be embarrassed to be in a cast and be seen by others.

Client Need: Psychosocial Integrity

6 - 3 8

Fill in the blank correct answer:

<u>Swing-through gait</u>

The swing-through gait is used by clients who have paralysis of the legs and hips. Both crutches are moved forward together. The client then lifts the body weight with the arms and swings through the beyond the crutches. The 3-point, 4-point, and 2-point gaits require weight bearing (partial or full) on one or both feet.

Client Need: Physiological Integrity

6 - 3 9

④ Traction is not applied to provide for comfort. In fact, traction is often uncomfortable.

1, 2, and 3. When a client is placed in 90-90 traction for a fractured femur, the purpose of the traction is to reduce dislocation, immobilize the leg, and decrease muscle spasms. Traction can realign the bone, prevent deformity, maintain alignment, and provide rest for the extremity.

Client Need: Physiological Integrity

6 - 4 0

Fill in the blank correct answer:

<u>vastus lateralis</u>

The vastus lateralis is the preferred site for an intramuscular injection in infants. This muscle is the best developed and relatively free of blood vessels and major nerves. The deltoid muscle is not large enough in an infant for intramuscular injection and an injection there would probably cause an abscess. The dorsogluteal muscle is not as large as the vastus lateralis in an infant. The dorsogluteal can be used for intramuscular injections when the child has been walking for approximately 1 year and the muscle has developed. The ventrogluteal muscle will not be developed enough for intramuscular injections until a child is approximately 18 months of age.

Client Need: Health Promotion and Maintenance

6 - 4 1

③ Fever and complaints of fatigue are common manifestations in clients who are experiencing acute rheumatoid arthritis. With an acute onset of rheumatoid arthritis, numerous joints suddenly become painful and swollen and the client also experiences chills and prostration.

1, 2, and 4. Pedal edema, generalized erythema, bradycardia, and slow respirations are not common manifestations of rheumatoid arthritis.

Client Need: Physiological Integrity

6 - 4 2

② Inadequate blood supply may occur following a dislocation. A lack of blood supply will cause necrosis if the dislocation is not treated.

1. Shock is not likely to occur following a dislocation. However, hypovolemic shock is a potential problem when bone fragments and lacerated vessels are involved.

3. Fat emboli is a complication of fractured bones, not dislocations.

4. It is not until after a dislocation has been reduced that attention is turned toward tissue healing and the prevention of contractions.

Client Need: Health Promotion and Maintenance

6 - 4 3

① A client who has had an above-the-knee (AK) amputation should have the affected limb placed in a position of extension to prevent contracture.

2, 3, and 4. Flexion, internal rotation, and external rotation will lead to the development of contractures in the affected limb.

Client Need: Health Promotion and Maintenance

6 - 4 4

① **The nurse will anticipate a prescription for the tensilon test. Myasthenia gravis is caused by an inadequate amount of acetylcholine at the myoneural junction. Administration of edrophonium (Tensilon), a short-acting cholinesterase inhibitor, can help to diagnose myasthenia gravis. When the client's strength improves after receiving Tensilon, the diagnosis of myasthenia gravis is confirmed.**

2. A cold stimulation test may be scheduled to confirm Raynaud's syndrome, not myasthenia gravis.

3. Magnetic resonance imaging (MRI) is helpful in confirming diagnoses such as cerebral infarction, tumor, abscesses, edema, hemorrhage, and nerve fiber damage and demyelination, not myasthenia gravis.

4. Electroencephalography (EEG) is valuable in assessing clients with symptoms of brain tumors, abscesses, and cerebral damage.

Client Need: Physiological Integrity

6 - 4 5

① ③ ④ **and** ⑤ **Good sources of dietary calcium include milk, yogurt, cheese (not cottage cheese), calcium-fortified orange juice, canned salmon, sardines, green leafy vegetables (especially broccoli and turnip greens), rhubarb, almonds, and figs.**

2. Cottage-cheese is not a good source of calcium.

Client Need: Health Promotion and Maintenance

6 - 4 6

Fill in the blank correct answer:

<u>Estrogen</u>

A deficiency in estrogen after menopause is the leading factor in osteoporosis among aging women.

Client Need: Health Promotion and Maintenance

6 - 4 7

① ③ and ④ **To treat or prevent constipation, a high-fiber diet is recommended. Foods contained in a high-fiber diet include bran and whole grains; legumes such as dried peas and beans; seeds and nuts, and fruits and vegetables (raw).**

2. Dairy products such as milk, yogurt, cheese as well as meat and meat substitutes (poached or boiled eggs) are low-residue and would be recommended to treat diarrhea, not constipation.

Client Need: Health Promotion and Maintenance

6 - 4 8

③ **It is usual, immediately following the amputation of a leg, to elevate the stump for 24 to 48 hours to prevent edema. After that time, it is necessary to place these clients in a prone position several times a day to prevent contractures.**

1. The original trauma to the leg, in addition to the amputation, would require longer than 8 to 12 hours of elevation to prevent edema.

2. It would take longer than 12 to 24 hours of elevation to prevent edema in the client's traumatized stump.

4. Elevating the stump longer than 48 hours is likely to contribute to the formation of contractures and is not recommended.

Client Need: Physiological Integrity

Practice Test 7

Neurological System and Special Senses/Pain

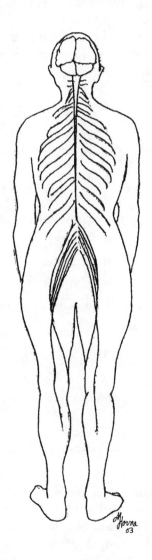

The Nervous System

OVERVIEW

The neurological system is composed of two divisions: the central nervous system (the brain and spinal cord) and the peripheral nervous system (the nerves). These two systems operate within an intricate complex of specialized tissues to regulate thoughts, actions, emotions, sensations, and basic body functions. Nerve cells operate constantly to synchronize our body's responses to various stimuli. The nervous system operates on both a conscious, or voluntary, basis and on an unconscious, or involuntary, basis.

CENTRAL NERVOUS SYSTEM

The central nervous system (CNS) is composed of the brain and the spinal cord. In the brain, the cerebrum controls thinking, reasoning, sensation, memory, and movement. The thalamus acts as a relay point for body sensations such as pain. The hypothalamus controls body temperature, appetite, sleep, and various emotions, and it also controls the pituitary gland. The cerebellum coordinates voluntary movements. The pons is a band of nerve fiber tracts that link the upper with the lower parts of the brain, and the medulla oblongata is a crisscross of nerve fibers that control involuntary activities such as heart rate, dilation of blood vessels, and respiratory function.

PERIPHERAL NERVOUS SYSTEM

The peripheral nervous system (PNS) includes 12 pairs of cranial nerves. They are the

- Olfactory
- Optic
- Oculomotor
- Trochlear
- Trigeminal
- Abducens
- Facial
- Acoustic
- Glossopharyngeal
- Vagus
- Accessory
- Hypoglossal

The peripheral nervous system also includes 31 pairs of spinal nerves, grouped as follows:

- 8 cervical
- 12 thoracic
- 5 lumbar
- 5 sacral
- 1 coccygeal

The nerves of the peripheral nervous system contain sensory and somatic motor fibers and the motor fibers of the autonomic nervous system.

AUTONOMIC NERVOUS SYSTEM

The autonomic nervous system (ANS) controls involuntary bodily functions. The ANS consists of motor nerves to visceral effectors: Smooth muscle; cardiac muscle; glands such as the salivary, gastric, and sweat glands; and the adrenal medulla. There are two divisions of the autonomic nervous system: the sympathetic and the parasympathetic. The sympathetic nerves stimulate the body in times of stress or crisis. They prepare the body for "fight or flight." For example, stimulation of the sympathetic nerves will increase heart and respiratory rates. On the other hand, stimulation of the parasympathetic nerves slows down respirations and heart rate. The parasympathetic nerves are in control when the body is relaxed. The functional and structural unit of the nervous system is called a neuron (nerve cell). A neuron consists of a cell body (perikaryon) and its processes (an axon and one or more dendrites). Neurons can initiate and conduct impulses. They can transmit impulses to other neurons or cells by releasing neurohormones into the bloodstream.

DISEASES/DISORDERS OF THE NEUROLOGICAL SYSTEM INCLUDE

Cerebral Aneurysm

A cerebral aneurysm is an abnormal dilatation of a blood vessel in the brain.

Cerebral Palsy

Cerebral palsy (CP) is associated with partial paralysis and deprivation of muscle coordination. CP is caused by damage to the cerebrum at the time of gestation or during the perinatal period.

Hydrocephalus

Hydrocephalus is the abnormal accumulation of cerebrospinal fluid (CSF) within the ventricle system in the brain. Treatment includes shunting the fluid into the peritoneal cavity.

Spina Bifida

Spina bifida is a defect in the walls of the spinal canal due to a lack of union between the laminae of the vertebrae. The membranes of the cord are forced through the opening.

Epilepsy

Epilepsy is a recurrent paroxysmal (convulsive) disorder occurring at the cerebral level. This condition is associated with a sudden attack of altered consciousness, motor activity, and sensory phenomena.

Alzheimer's Disease

Alzheimer's disease is a chronic progressive condition of the brain that leads to deterioration of intellectual function, personality changes, and communication problems.

Brain Abscess

A brain abscess is a collection of pus within the brain tissue. The usual source of infection is the entrance of pathogenic organisms from the ear, teeth, or mastoid process, or from a sinus infection.

Cerebrovascular Accident (CVA)

A cerebrovascular accident is also known as a stroke. It is associated with a lack of blood flow to the brain tissue. CVA is the third most common cause of death in the United States.

Meningitis

As the name implies, meningitis is the inflammation of the meninges, or membrane (the dura mater, arachnoid, and pia mater), that covers the brain and spinal cord. Symptoms include: Intense headache, fever, and nuchal rigidity.

Parkinson's Disease

Parkinson's disease is a chronic nervous disease associated with fine, slow, spreading tremors, muscle rigidity, and a shuffling gait.

Amyotrophic Lateral Sclerosis (ALS)

This is a syndrome associated with muscular weakness, atrophy, spasticity, and hyperflexia caused by the degeneration of the motor neurons of the spinal cord, medulla, and cortex. Progressive weakness leads to death. This is also known as Lou Gehrig's disease.

Multiple Sclerosis (MS)

MS occurs as a consequence of the destruction of the myelin sheath that covers the neurons in the central nervous system (CNS). The sheath is replaced by hard sclerotic tissue (plaque).

Bell's Palsy

Bell's palsy is characterized by unilateral facial paralysis. This condition is thought to involve the swelling of cranial nerve VII (the facial nerve).

Trigeminal Neuralgia

This disorder is associated with degeneration of or pressure on the trigeminal nerve, causing neuralgia (sharp, severe pain occurring along the course of a nerve).

DISEASES/DISORDERS OF THE EAR INCLUDE

External Otitis

External otitis affects the skin of the external ear and the ear canal. It is associated with inflammation or infection on the epithelium of the auricle (that part of the external ear not contained within the head) and the ear canal. A common cause of this condition is the introduction of flora during swimming. External otitis is also known as swimmer's ear.

Cerumen in the External Ear Canal

Impacted cerumen, commonly known as earwax, can become so tightly wedged that it causes pain and hearing loss. Other symptoms of cerumen impaction include: Tinnitus (ringing in the ears) and vertigo (dizziness).

Infectious Myringitis

Myringitis is the inflammation of the tympanic membrane (eardrum).

Mastoiditis

Mastoiditis is inflammation of the cells of the mastoid process. Clients experience fever, chills, and tenderness over the emissary vein (a tiny vein that pierces the skull and carries blood from the sinuses within the skull to the veins outside it).

Otitis Media

The most common problem of the middle ear is acute otitis media. This disorder is associated with childhood infections involving colds, sore throats, and blockage of the eustachian tube. The eustachian tube in children is short, wide, straight, and at an angle that makes it very easy for microorganism to enter the middle ear. In children with this condition, tympanostomy tubes may be necessary.

Acoustic Neuroma

Acoustic neuroma, also known as vestibular schwannoma, is a benign tumor that develops where the acoustic nerve (cranial nerve VIII) enters the internal auditory canal from the brain. Symptoms include: Progressive hearing loss, tinnitus, and intermittent vertigo. Surgery is the treatment of choice.

Labyrinthitis

Labyrinthitis is an inflammation of the inner ear that affects the cochlear and/or the vestibular portion of the labyrinth. This condition is easily treated with anti-infectives. More involved infections of the labyrinth (suppurative labyrinthitis) may cause complete destruction of the cochlea and labyrinth, resulting in permanent hearing loss.

Ménière's Disease

The three symptoms associated with inner ear problems are all present in clients who experience Ménière's disease; namely, vertigo (a whirling sensation), tinnitus (ringing in the ears), and episodic fluctuating sensorineural hearing loss. The cause of this condition is unknown and may eventually lead to permanent hearing loss.

DISEASES/DISORDERS OF THE NOSE INCLUDE

Cleft Lip and Palate

Cleft lip is a vertical cleft or clefts in the upper lip caused by a congenital condition resulting in faulty fusion. The condition may be unilateral or bilateral. Some incidences of cleft lip and palate are caused by other than genetic factors. Cleft palate is a congenital fissure in the roof of the mouth, which may be unilateral or bilateral.

Nasal Polyps

Nasal polyps are benign edematous projections originating from the mucous membrane that develop in association with repeated inflammation of the sinuses or nasal mucosa. Polyps can enlarge to the point that the airway is compromised. They can be removed surgically.

Sinusitis

Sinusitis is the inflammation of a sinus, in particular a paranasal sinus (located near or along the nasal cavities). Sinusitis may be caused by allergy, various bacteria, and viruses. A factor that underlies sinusitis is a lack of adequate sinus drainage.

DISEASES/DISORDERS OF THE THROAT INCLUDE

Laryngitis

Laryngitis is the inflammation of the larynx. Symptoms include: Hoarseness and aphonia (loss of speech sounds from the larynx). Treatment includes voice rest, liquid or soft diet, and inhalation of steam to loosen secretions. If the infection is bacterial, appropriate anti-infectives will be administered.

Pharyngitis

Pharyngitis is inflammation of the pharynx that produces symptoms including: Malaise, fever, dysphagia (difficulty swallowing), and postnasal secretions. Treatments consist of gargles, lozenges, bed rest, and appropriate anti-infectives.

Tonsillitis

Tonsillitis is the inflammation of a tonsil, in particular the faucial or palatine tonsil. This disease is thought to be caused by Group A beta-hemolytic streptococci. Sequelae (conditions that follow as the result of a disease) include: Rheumatic fever, carditis, and nephritis.

DISEASES/DISORDERS OF THE EYE INCLUDE

Blepharitis

Blepharitis is the inflammation (including possible ulceration) of hair follicles and glands located along the edges of the eyelids. Symptoms include: Red, swollen, tender eyelids with sticky exudates and scales. Edema may cause the lids to invert and eyelashes may fall out. The ulcerative type of blepharitis is usually caused by infection with staphylococci. Clients should be encouraged to keep their hair and brows clean and to avoid touching their eyes. Warm saline compresses are helpful in removing exudate. The appropriate medication will also be administered.

Sty

A sty is a localized bacterial infection involving one or more of the sebaceous glands of the eyelid. Sties may also involve internal sebaceous glands under the eyelid. These tend to be more serious.

Ptosis

Ptosis is the drooping or sagging of the eyelid due to paralysis or weakness.

Conjunctivitis

Conjunctivitis, also known as pinkeye, is the inflammation of the conjunctiva and is treated with the appropriate medication. Clients should be taught to keep their hands away from their eyes.

Keratitis

Keratitis, or inflammation of the cornea, is characterized by decrease of visual acuity. Pain is the typical symptom. This disease is caused by microorganisms, trauma, and reactions to immune-mediated factors.

Cataract

A cataract is best described as opacity of the lens of the eye. Early symptoms are: Difficulty in night driving due to distortions and photosensitivity to oncoming car lights. Severe visual impairment develops as the cataract progresses. The treatment of choice is surgical replacement of the impaired lens with an artificial lens.

Retinal Detachment

We understand a person has experienced a retinal detachment when the inner sensory layer of the retina separates from the outer, pigmented epithelium. This can be brought on by trauma or diseases such as diabetes and sickle cell anemia. Symptoms include: Blurred vision, flashes of light, vitreous floaters, and loss of visual acuity.

Glaucoma

Glaucoma is a group of eye diseases characterized by increased intraocular pressure, the result of which, if untreated, causes visual impairment and blindness. This disease is the third most prevalent cause of blindness in the United States. Glaucoma is said to occur when the aqueous humor drains too slowly from the eye to keep up with production in the anterior chamber. Treatment typically consists of miotic medications. Operative treatment is also possible.

Practice Test 7

Questions

7 - 1

Which of these observations would be considered characteristic of a normal newborn?

1. random, jerky, uneven movements of the eyes
2. a high-pitched, shrill cry
3. bulging fontanels
4. a lethargic posture during a bath

7 - 2

After a lumbar diskectomy, postoperative discharge instructions are prescribed. Which one of the following situations would the client be instructed to report to the surgeon immediately?

1. drainage from the operative site
2. discomfort for the first 2 weeks postoperatively
3. continuing to be overweight
4. diminished sexual activity

7 - 3

Which of the following medications is useful in the treatment of Parkinson's disease?

1. vasopressin
2. levodopa
3. aminophylline
4. levothyroxine

7 - 4

A client with cancer is complaining of pain in the back. Which question will assess the severity of the client's pain?

1. "Do you have more pain in your back than you do in any other area of your body?"
2. "Did your pain begin in your back or did it originate elsewhere?"
3. "Would you say your pain is worse when you are in a sitting position or when you are lying down?"
4. "On a scale of 0 to 10 with 0 being no pain and 10 being a lot of pain, what is your pain?"

7 - 5

A client is admitted to the hospital with a ruptured lumbar intervertebral disk. Prescriptions include bed rest, moist, warm heat packs, and meperidine hydrochloride. Before applying moist heat to the client's lower back, it is essential for the nurse to take which of the following actions?

1. Place a plastic protective covering on the skin before applying the heat source.
2. Apply a thin layer of petrolatum on the skin before applying the heat source.
3. Check the temperature of the heat source.
4. Wrap the heat source in a towel.

7 - 6

A 3-month-old infant with hydrocephalus had a ventriculoperitoneal shunt replacement yesterday. The infant is irritable and you note the dressing on the infant's head is wet. Possible causes might be perspiration, saliva, emesis, or cerebrospinal fluid. To determine whether the drainage is from cerebrospinal fluid, the nurse will test the fluid for:

1. pH.
2. chloride.
3. culture.
4. glucose.

7 - 7

A newborn is diagnosed with hydrocephalus. Which of the following measures should the nurse include in the care plan?

1. Measure the abdominal girth daily.
2. Change the infant's position every 2 hours.
3. Feed the infant on an established schedule.
4. Place the infant so the head is lower than the rest of the body.

7 - 8

Your client has Alzheimer's disease and frequently becomes agitated. Which of the following measures would be best to include in the client's plan of care?

1. Keep the client's room dimly lit, the side rails up, and stimulation at a minimum.
2. Place the client in a wheelchair at the nurses' station and give small simple tasks that are repetitious in nature.
3. Apply restraints and monitor the client daily.
4. Move the client close to the nurses' station, turn on a radio to soothing music, and check the client frequently.

7 - 9

A professional football player is hospitalized following a cervical 6 injury to the spinal cord. The client was placed on a mechanical ventilator immediately after the injury and is in skeletal traction. During the first 24 hours after the injury, the priority nursing diagnosis is:

1. impaired skin integrity.
2. decreased cardiac output.
3. ineffective individual coping.
4. impaired gas exchange.

7 - 1 0

A client has a grand mal seizure. A prescription for 1000 mg phenytoin intravenously is to be given. You will:

1. give the medication in a rapid intravenous push.
2. give concurrent nitroglycerin for the anticipated hypertension.
3. mix the medications in D5NS.
4. monitor the pulse and blood pressure throughout the infusion.

7 - 1 1

A client 69 years old has Parkinson's disease and is admitted to a long-term care facility. Admission prescriptions include diet and activity as tolerated. Prior to developing the client's nursing care plan, to which of these measures should the nurse give priority?

1. Explain to the client the roles of various nursing personnel.
2. Introduce the client to other long-term ambulatory clients.
3. Find out about the client's routines for care at home.
4. Evaluate how much the client knows about Parkinson's disease.

7 - 1 2

Which of the following observations by the nurse would indicate increased intracranial pressure in a client?

1. oliguria
2. pallor
3. lethargy
4. hypothermia

7 - 1 3

A client who is experiencing intractable pain in the head, neck, and arms may have which of the following procedures performed in order to relieve the pain?

1. cingulotomy
2. cordotomy
3. thalamotomy
4. rhizotomy

7 - 1 4

When talking to the parents of a child recently diagnosed with epilepsy, the most appropriate statement is:

1. "Medications used to treat seizures may cause problems with behavior."
2. "Your child should be able to participate in extracurricular activities."
3. "Be careful, since children die from head injuries during seizures."
4. "Avoid making your child cry since that can cause a seizure."

7 - 1 5

A client is diagnosed with herpes zoster involving the trigeminal nerve on the right side of the face. The client complains of itchiness on the right side of the face. Which procedure should the nurse include in the plan of care?

1. application of cool compresses
2. cleansing the area tid
3. removing any scales that may appear
4. applying petrolatum jelly qid

7 - 1 6

A child has tympanostomy ventilating tubes surgically implanted in both ears. Which of the following is an especially important preventive measure against infection following the insertion of the tubes?

1. Clean ear canal with alcohol solution daily.
2. Use earplugs when swimming or bathing.
3. Blow bubbles daily to keep the tubes patent.
4. Administer a mild decongestant.

7 - 1 7

A client has been hospitalized for an acute exacerbation of multiple sclerosis and is to be discharged on prednisone. The client has been instructed to continue taking the medication for 4 more weeks. The nurse is planning discharge teaching about the medication. Which instruction is essential for the client to know about prednisone?

1. The dosage of prednisone should be tapered off gradually.
2. The client is to take the same dose each day until the prescription is finished.
3. The drug should be taken before meals on an empty stomach.
4. The client will need to increase salt intake to prevent sodium depletion.

7-18

Assessment of a 30-year-old client reveals a positive Babinski reflex. What does this assessment indicate?

1. cerebellar dysfunction
2. increased intracranial pressure
3. central nervous system disease of the motor system
4. interruption of the peripheral nervous system

7-19

Which medication would be the drug of choice for a client experiencing a grand mal seizure?

1. Ativan
2. Dilantin
3. Klonopin
4. prednisone

7-20

During your morning assessment of a client with paraplegia, you notice a marked increase in blood pressure. The client complains of a headache and blurred vision. You notice that the client's upper body and head are diaphoretic. An appropriate intervention would be to:

1. administer acetaminophen po for the headache and explain that this is inevitable in a paraplegic.
2. reassure the client that this is a typical emotional response to stress.
3. quickly and vigorously palpate the chest and abdomen for any nodules.
4. assist the client to a sitting position very slowly and notify the physician.

7-21

A 9-year-old is admitted to the pediatric unit. Both eyes are bandaged because of an accidental eye injury. The child is scheduled for surgery the next day. The client's plan of care is least likely to include instructions:

1. for all personnel to speak as they enter the child's room.
2. allowing the child to take a favorite stuffed toy to the operating room.
3. to explain about equipment in use such as the intravenous infusion.
4. to explain what the operating room will look like.

7-22

Which of the following medications would be administered for the treatment of tonic-clonic seizure activity?

1. valproate
2. ranitidine
3. digoxin
4. captopril

7-23

A newly admitted client has a hearing impairment. Which nursing intervention will be the most useful in helping the nurse to communicate?

1. Use visual cues.
2. Refer the client to the speech therapist.
3. Speak slowly and articulate clearly.
4. Allow time for understanding and a response.

7-24

A client with hyperthyroidism is experiencing exophthalmos. Which nursing intervention is appropriate?

1. Keep the head of the bed flat.
2. Provide a high-calorie diet.
3. Instill methylcellulose eyedrops qid.
4. Place the client in a room away from high traffic.

7-25

Your client is experiencing severe depression that has not been alleviated by medication. The client is scheduled for electroconvulsive therapy. Nursing interventions appropriate for this therapy include:

1. informing the client that post-procedure memory loss is permanent.
2. discussing with the client and family that only 1 treatment may be given safely in a month.
3. describing the intended cardiac arrhythmias, including ventricular fibrillation, which occur during these treatments.
4. monitoring vital signs and airway patency after the treatment.

7-26

Your client has a head injury and is exhibiting signs of diabetes insipidus. Because of this development, you know you must monitor this client very closely for:

1. agitation and confabulation.
2. congestive heart failure.
3. hyperglycemia and metabolic acidosis.
4. dehydration and hypovolemia.

7-27

The following preoperative medications are prescribed for a child: meperidine 8 mg, atropine sulfate 0.06 mg. The medications are available as follows: meperidine 50 mg/cc, atropine sulfate 0.40 mg/cc. To administer the prescribed doses, the nurse should prepare:

_____
Fill in the blank

7-28

To assess for blockage in the vertebral canal, the Queckenstedt's test was performed during a lumbar puncture procedure. A rapid rise in cerebrospinal fluid pressure while pressing the neck veins indicates:

1. a blockage is present in the vertebral canal.
2. the presence of a tumor in the vertebral canal.
3. an infection such as meningitis.
4. a normal finding.

7-29

A client with a spinal cord injury has a nursing diagnosis of impaired physical mobility related to central nervous system injury. Your goal is to have the client gain mobility within the limits imposed by the injury. What assessment finding indicates that this goal has been met?

1. skin dry and intact
2. absence of contractures
3. seeks diversional activity
4. relaxed facial expression

7-30

You are using the Glasgow Coma Scale as part of your assessment of a client with a head injury. During your assessment, you observe the following: Eyes open to speech, motor response appropriate, client obeys commands, and conversation is confused. You will assign the client a score of:

1. 1 to 2
2. 4 to 5
3. 12 to 13
4. 19 to 20

7-31

A client diagnosed with acute hypothyroidism has just sustained a fracture of the left humerus. Morphine sulfate is prescribed for pain. The prescription reads: morphine sulfate 5 mg intramuscularly every 6 hours prn for pain. In response to your client's complaint of pain, the most appropriate action would be to:

1. administer the morphine as prescribed.
2. notify the physician and discuss non-narcotic options.
3. administer no analgesia.
4. administer the morphine intravenously because it will act faster.

7-32

A 76-year-old has cataracts in both eyes and is scheduled through the day-surgery clinic for a left cataract extraction. Instillation of mydriatic drops is prescribed preoperatively. Preoperative assessment of the client's vision by the nurse would reveal which of the following findings?

1. loss of visual acuity
2. the presence of double vision
3. complaints of visual fatigue
4. presence of floating filaments

7-33

A client was admitted to your unit with a medical diagnosis of cerebrovascular accident. You are concerned about your client developing increased intracranial pressure. What assessment finding is an early indication of this occurrence?

1. drowsiness
2. vomiting
3. hemiplegia
4. widened pulse pressure

7-34

An adult client complains of periodic episodes of blindness in the right eye. The physician is concerned that the oculomotor nerve has been damaged. Which assessment technique will verify this?

1. Inspect the retina with an ophthalmoscope.
2. Assess visual acuity with the Snellen chart.
3. Shine a penlight directly into the right eye and observe pupillary response.
4. Shine a penlight on the bridge of the nose and note where reflection is on each eye.

7-35

Which of these findings would not be suggestive of otitis media in your 3-year-old client?

1. tugging at the earlobe
2. temperature of 104° F
3. pain behind the ear
4. turning the head from side to side

7 - 3 6

A 5-year-old child is admitted with a possible cerebellar brain tumor. Which of the following neurological tests is most likely to be abnormal preoperatively?

1. pupil reflexes
2. deep tendon reflexes
3. number recall test
4. standing balance

7 - 3 7

A 6-year-old child with hydrocephalus is admitted for a possible ventriculoperitoneal shunt revision. The most likely assessment finding would be:

1. sunset eyes.
2. diplopia.
3. Macewen sign.
4. a high-pitched cry.

7 - 3 8

An infant born with a myelomeningocele experienced a successful closure soon after birth. The child is now 15 months old. The most appropriate nursing diagnosis at this time is:

1. altered urinary elimination.
2. impaired verbal communications.
3. bowel incontinence.
4. altered growth and development, gross motor.

7 - 3 9

Your client had a laminectomy performed under general anesthesia. After recovery, the client is returned to the unit. Vital signs include blood pressure 130/80, pulse rate 80 beats per minute. Which of the following vital signs would indicate the development of shock?

1. blood pressure 100/60, pulse 120
2. blood pressure 120/80, pulse 74
3. blood pressure 140/100, pulse 100
4. blood pressure 150/90, pulse 60

7 - 4 0

An infant is diagnosed with bacterial meningitis. Which of the following nursing interventions would be most appropriate at this time?

1. measure weight and head circumference each shift
2. monitor behavior at each encounter
3. evaluate Kernig's sign each shift
4. monitor fontanel tenseness daily

7 - 4 1

A client who has experienced a battery acid splash on the face and in the eyes should have his eyes treated immediately with:

1. copious water irrigation.
2. sodium bicarbonate irrigation.
3. lidocaine ointment.
4. atropine sulfate solution.

7 - 4 2

The most appropriate assessment to perform on a preschool-age child admitted for a possible brain tumor is:

1. walking ability.
2. head circumference.
3. skin color and capillary refill.
4. vocabulary size and use.

7 - 4 3

A client comes to the emergency department with slurred speech and a sudden onset of left-sided weakness. Prior to the administration of heparin sodium intravenously, a computer tomography of the head is prescribed. A lumbar puncture is also to be performed after the results of the computer tomography came back as "inconclusive for cerebral bleed." You know that the purpose of the lumbar puncture is to:

1. relieve pressure on the brain by draining cerebrospinal fluid.
2. test for fungal infection.
3. use as an access for the administration of the heparin sodium.
4. test for the presence of blood.

7 - 4 4

A 75-year-old is seen at a local clinic and receives a tentative diagnosis of herpes zoster involving the trigeminal nerve on the right side of the face. The client has vesicles and a rash on the right cheek. In developing a nursing assessment of the client, it would be important for the nurse to obtain the answer to which of the following questions?

1. Has the client had chickenpox?
2. Does the client have a history of canker sores?
3. Is the client using a new shaving cream?
4. Has the client ever had a dermatologic reaction to food?

7 - 4 5

Which of the following would be most appropriate for the nurse to include in the care plan for a client who is experiencing organic brain syndrome?

1. Carry our activities in the same order each day.
2. Encourage the client to focus conversation on present events.
3. Provide a variety of activities for the client.
4. Introduce the client to all the nursing staff.

7-46

A client has right-sided homonymous hemianopsia. How will you help the client cope with this deficit?

1. Approach the client from the right side at all times.
2. Place all objects on the right side of the client's bed.
3. Teach the client to turn the head toward the right.
4. Teach the client how to use the left hand to move the right arm.

7-47

A client with a seizure disorder is scheduled for an electroencephalogram in the morning. What nursing action, if any, is appropriate prior to the examination?

1. Withhold diazepam for 4 hours.
2. Nothing by mouth for 12 hours.
3. Omit coffee for 24 hours.
4. No special nursing actions are needed.

7-48

Which nursing action can help keep intracranial pressure down?

1. Keep the head of the bed flat.
2. Place a pillow under the knees.
3. Encourage deep breathing.
4. Administer 5% dextrose in water at 50 cc/hour.

7-49

Your pediatric client has otitis media. Amoxicillin is prescribed 20 mg/kg po daily in 3 divided doses every 8 hours. Your client weighs 60 lbs. How much of the medication will 1 dose contain?

Fill in the blank

7-50

Which prescription would you question for a client who has a diagnosis of acute hemorrhagic stroke?

1. dipyridamole 25 mg po daily
2. diazepam 10 mg prn intravenously for agitation
3. phenytoin sodium 100 mg po
4. dexamethasone 60 mg intravenously every 6 hours

7-51

Upon arrival at the emergency department, a client experiences diminished touch sensation in the lower extremities following a motor vehicle accident. The nurse should anticipate and assess related neurological deficits including:

1. pupil size and reaction.
2. distension of urinary bladder.
3. respiratory distress.
4. presence of headache and nausea.

7 - 5 2

A newborn with a myelomeningocele is to have a surgical repair 24 to 48 hours post-birth. The most important ongoing assessment in the preoperative period is assessment for:

1. fontanel status.
2. hip dysplasia.
3. bowel incontinence.
4. pain sensation below the defect.

7 - 5 3

Your client has trigeminal neuralgia (tic douloureux) and is experiencing acute pain. To help prevent an attack, the nurse will teach the client to:

Select all that apply by placing a ✔ in the square:

❐ 1. maintain a constant cool to cold environment.
❐ 2. avoid touching the affected area.
❐ 3. refrain from chewing gum.
❐ 4. avoid the vibration created by music.
❐ 5. brush teeth often to maintain good oral hygiene.

7 - 5 4

A 55-year-old mother of two, ages 32 and 34, has Huntington's disease. You will inform the family about this disorder. Which comments by the client's children suggest they understand the information given?

Select all that apply by placing a ✔ in the square:

❐ 1. "We can be tested to see if we will develop Huntington's disease."
❐ 2. "We feel helpless knowing our mother cannot be cured."
❐ 3. "Now we understand why our mother is experiencing nausea and vomiting."
❐ 4. "At first we thought our mother had Alzheimer's disease because of her memory loss and inability to concentrate."
❐ 5. "We are thankful that drugs are available that will minimize muscular contractures and jerking."

7 - 5 5

Your client has a brain abscess. You expect your assessment to reveal:

1. a decrease in the white blood cell (WBC) count.
2. a decrease in intracranial pressure (ICP).
3. general malaise and muscle weakness.
4. hypothermia.

Practice Test 7

Answers, Rationales, and Explanations

7 - 1

① **Random, jerky, uneven movements of the eyes (nystagmus) is a normal finding in the newborn, who has not learned to focus.**

2. A high-pitched, shrill cry is associated with neurological disorder.

3. Bulging fontanels are associated with increased intracranial pressure.

4. A lethargic posture during a bath is associated with a central nervous system disorder. The infant should have symmetric movement and strength in all extremities.

Client Need: Health Promotion and Maintenance

7 - 2

① **The client should be told to report any drainage from the operative site immediately. Drainage may indicate infection and needs immediate attention.**

2. Discomfort for the first 2 weeks should be brought to the attention of the surgeon, but it is not the immediate concern.

3. There is no indication that the client is overweight.

4. Diminished sexual activity can be addressed later.

Client Need: Health Promotion and Maintenance

7 - 3

② **Levodopa is an effective medication (dopaminergic) for the treatment of Parkinson's disease. Parkinson's disease is caused by a degeneration of a portion of the nervous system. Levodopa (Larodopa) augments the body's dopamine level. Dopamine is essential for neurotransmission.**

1. Vasopressin (ADH) is an antidiuretic hormone replacement and does not affect neurotransmission.

3. Aminophylline (Somophyllin) is a bronchodilator and does not affect neurotransmission.

4. Levothyroxine (Levothroid) is a hormone replacement and does not affect neurotransmission.

Client Need: Physiological Integrity

7 - 4

④   **Asking the client to evaluate pain on a 1 to 10 scale will help to identify the severity of the pain.**

1.   Asking the client if there is more pain in the back than any other place in the body will identify the location of the pain, not the severity of the pain.

2.   Asking if the pain began in the back or some other area will identify the origin of the pain, not the severity of the pain.

3.   Asking the client if the pain is worse when sitting or lying down will help to identify aggravating factors, not the severity of the pain.

Client Need: Safe, Effective Care Environment

7 - 5

③   **It is essential that the nurse check the temperature of the heat source prior to application. If the heat source is too hot, it may burn the client. Warm, moist heat packs are applied to the lower back several times a day for 10 to 20 minutes at a time to relax spastic muscles.**

1.   Once a moist compress is applied to the client's lower back, it should be covered with a piece of plastic to retain the heat.

2.   Petrolatum jelly is applied to the skin if the compress solution is irritating to tissues. This client's compresses are moist, warm water packs and would not be irritating to the skin.

4.   Warm, moist heat packs are not wrapped in a towel. An example of a heat source that should be wrapped in a towel would be a hot-water bottle.

Client Need: Physiological Integrity

7 - 6

④   **To determine whether the drainage is from cerebrospinal fluid, the nurse will test the fluid for glucose. Glucose is present in cerebrospinal fluid (CSF) but not in perspiration or saliva. Glucose is present only in food that might be in emesis.**

1.   The pH of CSF is not very distinct in comparison to many other body fluids except stomach contents.

2.   The chloride level is not a marker of CSF.

3.   A culture could only grow organisms, and this would not help to identify what the drainage is.

Client Need: Health Promotion and Maintenance

7 - 7

② **The nursing-care plan for a child with hydrocephalus will include changing the infant's position every 2 hours. It is important to change the infant's position at regular intervals to prevent the development of pressure areas on the baby's head.**

1. The infant's head circumference, not abdominal girth, should be measured at least once a day. Measurements should be recorded and plotted on a graph.

3. The infant's feeding schedule should be flexible enough to accommodate diagnostic procedures.

4. Placing the infant's head lower than the body will increase intracranial pressure and is contraindicated.

Client Need: Health Promotion and Maintenance

7 - 8

④ **The client should be moved closer to the nurses' station, where frequent checks can be made and soothing music can be heard. Current thoughts on Alzheimer's disease indicate that overstimulation increases agitation in clients. Yet some stimulation is necessary to provide reality orientation.**

1. Clients with Alzheimer's should be placed in brightly lighted rooms during the day and in sufficient light at night to help them identify surroundings.

2. Placing the client in a wheelchair will limit mobility and can increase agitation. Having the client engage in repetitious tasks is not recommended because of the short attention span.

3. Restraints are not recommended. They tend to increase agitation.

Client Need: Psychosocial Integrity

7 - 9

④ **During the first 24 hours after a cervical injury, maintenance of adequate respiratory function is critical to survival. Oxygen is administered to maintain a high arterial PO_2 since anoxemia can create or worsen neurological damage to the spinal cord.**

1. The client probably does not have significantly impaired skin integrity at this time. Measures need to be started to prevent skin breakdown, but this is not the priority.

2. Although decreased cardiac output is important, you must first of all have oxygen for the heart to circulate blood around the body.

3. The client is understandably frightened and attempting to cope with the enormity of the injuries. This must be dealt with, but first you must make sure that the client survives the injury.

Client Need: Physiological Integrity

7 - 1 0

④ **Clients receiving intravenous phenytoin (Dilantin) should be monitored for bradycardia and hypotension. These are two frequently occurring side effects associated with this medication.**

1. The rate of administration of phenytoin should not exceed 50 mg/min.
2. Phenytoin (Dilantin) administered intravenously may cause hypotension, not hypertension.
3. This medication is to be mixed with normal saline only. Mixing Dilantin with other solutions will cause precipitation.

Client Need: Physiological Integrity

7 - 1 1

③ **Before developing a nursing-care plan for a client hospitalized with Parkinson's disease, the nurse should determine what the client's routines are for care at home. The nurse will want to simulate these as much as possible. This will minimize anxiety generated by unexpected routines or demands. Interviewing the client is one method of collecting data for the development of the nursing-care plan. The client is usually the best source for information about patterns of coping with the activities of daily living.**

1. The nurse should explain the roles of various nursing personnel to all clients, not just those with Parkinson's disease.
2. Introducing the client to other long-term ambulatory clients will not influence the development of a nursing-care plan.
4. How much the client knows about Parkinsonism is not likely to affect the nursing-care plan. However, knowing the client's daily home routine of care will be most helpful, since the nurse will simulate these routines.

Client Need: Safe, Effective Care Environment

7 - 1 2

③ **Lethargy is a sign of increased intracranial pressure that may be observed by the nurse. Other clinical signs of increased intracranial pressure include: headache; vomiting; decrease in level of consciousness, motor function, and respiration; abnormal eye movements; changes in pupil size and reaction to light; widening pulse; bradycardia; irregular respiratory pattern; and decreases in motor functioning.**

1, 2, and 4. Oliguria, pallor, and hypothermia are not associated with increased intracranial pressure.

Client Need: Physiological Integrity

7 - 1 3

③   **Clients experiencing intractable pain in the head, neck, and arms may have a thalamotomy (a surgery designed to selectively destroy specific groups of cells in the thalamus
for relief of pain).**

1.   A cingulotomy (frontal white matter interruption) is performed on clients with intractable pain
associated with an extreme psychogenic component.

2.   A cordotomy interrupts the lateral spinothalamic tract in either the cervical or thoracic areas. It
may be used to relieve the severe pain associated with terminal cancer.

4.   A rhizotomy is performed for traumatic nerve injury. The surgery interrupts the posterior
nerve roots as they enter the spinal cord proximally to the posterior cell. This interrupts the
cranial nerve at its entrance into the brain stem. This surgery is used to control the severe chest
pain of lung cancer and for pain relief involving head and neck malignancies.

Client Need: Physiological Integrity

7 - 1 4

②   **An appropriate statement to make to the parents of a child recently diagnosed with
epilepsy would include the need for the child to continue participating in all activities.**

1.   Medications used to treat seizures may cause drowsiness at first, but that will soon subside.

3.   Telling parents that children die from head injuries during seizures is inappropriate. The parents should be taught to take precautions, but should not be taught in such a way that they fear
for their child's life.

4.   Disciplinary problems could occur as a consequence of the nurse telling parents that they
should avoid making their child cry because crying may cause a seizure. Crying rarely precipi-
tates a seizure.

Client Need: Health Promotion and Maintenance

7 - 1 5

①   **The application of cool compresses is recommended for clients with herpes zoster who
are experiencing itchiness. Herpes zoster (shingles) is an infection caused by the reacti-
vation of the varicella virus in clients who have experienced chickenpox. Acyclovir
(Zovirax) is an antiviral medication frequently administered to treat this condition.
Treatment focuses on relief of pain and avoidance of complications. The nursing-care
plan should include the application of cool compresses to the affected area. Cool compresses will relieve the itching by contracting the blood vessels.**

2.   Cleansing the affected area is not recommended, since touching causes pain.

3.   Scales are not associated with herpes zoster. Vesicles do form and may leave crusts when they
rupture.

4.   Applying Vaseline to the affected area is not recommended, since doing so stimulates the
affected area.

Client Need: Physiological Integrity

7 - 1 6

② **Earplugs for a child with tympanostomy ventilating tubes can defend against infection by preventing water from entering the external ear canal and going into the middle ear. Contaminated lake and bathwater in the ear canal increases the risk for infection.**

1. An effective method for preventing otitis externa is to place a combination of white vinegar and rubbing alcohol (50/50) in the ear canals in the morning, at night, and after swimming. However, this treatment is not recommended following tube insertion.

3. Having the child "blow bubbles" will increase pressure in the eustachian tube, which in turn will increase the pressure in the middle ear and possibly disrupt the integrity of the tympanostomy tubes.

4. There is not a strong link between the use of mild decongestants and the prevention of infection following the implantation of tympanostomy ventilating tubes.

Client Need: Health Promotion and Maintenance

7 - 1 7

① **Discharge instructions for clients receiving prednisone should emphasize the need to taper off the dosage gradually. Abrupt discontinuation of prednisone could lead to adrenal insufficiency. Prednisone is a hormone whose production and release is normally controlled by the adrenal gland. When exogenous prednisone is taken, usually for more than 2 weeks, the adrenal gland ceases its own release of hormone. Therefore, abrupt cessation leads to extreme steroid imbalance until the adrenal gland can resume its normal function.**

2. Rapid withdrawal of the drug could lead to adrenal insufficiency and should be avoided.

3. Prednisone causes gastrointestinal irritation and gastric ulcers. It should be taken with food.

4. Prednisone causes potassium (K) depletion and sodium (Na) retention. A Na-restricted diet with potassium supplements should be prescribed for clients receiving prednisone.

Client Need: Health Promotion and Maintenance

7 - 1 8

③ **A positive Babinski reflex in a client 30 years old indicates central nervous system disease of the motor system. The Babinski reflex is normally seen in infants under the age of six months. The Babinski reflex is characterized by the extension of the great toe and the spreading out of the outer toes when the lateral aspect of the sole is stroked.**

1. Cerebellar dysfunction would be manifested by ataxia and incoordination.

2. Increased intracranial pressure (ICP) is manifested by changes in level of consciousness (LOC), increased blood pressure, and decreased heart rate.

4. Interruption of the peripheral nervous system is manifested by numbness, tingling, and possible loss of sensation.

Client Need: Physiological Integrity

7-19

(2) **Phenytoin (Dilantin) is the drug of choice for the treatment of grand mal seizures.**

1. Lorazepam (Ativan) is indicated when a client is experiencing status epilepticus.

3. Clonazepam (Klonopin) is utilized for absence (petit mal).

4. Prednisone (Meticorten) is an anti-inflammatory corticosteroid preparation and does not impact on seizures.

Client Need: Physiological Integrity

7-20

(4) **Appropriate interventions for a client experiencing autonomic dysreflexia would include assisting the client to a sitting position and notifying the physician. This client is exhibiting the classic signs of autonomic dysreflexia caused by the stimulation of the nerves below the level of the spinal injury. This may cause cardiac arrhythmias and can be life threatening. By having the client sit up, the extreme hypertension associated with this condition is decreased momentarily, until the physician can be notified and an appropriate medication such as diazole (Hyperstat) can be given.**

1. Although acetaminophen may treat headaches, this client is exhibiting classic signs of autonomic dysreflexia, which requires immediate attention.

2. This client is exhibiting the classic signs of autonomic dysreflexia.

3. This client is exhibiting the classic signs of autonomic dysreflexia. Palpating the chest and abdomen would be inappropriate.

Client Need: Physiological Integrity

7-21

(4) **The least likely plan of care for a child scheduled for surgery who cannot see would be an explanation that describes the operating room. Because the child is unable to see, explaining what the operating room looks like is unimportant. Explaining the sounds, smells, and kinesthetics would be important.**

1. Speaking as you enter the room will let the child know someone is present. This will minimize fear and establish mutual respect and trust.

2. Having a security item such as a stuffed toy is very important during traumatic situations for toddlers, preschoolers, and young school-age children.

3. Equipment that can be sensed by the senses other than vision should be explained.

Client Need: Psychosocial Integrity

7 - 2 2

(1) Valproate (Depakote) is a medication that may be administered to treat clonic-tonic seizure activity. Depakote is an anticonvulsant medication whose impact on neural transmission makes it a very effective anticonvulsant agent.

2. Ranitidine (Zantac) is an anti-ulcer medication.

3. Digoxin (Lanoxin) is a cardiac glycoside.

4. Captopril (Capoten) is an antihypertensive.

Client Need: Physiological Integrity

7 - 2 3

(3) For the hearing-impaired client, it is imperative that the nurse speak slowly and articulate clearly. The nurse should also speak toward the client's best ear, reduce background noise, and make sure, if the client is wearing a hearing aid, that it is functioning properly.

1. Visual cues are not necessary if the nurse speaks slowly and distinctly.

2. There is no reason to refer the client to a speech therapist. The problem has to do with the client hearing the nurse.

4. The nurse should always allow clients, including the hearing-impaired, time to consider what has been said before expecting a response. However, the client must hear what is being said before she can respond.

Client Need: Health Promotion and Maintenance

7 - 2 4

(3) Administration of methylcellulose eyedrops qid helps reduce eye irritation for clients who have exophthalmos. Protrusion of the eyeballs (exophthalmos) occurs with hyper-thyroidism due to increased deposits of fats and fluid in the retro-orbital tissues. Because of this, there is a potential for injury to the cornea due to dryness and irritation.

1. To prevent increased intraocular pressure, the head of the bed should be elevated, not flat.

2. A high-calorie diet would be appropriate in meeting the client's increasing needs for calories, but this would not affect the exophthalmos.

4. Clients with hyperthyroidism do not need the additional stimuli that would be experienced by placing them in a high-traffic area.

Client Need: Health Promotion and Maintenance

7-25

④ The nurse will monitor the client's airway patency and vital signs following an electroconvulsive treatment. Nursing interventions prior to electroconvulsive therapy include the administration of a sedative. Therefore, monitoring vital signs and airway patency after the treatment is essential.

1. Memory loss is common, though transient.
2. Treatments may be given 3 times a week.
3. No cardiac arrhythmia is intended.

Client Need: Safe, Effective Care Environment

7-26

④ The nurse should observe the client who has diabetes insipidus for signs of dehydration and hypovolemia. Decreased levels of antidiuretic hormone that may result from an injury to the hypothalamus will tend to cause marked diuresis and potential dehydration.

1. Agitation and confabulation are not typical signs of diabetes insipidus. Typical signs of diabetes insipidus include polyuria and dehydration.
2. Clients who experience diabetes insipidus tend to present with dehydration due to polyuria, not fluid overload.
3. Hyperglycemia and metabolic acidosis are typical of diabetes mellitus, not diabetic insipidus.

Client Need: Health Promotion and Maintenance

7-27

Fill in the blank correct answer:

<u>meperidine 0.16cc and atropine 0.15cc</u>

To obtain 8 mg of meperidine:

$$\frac{50 \text{ mg}}{8 \text{ mg}} = \frac{1 \text{cc}}{X}$$

$$50X = 8 \text{ mg}$$

$$X = 0.16 \text{ cc}$$

To obtain 0.06 mg of atropine:

$$\frac{0.40 \text{ mg}}{0.06 \text{ mg}} = 0.15 \text{ cc}$$

Client Need: Physiological Integrity

7-28

④ A rapid rise in the cerebrospinal fluid pressure while pressing on the neck veins indicates a normal finding. To assess for blockage in the vertebral canal, the Queckenstedt's test (compression of the veins in the neck) is performed during a lumbar puncture.

1, 2, and 3. A blockage in the vertebral canal, presence of a tumor, or an infection such as meningitis will result in a minimal increase or no change in the cerebrospinal fluid pressure.

Client Need: Physiological Integrity

7-29

② The goal of mobility within the limits imposed by the injury will be met by absence of contractures.

1. Intact, dry skin would meet the goal for the nursing diagnosis of impairment of skin integrity related to sensory loss and immobility.

3. Seeks diversional activity would meet the goal for the nursing diagnosis of ineffective individual coping related to impact of dysfunction on daily living.

4. A relaxed facial expression would meet the goal for the nursing diagnosis of pain and discomfort related to treatment and prolonged immobility.

Client Need: Health Promotion and Maintenance

7-30

③ The nurse will assign the client a score of 12 to 13. A score on the Glasgow Coma Scale (GCS) of 12 to 13 is a relatively high score indicating a relatively high level of consciousness.

1. The Glasgow Coma Scale doesn't go as low as 1 to 2. The lowest score is a 1 for each of the three areas observed.

2. A score of 4 to 5 is very low, more appropriate for a client with no verbal response, abnormal flexion, and no eye opening.

4. The maximum score on the GCS is 15.

Client Need: Health Promotion and Maintenance

7-31

② The physician should be notified for the purpose of discussing a nonnarcotic option for a client who has hypothyroidism and is in pain. Clients with hypothyroidism tend to have lower metabolic functioning. They are very susceptible to the effects of narcotics and have an increased risk of respiratory depression. It is prudent to avoid the use of narcotics in clients with acute hypothyroidism.

1. This prescription should be verified, since this client is at risk for respiratory depression due to hypothyroidism.
3. Analgesia should be administered for pain.
4. The route should not be altered in a medication prescription.

Client Need: Physiological Integrity

7-32

① Nursing assessment of the client's vision prior to surgery would reveal loss of visual acuity. Dense cataracts appear as gray opacity of the lens and impede visual acuity.

2. Cataracts do not cause diplopia (double vision).
3. Visual fatigue is not associated with cataracts.
4. Floating filaments (floaters) are associated with retinal detachment, not cataracts.

Client Need: Physiological Integrity

7-33

① Drowsiness is an early indication of increased intracranial pressure (ICP).

2, 3, and 4. Vomiting, hemiplegia, and widening pulse pressure are later signs of increased intracranial pressure.

Client Need: Physiological Integrity

7 - 3 4

③ The assessment technique that determines oculomotor nerve (CNIII) damage involves shining a penlight directly into the right eye and observing pupillary responses of both eyes. Direct and consensual pupillary responses should be observed. The lack of direct and consensual responses suggests oculomotor damage.

1. The ophthalmoscope is used for assessing the ocular media and for examination of the retina. However, this would not give any information about the oculomotor nerve.

2. The Snellen chart assesses visual acuity but does not give information about the oculomotor nerve.

4. Shining a penlight on the bridge of the nose and noting where reflection is on each eye will assess the anterior chamber of the eye for normal transparency, not oculomotor damage.

Client Need: Physiological Integrity

7 - 3 5

③ Pain behind the ear is indicative of mastoiditis, not otitis media.

1, 2, and 4. Common behaviors of young children with otitis media include tugging at the earlobes and turning the head from side to side. Otitis media is not unusual in young children because their eustachian tubes are short, wide, and straight—characteristics that contribute to the spread of inflammation.

Client Need: Physiological Integrity

7 - 3 6

④ The child with a brain tumor is most likely to have signs of increased intracranial pressure and problems with balance and coordination because most brain tumors in children are located in the cerebellum.

1, 2, and 3. Abnormal results of pupil reflexes, deep tendon reflexes, and the number recall test are related to cranial nerves and memory. Most brain tumors in children are in the cerebellum and therefore cause increased intracranial pressure and problems with balance and coordination.

Client Need: Physiological Integrity

7 - 3 7

② The most likely assessment finding for a child admitted for a possible ventriculoperitoneal shunt revision would be diplopia. Strabismus (crossed eyes) and diplopia (double vision) may occur, not cranial enlargement. Signs of the condition are related to the increased intracranial pressure associated with hydrocephalus.

1. The cranial sutures are closed in a 6-year-old. Therefore, the skull cannot enlarge to cause sunset eyes.

3. This is a "cracked pot" sound upon skull percussion when the skull is enlarged. This child is 6 years old and the cranial sutures are closed.

4. A high-pitched cry is most often associated with brain damage. There is no reason to believe that this child has brain damage.

Client Need: Health Promotion and Maintenance

7 - 3 8

④ The most appropriate nursing diagnosis for a 15-month-old who has had a myelomeningocele repair would be: altered growth and development, gross motor. At 15 months of age, a child is in a stage of active gross motor learning. Paralysis of the legs would interfere in this process.

1. Fifteen months of age is too early for normal bladder continence.

2. Impaired verbal communication is not a problem with children who have had myelomeningocele repair.

3. Fifteen months of age is too early for normal bowel continence.

Client Need: Physiological Integrity

7 - 3 9

① Shock is characterized by a dropping blood pressure and a rising pulse rate. Therefore, a blood pressure of 100/60 and a pulse of 120 would signal shock in the client whose baseline blood pressure and pulse were 130/80 and 80.

2. Signs of developing postoperative shock would include an increase in pulse rate, not a decrease. Also, the blood pressure would drop significantly.

3. Signs of developing postoperative shock would include a decrease in the blood pressure, not an increase.

4. Signs of developing postoperative shock would include a decrease in blood pressure, not an increase. Also, the pulse rate would increase, not decrease.

Client Need: Physiological Integrity

7 - 4 0

---

② An infant who has bacterial meningitis should have behavior monitored at each encounter. Meningitis is an inflammation of the meninges of the brain caused by bacteria or viruses. Behavior is a good indicator of intracranial pressure and is often an early sign of changes in intracranial pressure.

1. Weight and head circumference should be assessed daily, not every 8 hours.

3. Kernig's sign (pain in the 3 hamstring muscles when attempting to extend the leg after flexing the thigh upon the abdomen) needs to be evaluated for initial diagnosis only.

4. Fontanels should be evaluated at least once every 8 hours. Evaluating fontanels only once in 24 hours would not be adequate due to the possibility of increased intracranial pressure.

Client Need: Physiological Integrity

7 - 4 1

---

① Flushing the eyes with copious amounts of water is a first-aid measure and is very effective in reducing eye damage. Strong chemicals may injure the eyes. Removal of the hazardous chemical is the first priority.

2 and 3. Neither sodium bicarbonate irrigation nor Lidocaine ointment are indicated to treat chemical splashes to the eye.

4. Atropine solution is used to dilate the pupil for examination or procedure purposes.

Client Need: Physiological Integrity

7 - 4 2

---

① Walking ability is the most appropriate assessment to perform on a preschool child who is suspected of having a brain tumor. Most brain tumors in children are in the cerebellum brain stem. Pressure on the cerebellum will affect balance and coordination.

2. The head will not enlarge in the preschool child in response to increased intracranial content since the cranial sutures are closed.

3. Circulation and oxygenation are not affected.

4. Vocabulary is a function of the cerebrum and most brain tumors in children are located in the cerebellum.

Client Need: Health Promotion and Maintenance

7 - 4 3

④ **The purpose for a lumbar puncture in this situation is to test for the presence of blood. Blood in the CSF indicates a cerebral bleed. Therefore, the initiation of heparin therapy may be based on these results.**

1. Elevation of intracranial pressure is usually treated with medications.

2. Although the cerebral spinal fluid (CSF) may be tested for many things, the purpose in this situation is to test for the presence of blood prior to the initiation of heparin therapy.

3. Administering heparin via lumbar puncture is inappropriate.

Client Need: Health Promotion and Maintenance

7 - 4 4

① **The nurse should determine if the client ever had chickenpox. The virus that causes herpes zoster also causes chickenpox.**

2. Ulceration of the mouth and lips is not associated with herpes zoster.

3. A new shaving cream might be associated with contact dermatitis, not herpes zoster.

4. Food allergies are not associated with herpes zoster.

Client Need: Physiological Integrity

7 - 4 5

① **Activities should be performed in the same order each day for clients experiencing organic brain syndrome. A stable, predictable environment is crucial in minimizing the confusion that comes with memory loss.**

2 and 4. Clients with organic brain syndrome have difficulty remembering recent events and new faces. It would be best to converse with the client about events and people that are remembered from the past.

3. Providing a variety of activities for clients who have difficulty remembering recent events would not be helpful. It is likely to increase the client's confusion.

Client Need: Health Promotion and Maintenance

7 - 4 6

③ **Individuals who are experiencing right-sided homonymous hemianopsia should be taught to compensate by turning the head to the right. This will help minimize the deficit. When clients experience right-sided homonymous hemianopsia, they are unable to see out of the right side of each eye.**

1. Clients with right-sided homonymous hemianopsia cannot see out of the right side of either eye. Therefore, the client would not be able to see a nurse approaching from the right side.

2. Clients with right-sided homonymous hemianopsia would not be able to see objects that are placed on the right side of the bed.

4. Homonymous hemianopsia does not affect hand and arm movements.

Client Need: Health Promotion and Maintenance

7 - 4 7

③ **Clients who are scheduled for an electroencephalography (EEG) should be told not to drink fluids that contain caffeine, such as coffee and cola drinks. Caffeine is a central nervous system stimulant and could distort the electroencephalography results.**

1. Anticonvulsants, tranquilizers, barbiturates, and other sedatives such as diazepam (Valium) should be withheld for 24 to 48 hours (not 4 hours) prior to the EEG because they can alter the brainwave pattern.

2. There is no need to restrict food or fluids prior to an EEG unless they contain caffeine.

4. The nurse should explain the procedure and advise the client against consuming anything that contains caffeine.

Client Need: Health Promotion and Maintenance

7 - 4 8

③ **Encouraging deep breathing can help keep intracranial pressure down. Carbon dioxide (PaCO₂) causes cerebral vasodilation and increases intracranial pressure. To lower carbon dioxide levels, the client should be encouraged to deep breathe. Hyperventilation lowers carbon dioxide levels.**

1 and 2. Keeping the head of the bed flat and placing a pillow under the knees increases intracranial pressure.

4. Administering 5% dextrose in water at 50 cc per hour will increase circulating fluid volume and thereby increase intracranial pressure.

Client Need: Physiological Integrity

7 - 4 9

Fill in the blank correct answer:

<u>182 mg</u>

One dose of amoxicillin will contain 180 mg.

$$\frac{60 \text{ lbs}}{3 \text{ doses}} \times \frac{1 \text{ kg}}{2.2 \text{ lbs}} \times \frac{20 \text{ mg}}{1 \text{ kg}} = \underline{181.8 \text{ mg}}$$

Client Need: Physiological Integrity

7 - 5 0

① A prescription for dipyridamole (Persantine) should be questioned for a client experiencing an acute hemorrhagic stroke. Dipyridamole (Persantine) is an antiplatelet agent that could promote further bleeding in the client with an acute hemorrhagic stroke.

2, 3, and 4. Diazepam (Valium), phenytoin (Dilantin), and dexamethasone (Dexadron) are all appropriate medications to administer.

Client Need: Physiological Integrity

7 - 5 1

② The nurse will anticipate related neurological deficits such as distension of the urinary bladder. Diminished sensation in the lower extremities following a motor vehicle accident is indicative of a neurological deficit related to spinal cord injury involving the lumbar and sacral regions.

1, 3, and 4. Pupil size and reaction, respiratory distress, and the presence of a headache and nausea are signs of head injury unrelated to the presenting neurological symptom of decreased sensation in the lower extremities.

Client Need: Physiological Integrity

7 - 5 2

① Preoperative assessment of an infant prior to the surgical repair of a myelomeningocele should include ongoing fontanel status. Hydrocephalus is a common condition that may develop pre- or postoperatively with children who have a myelomeningocele. Ongoing fontanel assessment along with measurement of the head circumference would help monitor for hydrocephalus.

2, 3, and 4. Hip dysplasia, bowel incontinence, and pain sensation below the defect are conditions which may be present at birth but do not need immediate attention and are not life threatening. Assessment does not need to be ongoing.

Client Need: Physiological Integrity

7 - 5 3

---

②③ and ④ Triggers that initiate attacks (nerve pain) include a cold environment, touching the affected area, chewing gum, the vibration created by music, brushing teeth, talking, smiling, and a passing breeze. Trigeminal neuralgia (nerve pain) affects the fifth cranial nerve, which has three major branches: namely, the mandibular, maxillary, and ophthalmic. Trigeminal neuralgia is thought to be caused by compression of the nerve root.

1. A cool/cold environment is among the triggers that can initiate nerve pain. A constant moderate temperature in the environment is recommended.

5. Brushing the teeth can trigger nerve pain. There is no need to emphasize scrupulous mouth care in this condition.

Client Need: Physiological Integrity

7 - 5 4

---

① Huntington's disease is a hereditary disorder. The children of a parent with this disease can learn if they will develop the disease through DNA testing.

② There is no cure for Huntington's. It is treated symptomatically.

④ Some of the same symptoms seen in clients who have Alzheimer's disease are seen in clients who have Huntington's disease, such as loss of memory and inability to concentrate.

⑤ Drugs such as haloperidol (Haldol) and risperidone (Risperdol) may be administered to treat dyskinesias.

3. Nausea and vomiting are not symptoms associated with Huntington's disease.

Client Need: Physiological Integrity

7 - 5 5

---

③ Symptoms associated with a brain abscess include fever, an increase in intracranial pressure, headache, paralysis, seizures, muscle weakness and general malaise. Also, an elevated white blood cell count is expected.

1. A brain abscess occurs as a result of an infection. Therefore, an elevated white blood count (WBC) is expected.

2. Because a brain abscess takes up space, an increase in intracranial pressure (ICP) is anticipated.

5. Fever is expected due to infection.

Client Need: Physiological Integrity

Practice Test 8

Renal System with Fluids and Electrolytes

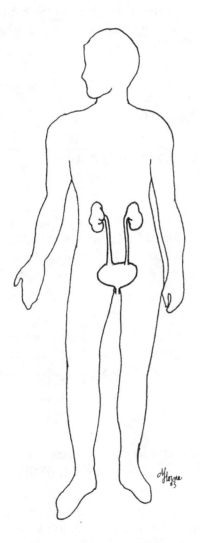

The Male Renal System

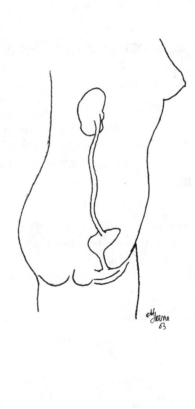

The Female Renal System

OVERVIEW

The major function of the urinary system is to remove urea (the end product of protein metabolism) from the bloodstream. If urea accumulates in the bloodstream rather than being excreted, a highly toxic condition known as uremia results.

Urea is formed in the liver from ammonia. It comes from the breakdown of simple proteins, called amino acids, in the body cells. Urea is carried in the bloodstream to the kidneys, where it passes, with water, salts, and acids, out of the bloodstream and into the kidney tubules as urine. Urine makes its way down the ureters into the bladder and out of the body.

Kidneys also function to maintain the proper balance of water, salts, and acids in body fluids. Salts, such as sodium (Na+) and potassium (K+), and some acids, are called electrolytes. Electrolytes are small molecules that conduct an electrical charge. Electrolytes help to maintain proper functioning of muscle and nerve cells. The kidneys are great "adjustors." They adjust the amounts of water and electrolytes in the body by secreting some substances into the urine and retaining other substances in the bloodstream for use in the body. The kidneys also act as endocrine organs by secreting substances into the bloodstream that act at distant sites in the body. For example, they secrete

- Renin, an enzyme that helps control blood pressure
- Erythropoietin, a hormone that stimulates production of red blood cells
- Vitamin D, a vitamin necessary for the absorption of calcium from the intestines

DISEASES/DISORDERS OF THE RENAL AND URINARY SYSTEM INCLUDE

Obstructive Disorders

NEPHROLITHIASIS (RENAL CALCULI) This condition is commonly known as kidney stones. A calculus (stone) in the kidney can obstruct the flow of urine. A stone wedged in the ureters causes sudden, severe pain, renal colic, chills, fever, hematuria (blood in the urine), and urinary frequency. Kidney stones can be dissolved by drugs or disintegrated ultrasonically.

NEUROGENIC BLADDER Neurogenic bladder is characterized by involuntary retention of urine and distended (bulging) bladder. Clients experience chills, fever, and a burning sensation.

TUMORS (RENAL CELL CARCINOMA) Most kidney tumors are malignant and usually block the flow of urine. Hematuria (blood in the urine) is the most common symptom. Renal cancers most often metastasize (spread) to the lungs and bone tissue. As these cancers progress, clients experience pelvic pain and urinary obstruction.

Inflammatory Disorders

URETHRITIS (URINARY TRACT INFECTIONS) Urethritis is the inflammation of the urethra. This disease is often associated with a bacterial infection such as gonorrhea. Nongonococcal urethritis (NGU) includes chlamydia and herpes simplex infections.

CYSTITIS Cystitis refers to inflammation of the bladder. The condition may be caused secondary to an ascending urinary infection. It occurs more frequently in women because in women the urethra is short and the urethral opening is close to the anus. Symptoms include: Urinary frequency, pelvic pain, and hematuria.

PYELONEPHRITIS Pyelonephritis is inflammation of the renal pelvis and the connective tissues of the kidney. This condition is usually caused by bacterial infections; however, it may be associated with a viral infection, calculi, tumors, or pregnancy.

Nephrotic Syndrome

Nephrotic syndrome is a glomerular disorder associated with a collection of signs and symptoms characterized by: Proteinuria (presence of protein in the urine), hypoalbuminemia (low albumin in the blood), and edema (generalized swelling in the tissues).

Kidney Failure

As the name implies, kidney failure occurs when the kidneys are no longer able to properly perform their essential functions; i.e., removing urea from the body and regulating electrolyte and water balance. Renal failure may be acute (abrupt reduction of kidney function) or chronic (slow but progressive failure associated with gradual loss of nephrons).

STAGES OF CHRONIC RENAL FAILURE

Stage 1 This stage is characterized by some loss of nephrons. The condition at this point is asymptomatic and may last for years.

Stage 2 This stage is known as renal insufficiency. Existing nephrons are able to handle the load, but the BUN (blood urea nitrogen) is increasing and kidney function is decreasing.

Stage 3 The final stage of chronic renal failure is called uremia. The BUN is very high. The client experiences hypertension. Unless there is an intervention, such as a kidney transplant, the client will die.

Practice Test 8

Questions

8 - 1

Which electrolyte imbalance is often associated with hypocalcemia?

1. hyperkalemia
2. hypoglycemia
3. hyperglycemia
4. hypomagnesemia

8 - 2

A 55-year-old female client has had frequent urinary tract infections. Which statement by the client indicates a need for further teaching?

1. "I will drink plenty of fluids."
2. "I will use bubble bath when bathing."
3. "I will wash my hands after going to the bathroom."
4. "I will wipe from the front to the back after having a stool."

8 - 3

A 4-year-old child is being treated for a urinary tract infection. Ampicillin by mouth 4 times a day has been prescribed. The most appropriate teaching about this medication when prescribed for the treatment of a urinary tract infection is:

1. A full glass of water should be given with each dose.
2. Doses should be administered every 6 hours.
3. Chewable tablets are as effective as capsules and are easier for a child this age to take.
4. Allergy is more likely to occur when penicillin is given 4 times daily rather than twice daily.

8 - 4

A client with a long history of diabetes has developed renal failure secondary to diabetes. The physician has prescribed an 1800 k-calorie renal diet. This diet consists of:

1. k-calories (1800) with sodium and potassium restriction.
2. sodium (1800 mg) with potassium restriction.
3. k-calories (1800) with 4 g sodium.
4. k-calories (1800) with low sodium and high protein.

8 - 5

A client is scheduled for an intravenous pyelogram. Which of the following data would be most important for the nurse to know and record before this procedure is carried out?

1. Is the client's urine negative for sugar and acetone?
2. Does the client have a history of allergies?
3. Has the client received a recent thyroid scan?
4. Does the client have frequency of urination?

8 - 6

A 33-year-old is seen in the clinic and diagnosed with acute pyelonephritis. The client is placed on bed rest and given fluids ad lib. The client asks the nurse why it is necessary to stay in bed. You will teach the client that bed rest will:

1. prevent respiratory infection by reducing the client's contact with other people.
2. ensure safety while the client has toxins in the bloodstream.
3. assist the client's body defenses in combating infection.
4. control ascending urinary infection by maintaining a horizontal position.

8 - 7

When teaching a client who is experiencing end stage renal disease how to diminish the irritating effects of pruritus, the nurse will instruct the client to:

1. take frequent warm baths.
2. take tepid baths with emollients.
3. gently rub the skin with the palmar surface of the hands.
4. apply antihistamine cream to the skin every 8 hours.

8 - 8

A routine urinalysis was requested by the physician. To prevent contamination during the collection of the specimen, the nurse should:

1. wear gloves when handling the urine specimen.
2. wash the hands before handling the specimen.
3. collect the specimen in a prelabeled container.
4. use sterile specimen containers only.

8 - 9

A client is receiving an intravenous infusion of D5W in 0.45% normal saline at 125 ml per hour through an infusion pump. Which of the following actions by a new graduate nurse needs further attention from the charge nurse?

1. ensuring that the volume infused coincides with the time tape on the intravenous bottle
2. adjusting the height of the pump attachment to ensure that the intravenous fluid flows by gravity
3. ensuring that the intravenous tubes are not pinched or kinked
4. including the infusion device used in the documentation of the intravenous therapy

8 - 1 0

A child with acute glomerulonephritis may experience all of the following manifestations. Which one indicates a possible complication?

1. hematuria
2. periorbital edema
3. headache
4. anorexia

8 - 1 1

A 2-year-old is in the acute phase of nephrotic syndrome. Which observation would be most important for the nurse to report to the child's health-care provider?

1. a cloudy nasal discharge
2. ate only a few bites of each meal yesterday
3. lethargic and easily fatigued
4. edema in the genital area

8 - 1 2

Your client is receiving a continuous infusion of the antineoplastic agent doxorubicin via a peripheral intravenous line. You observe a bleb at the infusion site of the client's intravenous infusion. Which of the following interventions will you take initially?

1. Lower the height of the infusion container.
2. Stop the fluid infusion
3. Flush the infusion tubing with isotonic saline solution.
4. Slow the infusion rate.

8 - 1 3

When developing a plan of care for an older client following a perineal prostatectomy, the nurse should include gradual supervised ambulation to:

1. shift the center of gravity forward in the body.
2. promote use of extensor rather than flexor muscles.
3. minimize the response to orthostatic reflex stimulation.
4. deter ossification of the long bones.

8 - 1 4

Your client had a perineal prostatectomy. Because the client was in a lithotomy position for the operative procedure, the nurse will perform which of the following measures during the early postoperative period?

1. Turn the client from side to side and place a pillow between the legs.
2. Encourage flexion and extension exercises of the legs and apply elastic stockings.
3. Elevate the foot of the bed to 15 degrees and put a pillow at the head of the bed.
4. Place the head of the bed up and the feet down and put a pillow at the foot of the bed.

8 - 1 5

The nurse is teaching a client who has an indwelling catheter how to help prevent bladder infections. The nurse will plan to emphasize which of the following?

1. Encourage the client to eat the diet that is provided.
2. Have the client drink liberal amounts of fluid.
3. Tell the client to drink one glass of cranberry juice each day.
4. Instruct the client to keep the drainage bag level with the top of the mattress.

8 - 1 6

A client with syndrome of inappropriate antidiuretic hormone is complaining of muscle cramps and weakness. The nurse will associate these complaints with:

1. hyponatremia
2. hyperkalemia.
3. hyperchloremia.
4. hypercalcemia.

8 - 17

An adult client with cancer has an implanted venous access device. You are preparing to insert a specially designed needle to institute a prolonged continuous infusion of fluids. At what angle should you insert this needle?

1. 15 degrees
2. 30 degrees
3. 45 degrees
4. 90 degrees

8 - 18

During a hemodialysis, a client is receiving antibiotics. How can air be prevented from getting into the mechanical kidney?

1. Place the client with the head lower than the legs and feet.
2. Establish an intermittent infusion cap to administer the antibiotic.
3. Check the administration set every 5 minutes.
4. Aspirate all air from the intravenous bag prior to administration.

8 - 19

Your client is experiencing incontinence due to a reflex bladder ("spastic" bladder). The anticholinergic, spasmolytic drug Ditropan has been prescribed. Which of the following historical information will alert the nurse to potential complication?

1. history of peptic ulcers
2. seizure disorders of unknown causes
3. migraine headaches
4. untreated glaucoma

8 - 20

The nurse is preparing a client for an abdominal paracentesis. It is essential for the nurse to take which of the following actions?

1. Instruct the client about how to participate in the procedure.
2. Withhold oral intake for at least 24 hours before the procedure.
3. Have the client empty the bladder immediately prior to the procedure.
4. Provide the client with a rolled blanket to place against the back to maintain a sitting position during the procedure.

8 - 21

A client's intravenous fluids contain potassium chloride, which is being given to replace potassium chloride that has been lost during gastric suctioning. The nurse will observe the client for symptoms of potassium deficiency including:

1. abdominal muscle spasticity.
2. labored respirations.
3. leg muscle weakness.
4. hypertension.

8 - 22

A client 82 years old is admitted to the hospital with benign prostatic hypertrophy. Which of the following questions would be appropriate for the nurse to ask when assessing the client's symptoms?

1. "Do you have difficulty in voiding?"
2. "Is there a discharge from your penis?"
3. "Is there swelling in your groin?"
4. "Do you have tenderness in your scrotum?"

8 - 2 3

A 46-year-old is admitted to the hospital with a diagnosis of renal calculi. Which of the following actions would be most important for the nurse to initiate for the client?

1. Provide a quiet environment.
2. Strain all urine.
3. Tell the client not to eat or drink anything.
4. Advise the client to remain in bed.

8 - 2 4

A client who has been scheduled for dialysis has a blood urea nitrogen of 63 mg/dl, a creatinine of 4.5 mg/dl, and a potassium of 7.4 mEq/l. A kayexelate enema is prescribed. You know the purpose of the enema is to:

1. empty the bowel prior to the dialysis.
2. lower the blood urea nitrogen level.
3. lower the potassium level.
4. increase the creatinine level.

8 - 2 5

Which of the following microorganisms is responsible for the majority of urinary tract infections in female clients?

1. Escherichia coli
2. Nesseria gonorrhea
3. Corpus albicans
4. Haemophilus influenzae

8 - 2 6

Your client has had a nephrectomy for removal of a Wilms' tumor. The least appropriate nursing intervention for a child who has had a nephrectomy for removal of a Wilms' tumor is:

1. monitoring urine for gross and microscopic hematuria.
2. monitoring bowel sounds and abdominal distention.
3. monitoring vital signs, including blood pressure.
4. encouraging deep breathing and coughing often.

8 - 2 7

A client has developed an acute renal insufficiency following antibiotic therapy. Dopamine intravenous infusion was prescribed to restore renal function. Dopamine's therapeutic action includes:

1. increasing renal function.
2. lowering blood pressure.
3. increasing cardiac output.
4. decreasing serum potassium levels.

8 - 2 8

An infant who is on intake and output measurements spits up all over the bib and nightgown. Which action is indicated?

1. Caution the parents to be more observant and catch all emesis in a basin.
2. Weigh the soiled items before and after laundering to estimate fluid loss.
3. Suggest that the parents call for assistance the next time vomiting occurs.
4. Provide a bath basin to catch any vomitus.

8 - 2 9

A client with chronic obstructive pulmonary disease developed a respiratory infection that was successfully treated with gentamicin sulfate. The client is now complaining of nausea and anorexia. Blood work reveals a potassium of 4.8 mmol/l, blood urea nitrogen of 36 mg/dl, creatinine of 3.2 mg/dl, sodium of 148 mEq/l, and a glucose of 116 mg/dl. Which problem is suggested by these results?

1. acute renal failure
2. hypokalemia
3. dehydration
4. hypoglycemia

8 - 3 0

Your client is to receive 1000 cc of D5W over a 6-hour period. The drop factor on the infusion set is 15. The nurse will infuse the fluids at:

_____.

Fill in the blank

8 - 3 1

A client is admitted with a provisional diagnosis of benign prostatic hypertrophy. To assist in assessing urinary status, the physician writes a prescription: "Catheterize for residual urine." To administer this prescription, the nurse should explain the procedure and:

1. insert an indwelling urinary catheter, record 24-hour output, then remove the indwelling catheter.
2. ask the client to void, insert a straight catheter, drain the bladder and measure output, remove catheter, and record.
3. insert an indwelling urinary catheter, drain the bladder, instill 500 cc of sterile saline into the bladder, and have the client void.
4. ask the client to void, insert straight catheter, instill methylene blue solution into the bladder, have the client void, and record.

8 - 3 2

A client is experiencing acute renal failure that is postrenal in nature. You know that this is probably due to:

1. hypovolemia.
2. cardiogenic shock.
3. nephrototoxicity.
4. urethral obstruction.

8 - 3 3

Your client is experiencing dependent edema and has been receiving furosemide 20 mg intravenously bid for the past 3 days. An appropriate nursing intervention would be to:

1. encourage po fluid intake.
2. keep the room dimly lit.
3. monitor electrolytes.
4. avoid and discourage high potassium.

8 - 3 4

A client is scheduled for a nephrectomy. You will plan to give the client's preoperative medication:

1. prior to morning care to allow for observations of the client's reaction to the medication.
2. prior to morning care to promote optimal relaxation for the client.
3. after morning care to prevent disturbing the client until surgery.
4. after morning care because the medication would otherwise interfere with the care.

8 - 3 5

A client has a vulvectomy and returns to her room with an indwelling urethral catheter attached to gravity drainage and a perineal dressing held in place with a T-binder. When performing an initial postoperative assessment, the nurse will expect the urine to appear:

1. bright red.
2. cloudy.
3. blood-tinged.
4. amber.

8 - 3 6

A client has just returned from a cystoscopy. An essential nursing intervention at this time would be to:

1. assess the color of the client's urine.
2. keep the client npo for 2 hours.
3. assess the client's gag reflex prior to feeding.
4. encourage the client to ambulate immediately following the examination.

8 - 3 7

A client is to receive 1500 ml of 5% dextrose in water over a period of 8 hours. The drop factor is 20 gtts/ml. The fluid should infuse at what rate?

Fill in the blank

8 - 3 8

Your client had a cystectomy for the purpose of removing a large tumor in the urinary bladder. An ileal conduit was performed. You know to record the client's urinary volume:

1. every hour.
2. every 30 minutes.
3. at each shift change.
4. every 2 hours.

8 - 3 9

Your client is receiving cortisone acetate 100 mg po and hydrochlorothiazide 50 mg po daily. You will monitor which of the following laboratory values?

1. elevated serum potassium
2. low serum potassium
3. low hemoglobin
4. low serum glucose

8 - 4 0

With which of the following conditions is dehydration least likely to occur?

1. pneumonia
2. meningitis
3. nephrotic syndrome
4. elevated blood sugar

8 - 41

After a transurethral prostatectomy, your client is returned to your unit from recovery. The client has an indwelling urethral catheter and is receiving continuous bladder irrigations with normal saline solution. When monitoring the irrigation, the nurse should:

1. clamp the flow from the irrigating solution for the specified time, then open to allow a designated amount of solution to flush the bladder.

2. infuse no more than 50 ml of irrigating solution, then apply a moderate amount of suction to withdraw the solution.

3. check to be sure that the solution outflow corresponds to the irrigation inflow and patency of the catheter is maintained.

4. warm the irrigating solution to body temperature and infuse at 100 cc per hour.

8 - 42

Your client is in renal failure and is being treated with hemodialysis. Because of an infected fistula, the decision has been made to initiate peritoneal dialysis. You explain to your client that this procedure:

1. requires the injection of dialysate into the digestive tract and allows electrolyte exchange to occur there.

2. may be used for a maximum of 2 exchanges.

3. utilizes the peritoneum as the semipermeable membrane.

4. is much quicker in resolving electrolyte imbalance than hemodialysis.

8 - 43

Sodium polystyrene sulfonate is prescribed for a client. When administering this medication, the nurse will expect the desired therapeutic effect to occur through which of the following actions?

1. shifts in intracellular potassium
2. decreased potassium intoxication
3. lower serum sodium levels
4. increased serum sulfate levels

8 - 44

Your client has received intravenous fluids for 3 days postoperatively. You plan to observe for any signs of fluid overload. You know that signs of fluid overload include:

1. weight loss.
2. decrease in blood pressure.
3. depressed inspiration rate.
4. coughing and wheezing.

8 - 45

A client enters the hospital in acute renal failure. The client complains of drowsiness and nausea and has Kussmaul's breathing. Laboratory tests indicate a serum potassium of 6.8 mEq/l, serum sodium 120 mEq/l, and a blood pH of 7.2. Which prescription should be questioned?

1. polystyrene sodium sulfonate 50 gm per rectum, as enema

2. a 2000-calorie, high-carbohydrate, high-protein diet when nausea subsides

3. hypertonic glucose (25%), 300 cc with 35 units of Regular insulin per intravenous infusion over 1 hour

4. limit po fluids per 8 hours to no more than 100 cc above the urinary output for the previous 8 hours

8 - 4 6

Which of the following information about nephrolithiasis is accurate?

1. The incidence of nephrolithiasis is greater in women than in men.
2. The incidence of nephrolithiasis is greatest in the African-American population.
3. Low urine volume will increase the risk of nephrolithiasis.
4. Nephrolithiasis will cause constant, aching pain.

8 - 4 7

Following a transurethral resection of the prostate, you perform an initial assessment and find vital signs stable, client alert and complaining of feeling a need to void; a 3-way #24 indwelling catheter with continuous normal saline irrigation is draining well, catheter drainage is pinkish-red with numerous tiny clots. Your first action will be to:

1. notify the physician of the urine color and the passage of clots.
2. palpate the suprapubic area gently for signs of bladder fullness.
3. position and anchor the catheter by taping it to lie horizontally across the upper thigh.
4. encourage the client to bear down slightly as if trying to void.

8 - 4 8

Your client is in renal failure. You anticipate changes in the client's serum values. You expect the client's serum:

1. calcium to be increased.
2. potassium to be decreased.
3. albumin to be increased.
4. uric acid to be increased.

8 - 4 9

You are assessing a client who has had a kidney transplant for possible rejection. Signs and symptoms of kidney transplant rejection include:

Select all that apply by placing a ✔ in the square:

❏ 1. edema.
❏ 2. polyuria.
❏ 3. increase in blood pressure.
❏ 4. increase in serum creatinine levels.
❏ 5. weight loss.

Practice Test 8

Answers, Rationales, and Explanations

8 - 1

④ Hypocalcemia is often associated with the electrolyte imbalance of hypomagnesemia. Magnesium is one of the electrolytes that affects parathyroid hormone levels. Low magnesium levels therefore have the tendency to lower calcium levels, too, since parathyroid hormone (PTH) directly affects serum calcium levels. An increase in serum magnesium will often cause a corresponding rise in serum calcium level.

1, 2, and 3. Neither serum potassium levels nor serum glucose levels directly influence serum calcium levels, unlike the association between magnesium and the parathyroid hormone.

Client Need: Physiological Integrity

8 - 2

② A woman with a urinary tract infection should be taught not to use bubble bath when bathing. Inflammation of the bladder and ureters can develop from exposure to ingredients contained in bubble baths and shampoos.

1, 3, and 4. Urinary tract infections can be treated and prevented by drinking plenty of water, washing the hands, and wiping from the front to the back after having a stool.

Client Need: Physiological Integrity

8 - 3

② The most appropriate teaching about ampicillin when prescribed for the treatment of a urinary tract infection is to administer the dosage every 6 hours. Administering ampicillin every 6 hours will assure a uniform therapeutic blood level of the drug. Maintaining a steady therapeutic blood level is necessary for effective treatment.

1. Fluids need to be given frequently, not just when administering the medication.

3. Ampicillin is not available in chewable tablets.

4. Allergy can occur at any time and dosing frequency does not contribute to allergy.

Client Need: Health Promotion and Maintenance

8 - 4

① An 1800 k-calorie renal diet consists of 1800 k-cal for calorie control. Sodium (Na) is 1–3 q/day and potassium (k+) is 60–70 mEq/day for management of renal failure.

2. The calories should be 1800, sodium should be 2 g rather than 1800 mg, and the potassium restriction is not specified.

3. The diet should contain 1800 k-calories and 2 g of sodium with potassium restriction.

4. Clients experiencing renal failure require protein restrictions because of poor ammonium clearance.

Client Need: Health Promotion and Maintenance

8 - 5

② A client should be assessed for a history of allergies before having an intravenous pyelogram. An intravenous pyelogram (IVP) requires an iodine radiopaque dye. The client may have an allergy to iodine and may therefore be allergic to the IVP dye. Clients are given a clear liquid diet on the evening before the procedure, since food in the stomach could obstruct the view of the urinary structure. The client is given only water until bedtime, and then is npo for 8 to 10 hours before the test. Usually laxatives are given the night before and an enema until clear in the morning before the test. The nurse should record the client's reaction to the dye, such as tingling, numbness, and palpitations. After the procedure, fluids are forced to remove the dye and relieve any dehydration.

1. It is not necessary that the urine be negative for sugar and acetone in order for the client to have an IVP.

3. The fact that a client may have received a recent thyroid scan would not interfere with an IVP. However, the reverse is not true. A recent IVP could interfere with the results of a thyroid scan.

4. Frequency of urination would not affect the results of an IVP.

Client Need: Safe, Effective Care Environment

8 - 6

③ Clients experiencing pyelonephritis (inflammation of the kidney) are placed on bed rest because bed rest will assist the body's defenses in combating infection by conserving energy and allowing the body to use its resources to combat infection.

1 and 2. This client has pyelonephritis. Bed rest will not prevent respiratory infections, nor will bed rest ensure safety while there are toxins in the body. Bed rest will help the body to combat infection in the kidneys.

4. Maintaining a horizontal position would worsen pyelonephritis by allowing bacterial infection to travel upward to the pelvis of the kidney (pyelonephritis results from the spread of infection from the lower urinary tract).

Client Need: Health Promotion and Maintenance

8 - 7

② Clients with end-stage renal disease (ESRD) may have pruritus (severe itching of the skin). Tepid baths with emollients are soothing and remove the bile salts that exude onto the surface of the skin.

1. Warm baths will cause further drying of the skin and contribute to pruritus.

3. Rubbing the skin may cause further skin irritation.

4. Creams are used as an adjunct, but they are costly.

Client Need: Physiological Integrity

8 - 8

① To prevent contamination during the collection of a urine specimen, the nurse should wear gloves when handling the specimen. Wearing gloves will prevent contamination of the specimen and the collector. This meets the requirements of the Occupational Safety and Health Administration (OSHA).

2. The nurse should wear gloves.

3. It is not necessary that the specimen container be prelabeled as long as the nurse wears gloves when handling the specimen.

4. It is not necessary to use a sterile container when collecting a routine urine specimen for urinalysis.

Client Need: Safe, Effective Care Environment

8 - 9

② A new graduate is in need of attention from the charge nurse if the graduate adjusts the height of the pump attachment. It is not necessary to adjust the height of the pump attachment to ensure that the intravenous fluid flows by gravity. Infusion pumps do not depend on gravity pressure. They can be placed at any level. Eye level is convenient for checking the pump's functioning.

1. The volume infused should coincide with the time tape on the intravenous bottle.

3. The intravenous tubing should not be pinched or have kinks.

4. Documentation should include the device used to infuse the fluids.

Client Need: Health Promotion and Maintenance

8 - 1 0

③ A possible complication associated with acute glomerulonephritis would be a headache. Headache may be an indicator of encephalopathy due to hypertension. Other key indicators include dizziness, abdominal discomfort, and vomiting. Grand mal seizures may also occur. The most common cause of acute glomerulonephritis is a previous infection by group A beta-hemolytic streptococcus.

1. Hematuria (blood in the urine) is a clinical manifestation of glomerulonephritis, not a complication. The presence of hematuria is essential for a diagnosis of glomerulonephritis. The degree of hematuria may range from severe to microscopic. The client's urine may be dark tea-colored.

2. Edema is a clinical manifestation of glomerulonephritis, especially around the eyelids (periorbital) and in the ankles.

4. Nausea and vomiting are clinical manifestations of glomerulonephritis, not complications.

Client Need: Physiological Integrity

8 - 1 1

① A cloudy nasal discharge from a child in the acute phase of nephrotic syndrome should be reported immediately to the child's health-care provider. A cloudy nasal discharge is an indicator of infection. Children with nephrotic syndrome (a kidney disorder manifested by proteinuria, hypoalbuminemia, and edema) are very susceptible to infection because of treatment with corticosteroids, loss of proteins, and generalized edema. Prompt treatment of infection is essential.

2, 3, and 4. Anorexia, lethargy, fatigue, and generalized edema are to be expected with this condition.

Client Need: Health Promotion and Maintenance

8 - 1 2

② The nurse should stop an intravenous fluid infusion immediately if extravasation (the escape of fluids into the surrounding tissues) is suspected. Doxorubicin (Adriamycin) is very vesicant (a caustic, blister-forming medication) when it escapes from the vein into surrounding tissues.

1, 3, and 4. The fluid should be stopped and the physician notified before any additional intervention is implemented.

Client Need: Safe, Effective Care Environment

8 - 1 3

③ **The nurse can minimize the older client's response to orthostatic reflex stimulation by supervised gradual ambulation. Postoperatively, older adults are more susceptible to orthostatic hypotension due to a decrease in the sensitivity of their baroreceptors to position change.**

1. The center of gravity affects balance but does not impact on orthostatic hypotension.
2. Promoting the use of extensor rather than flexor muscles is helpful when treating and preventing contractures. However, this will not affect orthostatic hypotension.
4. Gradual supervision of ambulation does not deter ossification of long bones.

Client Need: Physiological Integrity

8 - 1 4

② **The nurse will encourage clients who have assumed a lithotomy position to flex and extend their legs. Also, elastic stockings may be applied. The lithotomy position (client lying on back with feet in stirrups, the hips acutely flexed and the thighs separated) places the client at increased risk for deep vein thrombosis. Encouraging flexion and extension exercises of the client's legs and applying elastic stockings will prevent venous stasis and thrombophlebitis.**

1. Placing a pillow between the legs would be uncomfortable for a client who has had a perineal prostatectomy and would not prevent venous stasis and thrombophlebitis.
3. Elevating the head of the bed 15% is not as effective in preventing venous stasis and thrombophlebitis as flexion and extension exercises of the legs along with elastic stockings.
4. Clients may be placed with the head of the bed up and the feet down to treat increased intracranial pressure. This client does not require such a position.

Client Need: Safe, Effective Care Environment

8 - 1 5

② **The nurse will encourage the client who has an indwelling urinary catheter to drink liberal amounts of fluid. A high fluid intake will dilute the urine and decrease mucosal irritation. The increase in urine volume also facilitates maintenance of catheter patency.**

1. Encouraging a well-balanced diet helps to maintain good health generally. However, a specific action that should be encouraged to prevent infections associated with indwelling catheters is to consume liberal amounts of fluids.
3. One glass of cranberry juice daily will not provide enough consistent acidity to prevent urinary infections.
4. The drainage bag should be kept below the level of the client's bladder to prevent a backflow of contaminated urine into the client's bladder from the bag.

Client Need: Physiological Integrity

8 - 1 6

① The nurse will associate muscle cramps and weakness with hyponatremia. Hyponatremia (serum sodium below 135 mEq/l) will cause muscle cramps and weakness in clients experiencing syndrome of inappropriate antidiuretic hormone (SIDH). These clients have low urinary output with high specific gravity, a sudden weight gain, or a serum sodium decline. Excess antidiuretic hormone increases renal tubular permeability and the reabsorption of water into the circulation. This results in extracellular fluid expansion, followed by plasma osmolarity and serum sodium decline. Lastly, glomerular filtration rate rises and sodium levels decline.

2. Hyperkalemia (serum potassium levels above 5.5 mg/dl) is not associated with SIDH. Signs of hyperkalemia include muscle weakness and impaired muscle functions, tremors, twitching, cardiac dysrhythmias, and cardiac arrest. Disease processes associated with hyperkalemia include Addison's disease and renal failure.

3. Hyperchloremia (serum chloride levels above 390 mg/dl) is not associated with SIDH. Signs of hyperchloremia include developing stupor; rapid, deep breathing; and weakness that may lead to coma.

4. Hypercalcemia (serum calcium levels above 10.1 mg/dl) is not associated with SIDH. Signs of hypercalcemia include bone pain, flank pain due to renal calculi, and muscle hypotonicity.

Client Need: Physiological Integrity

8 - 1 7

④ For prolonged continuous infusions of fluids or chemotherapy, a 90-degree angled, specially designed needle (Huber needle) is used for top entry ports. Straight Huber needles are available for bolus injections and blood withdrawn from both top- and-side-entry ports. The angled bevel of the Huber needle prevents coring of the rubber septum of the port and permits repeated insertion. A dressing is applied over the 90-degree needle to secure the needle position and prevent infection.

1, 2, and 3. All are incorrect angles.

Client Need: Physiological Integrity

8 - 1 8

④ The nurse will aspirate all the air from the intravenous bag. Aspirating all air from the intravenous bag creates a vacuum, preventing air from entering the mechanical kidney.

1. Placing the client in the Trendelenburg position (head lower than the legs and feet) will not prevent air from entering the machine.

2. It is not necessary to establish an intermittent infusion cap.

3. Checking the administration every 5 minutes is not realistic.

Client Need: Safe, Effective Care Environment

8 - 1 9

④ **A client with a history of untreated glaucoma would be at risk for complications should oxybutynin chloride (Ditropan) be administered. Ditropan is contraindicated for clients with untreated glaucoma because it impairs outflow of aqueous humor and causes increased intraocular pressure. An acute attack of glaucoma could occur following the administration of an anticholinergic drug.**

1. A history of peptic ulcers would not interfere with the administration of Ditropan.
2. Clients with seizure disorders are not prohibited from taking Ditropan.
3. Clients who have a history of migraine headaches are not prohibited from taking Ditropan.

Client Need: Health Promotion and Maintenance

8 - 2 0

③ **It is essential that the nurse have the client empty the bladder immediately before an abdominal paracentesis. Having the client void will lessen the danger of accidentally piercing the bladder when the surgeon introduces the trocar through a stab wound below the umbilicus.**

1. The nurse should inform all clients about what is expected of them during any procedure, not just an abdominal paracentesis.
2. It is not necessary to withhold oral intake prior to an abdominal paracentesis.
4. The client can either remain in bed in an upright position (90 degrees) or sit in a chair with a supportive back. It is not necessary to place a rolled blanket against the client's back.

Client Need: Safe, Effective Care Environment

8 - 2 1

③ **Potassium depletion (hypokalemia) results in decreased muscular function, which is manifested by weakness, flaccid paralysis, shallow respirations, decreased intestinal motility, abdominal distension, paralytic ileus, and vomiting. Other signs include decreased neuromuscular irritability and cardiac dysrhythmia.**

1. Abdominal muscle spasticity is not associated with potassium depletion. However, abdominal distension may be experienced.
2. In severe cases of hypokalemia, shallow respirations and respiratory paralysis may occur, not labored breathing.
4. Hypotension, not hypertension, may occur with potassium depletion.

Client Need: Physiological Integrity

8 - 2 2

① **It would be appropriate for the nurse to ask if the client is experiencing difficulty voiding. As the prostate gland enlarges, it puts pressure on the urethra and causes urinary stasis, recurring infections, frequent urination, nocturia, and dysuria.**

2. A discharge from the penis is not associated with benign prostatic hypertrophy. However, discharge from the penis does occur with sexually transmitted diseases (STDs) such as gonorrhea.

3. Swelling in the groin is not associated with benign prostatic hypertrophy. However, swelling in the groin may be seen in conditions such as inguinal hernia.

4. Tenderness in the scrotum is associated with conditions such as testicular torsion.

Client Need: Safe, Effective Care Environment

8 - 2 3

② **All urine of a client suspected of having a renal or ureteral calculus should be strained in the event the stone is passed. Fluids are encouraged to assist stones in their downward passage and ambulation utilizes gravity in moving stones along.**

1. A quiet environment is not as important as straining all the client's urine for passage of renal stones.

3. Food and fluids are not restricted. In fact, fluids are encouraged in an attempt to flush out the calculi.

4. Clients with renal or ureteral calculi may assume any position they wish. They do not need to remain in bed. Ambulation may actually help the calculi to pass.

Client Need: Physiological Integrity

8 - 2 4

③ **A sodium polystyrene sulfonate (Kayexalate) enema is administered to lower the client's potassium. Kayexalate is an electrolyte modifier that exchanges sodium ions for potassium in the intestines. The normal serum potassium is 3.5 to 5.5 mEq/l. A potassium level above 5.5 mEq/l is considered hyperkalemic and requires treatment.**

1. The Kayexalate enema may empty the bowel. However, emptying the bowel is not the intended effect of the Kayexalate.

2. The normal blood urea nitrogen (BUN) value ranges from 8 to 20 mg/dl. A BUN of 63 mg/dl is abnormally high and suggests renal disease. Obtaining a BUN level also aids in the assessment of dehydration. A Kayexalate enema will have little if any effect on a client's BUN level.

4. A normal creatinine level is between 0.7 and 1.5 mg/dl. However, even though the client has a high creatinine level of 4.5 mg/dl, a Kayexalate enema would not have any effect on creatinine.

Client Need: Physiological Integrity

8 - 2 5

① *Escherichia coli* (*E. coli*) is a normal part of the intestinal flora and is responsible for the majority of urinary tract infections in the female. Because of the proximity of the urethra to the rectum, women are more prone to urinary tract infections caused by this bacterium. Over 80% of urinary tract infections in women are caused by *E. coli.*

2 and 3. *Nesseria gonorrhea* (*N. gonorrhea*) and *Corpus albicans* (*C. albicans*) typically produce vaginitis.

4. *Haemophilus influenzae* (*H. influenzae*) is associated with infections of the respiratory tract and ear.

Client Need: Physiological Integrity

8 - 2 6

① The least appropriate nursing intervention for a child who has had a nephrectomy for the removal of a Wilms' tumor is monitoring urine for gross and microscopic hematuria. The affected kidney has been removed. Therefore, hematuria should not be present. The remaining kidney is left intact and undisturbed. A large transabdominal incision is made to allow for easy removal of the involved kidney (and adjacent adrenal gland) and visualization of the uninvolved kidney. Follow-up includes radiation and chemotherapy with actinomycin D and vincristine.

2 and 3. In addition to experiencing the effects of general anesthesia, this client may develop adynamic ileus from the vincristine, edema in the abdomen from the radiation, and possibly infections.

4. The high, extensive abdominal incision contributes to a greater possibility of developing respiratory infections.

Client Need: Health Promotion and Maintenance

8 - 2 7

① Dopamine's therapeutic action includes increasing renal function. Dopamine hydrochloride (Intropin) affects both the alpha and beta adrenergic receptors of the sympathetic nervous system. At low doses (1 to 2 mcg/kg/min), Dopamine has a vasodilatory effect on the brain, kidneys, and other organs, thereby increasing renal perfusion and subsequent urinary output.

2. With improved renal function, blood pressure will return to normal as an indirect action of the Intropin.

3. Intropin does not directly improve cardiac output.

4. With improved renal function, water and electrolyte excretions will increase; however, this is not the primary action of Intropin.

Client Need: Physiological Integrity

8 - 2 8

②   **The nurse should weigh the soiled linens before and after laundering. Infants can dehydrate quickly, since their bodies are composed of approximately 80% water.**

1 and 3. It may not be possible for the nurse or the client's parents to account for all emesis by collecting it in a basin. Therefore, soiled bibs and nightgowns should be weighed before and after laundering.

4.   Even if the proper basins are available, vomiting may be sudden and unexpected and therefore not likely to be collected.

Client Need: Health Promotion and Maintenance

8 - 2 9

①   **The combination of a blood urea nitrogen (BUN) of 36 mg/dl (normal is 8 to 20 mg/dl) and a creatinine of 3.2 mg/dl (normal is 0.7 to 1.5 mg/dl) suggests renal failure. Renal failure occurs with gentamicin therapy because it is nephrotoxic.**

2 and 4. The client's serum potassium is within the normal range of 3.5 to 5.5 mmol/l, as is the glucose, whose normal is 60 to 120 mg/dl.

3.   Dehydration is often indicated by an elevated BUN but a normal creatinine.

Client Need: Physiological Integrity

8 - 3 0

Fill in the blank correct answer:

<u>**41 drops per minute**</u>

Formula:

$$\frac{\text{amount} \times \text{drop factor}}{\text{Time (in minutes)}} =$$

$$\frac{1000 \times 15}{6 \times 60} = \frac{15,000}{360} = 41 \text{ gtts/min}$$

Client Need: Safe, Effective Care Environment

8 - 31

② Urine remaining in the bladder after voiding is called residual urine. The amount is usually determined by catheterizing the client immediately after voiding. With normal, or near normal, bladder functioning, the volume of residual urine is 50 cc or less. An indwelling urinary catheter may be used if a large amount of residual urine is expected and the physician has indicated that an indwelling catheter is to be left in place if a specified volume of residual urine is exceeded.

1. Recording a 24-hour urine output is not the process one would follow to determine residual urine.

3. Placing sterile saline in the bladder may be initiated following a prostatectomy to relieve any obstruction that may cause discomfort. However, a sterile saline irrigation is not associated with the procedure for collecting residual urine.

4. Methylene blue helps to delineate the cause of a fistula. It is not associated with the procedure for collecting a residual urine.

Client Need: Health Promotion and Maintenance

8 - 32

④ Urethral obstruction is a typical cause of postrenal failure (obstruction of the urinary collecting system anywhere from the calyces to the urethral meatus). Urethral obstruction causes urine to back up and pressure in the kidneys to rise. Postrenal failure refers to any condition occurring below the level of the kidney.

1 and 2. Hypovolemic and cardiogenic shock may cause prerenal failure. Both cause systemic hypoperfusion and thus renal hypoperfusion.

3. Nephrotoxic substances (substances that damage kidney tissues) directly assault the nephron.

Client Need: Physiological Integrity

8 - 33

③ Clients receiving furosemide should have their electrolytes monitored. Potassium and sodium are excreted in the urine of clients receiving furosemide (Lasix). Therefore, fluids and electrolytes should be monitored carefully in clients experiencing dependent edema.

1. Encouraging fluids would be contraindicated for clients receiving diuretics.

2. Photosensitivity is not a common side effect of furosemide. There is no reason to keep the client's room dimly lit.

4. Persons on loop diuretics, such as Lasix, are at risk for hypokalemia. Therefore, you would encourage foods high in potassium.

Client Need: Health Promotion and Maintenance

8 - 3 4

③ **The purpose of a preoperative medication is to relax the client, alleviate anxiety, and permit a smooth induction of anesthesia prior to surgery. Therefore, the morning care should be completed before the preoperative medication is given to prevent disturbing the client.**

1 and 2. The preoperative medication is given to relax the client, allay anxiety, and to permit a smooth induction of anesthesia. The client should not be disturbed after preoperative medication is given.

4. The purpose for giving the preoperative medication after morning care is not because it would interfere with the care. It is given after morning care so that the client will not be disturbed while the medication take effect.

Client Need: Safe, Effective Care Environment

8 - 3 5

④ **Following a vulvectomy, urine from the indwelling catheter should be amber (the normal color) in the initial postoperative assessment.**

1. A bright red color would indicate possible hemorrhage and a complication of surgery.

2. Initially, a cloudy color would not be expected postoperatively because this would indicate an infection, which needs time to develop.

3. Blood-tinged urine would indicate possible hemorrhage and a complication of surgery.

Client Need: Physiological Integrity

8 - 3 6

① **An essential nursing intervention at this time would be to observe the client's urine to see if it is bloody or cloudy. A cystoscopy is a procedure in which the physician views the interior of the bladder and urethra with a cystoscope.**

2. The client should be encouraged to drink plenty of fluids. Intake and output should be monitored.

3. The gag reflex does not need to be assessed because the client's throat has not been anesthetized.

4. The client is usually kept on bed rest for the first 4 to 6 hours after the procedure.

Client Need: Physiological Integrity

8 - 3 7

Fill in the blank correct answer:

<u>63 gtts/min</u>

The fluid should infuse at 63 drops per minute.

Formula:

<u>Amount x drop factor</u>
Time (in minutes)

<u>1500 x 20</u> = <u>30,000</u>
  8 x 60   480   =   63 gtts/min

Client Need: Safe, Effective Care Environment

8 - 3 8

① The postoperative urinary volume should be checked every hour. Following surgery, the kidneys should produce a minimum of 30 cc of urine every hour. A minimum of 240 cc for an 8-hour period is expected.

2. Every 30 minutes is too frequent to make a correct evaluation since the kidneys normally produce a minimum of 30 cc of urine every hour.

3 and 4. Checking the urinary volume at each shift change or every 2 hours does not give an accurate recording of the urine being excreted every hour.

Client Need: Health Promotion and Maintenance

8 - 3 9

② The nurse will monitor closely for low serum potassium. Concurrent use of a thiazide diuretic such as hydrochlorothiazide (Ezide) may increase the potassium-wasting effect of cortisone acetate. Therefore, the client should be monitored for low serum potassium.

1. Concurrent use of these medications will tend to lower, not elevate, the serum potassium level.

3. Cortisone acetate and hydrochlorothiazide do not impact on hemoglobin.

4. Serum glucose tends to be higher than normal, not lower, when a client is on cortisone acetate.

Client Need: Physiological Integrity

8 - 4 0

③ **Dehydration is least likely to occur among clients who have nephrotic syndrome.**

1. Fluid loss and subsequent dehydration can occur among clients who have pneumonia due to tachypnea, fever, and anorexia.
2. Fluid loss and subsequent dehydration can occur among clients who have meningitis due to fever and vomiting.
4. Clients who have elevated blood glucose may become dehydrated. Fluid will be lost via the kidneys as excess glucose is excreted.

Client Need: Physiological Integrity

8 - 4 1

③ **When monitoring the irrigation, the nurse should check to be sure that the solution out-flow corresponds to the irrigation inflow and that patency of the catheter is maintained. Continuous bladder irrigations require a steady flow of fluids into the bladder. Fluid entering the bladder and fluid draining from the bladder should be in appropriate proportions (equal amounts).**

1. The bladder irrigation should be continuous.
2. The irrigations should be continuous and should flow by gravity.
4. The irrigating solution should be administered at room temperature.

Client Need: Physiological Integrity

8 - 4 2

③ **Peritoneal dialysis utilizes the peritoneum as a semipermeable membrane. The dialysate dwells in the abdominal cavity and exchange takes place through the peritoneum.**

1. The dialysate dwells in the abdominal cavity, which surrounds the intestines; it does not dwell in the intestines.
2. Peritoneal dialysis may be used indefinitely if it is successful and remains free of infection.
4. The complete peritoneal dialysis takes several times longer than hemodialysis and often requires several changes.

Client Need: Physiological Integrity

8 - 4 3

② When administering sodium polystyrene sulfonate, the nurse will expect the desired therapeutic effect to occur through decreased potassium intoxication. Sodium polystyrene (Kayexalate) is an ion-exchange resin that removes potassium (K+) from the gastrointestinal tract. The resins, which are not absorbed in the gastrointestinal tract, exchange sodium (Na+) and hydrogen (H+) for potassium (K+). Potassium is then excreted in the feces.

1. The desired therapeutic effect of sodium polystyrene sulfonate will not occur via shifts in intracellular potassium because the ion exchange is effective only in the gastrointestinal tract.

3 and 4. Serum sodium levels are not affected by Kayexalate administration.

Client Need: Physiological Integrity

8 - 4 4

④ The signs of fluid overload are coughing and wheezing. A cough and wheeze may be due to the buildup of fluid in the lungs that can occur if excess intravenous fluids are administered. Other signs and symptoms of fluid overload include headache, hyponatremia, distended neck veins, and rapid breathing.

1. Weight gain (not loss) would indicate fluid overload.

2. An increase (not decrease) in blood pressure would indicate fluid overload.

3. An increase (not decrease) in respiratory rate would indicate fluid overload. An increase in the respiratory rate would increase insensible loss of fluid and would be considered a compensatory mechanism in response to fluid overload.

Client Need: Physiological Integrity

8 - 4 5

② The nurse should question a 2000-calorie, high-carbohydrate, high-protein diet. Dietary protein is usually limited in acute renal failure to decrease nitrogenous metabolic waste products.

1. Polystyrene sodium sulfonate (Kayexalate) reduces serum potassium by exchanging sodium for potassium ions in the gastrointestinal tract. Because the client is hyperkalemic and hyponatremic, this is a reasonable prescription. Normal potassium is 3.5 to 5.5 mEq/l. Normal sodium is 135 to 145 mEq/l.

3. Hypertonic glucose and insulin promote movement of potassium into the cells. This will reduce hyperkalemia.

4. Fluid imbalance must be carefully monitored. Intake should be only slightly more than output per 24 hours. Intake is frequently based on prior 8-hour output.

Client Need: Safe, Effective Care Environment

8 - 4 6

③   A low urine volume will increase the risk of nephrolithiasis. Nephrolithiases (kidney stones) are formed from the salts of urine. The incidence is related to gender, race, diet, and geographic location.

1. Men are more prone to develop kidney stones than women.
2. Persons of European descent tend to have a higher incidence of kidney stones than persons of African descent.
4. Kidney stones are not associated with pain until they become lodged in a portion of the urinary tract.

Client Need: Physiological Integrity

8 - 4 7

②   Although the catheter appears to be draining well, gentle palpation can be used to further assess the client for bladder distention.

1. Pinkish-red urine with small clots is a normal finding at this time.
3. The catheter is usually positioned to pull the retention balloon into the prostatic fossa to provide hemostasis following a transurethral resection of the prostate.
4. Attempting to void around the catheter causes the bladder muscles to contract and produces painful bladder spasms. The client should be instructed not to bear down in an attempt to void around the catheter.

Client Need: Health Promotion and Maintenance

8 - 4 8

④   A client experiencing renal failure would have an increase in uric acid. In males, the normal uric acid is 3.6 to 8.5 mg/dl. In females, it is 2.3 to 6.6 mg/dl.

1. A client in renal failure would have a decrease in serum calcium. Normal calcium is 8.8 to 10mg/dl.
2. A client in renal failure would have an increase in serum potassium. Normal potassium is 3.5 to 5.0 mEq/l.
3. A client in renal failure would have a decrease in albumin.

Client Need: Physiological Integrity

8 - 4 9

① ③ and ④   Signs and symptoms associated with kidney transplant rejection include oliguria, edema, fever, increasing blood pressure, weight gain, swelling or tenderness over the transplanted kidney, and an increase in serum creatinine levels.

2. Oliguria, not polyuria, is a symptom of kidney transplant rejection. As kidney function deteriorates, smaller amounts of urine are produced.
5. Weight gain, not weight loss, is a symptom of kidney transplant rejection.

Client Need: Physiological Integrity

Practice Test 9

Female and Male Reproductive Systems

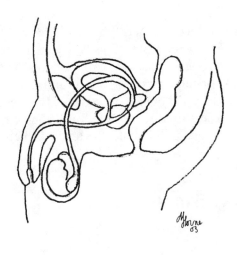

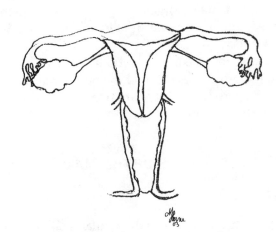

The Male Reproductive System   **The Female Reproductive System**

OVERVIEW

The male and female reproductive systems are specific for reproduction; their biological purpose is to produce offspring. The creation of a unique individual begins with the female sex cell (egg/ovum) and the male sex cell (sperm). Through the process of sexual intercourse, the egg and sperm unite (conception), forming a new and unique life. Male and female sex cells (gametes) each contribute half the number of chromosomes (23 of 46) that a normal body cell contains. Gametes are produced in organs known as gonads. In the female, gonads are called ovaries, and in the male, gonads are called testes.

THE FEMALE REPRODUCTIVE SYSTEM

After leaving the ovary, the egg travels down a duct (the fallopian tube) that leads to the uterus. If sexual intercourse has taken place, sperm will be waiting in the fallopian tube. It is at this time and place (the outer one-third of the fallopian tube) that union of the sperm and egg occurs. This is known as fertilization, and it produces a zygote. The zygote continues to progress by dividing over and over again. After approximately 7 days, the zygote will implant itself into the wall of the uterus. In 7 weeks, the zygote becomes known as an embryo and is receiving nutrients and oxygen through its umbilical cord from the placenta. At 2 months, the embryo becomes known as a fetus; and even though it is only the size of a walnut, all of the organs of a new human being are developing. The fetus will continue to grow and develop for a total of 9 months, at which time the mother will deliver the fetus (infant).

THE MALE REPRODUCTIVE SYSTEM

The primary function of the male reproductive system is to produce sperm cells (spermatozoa). Therefore, the primary organs of the male reproductive system are the testes. This is where sperm cells are formed. There are organs in the male reproductive system referred to as accessory organs. The epididymides serve as storage for sperm cells. The vas deferens, ejaculatory ducts, and urethra convey sperm cells to the outside of the body. Structures that aid the survival of sperm cells are: The seminal vesicles, the prostate gland, and the bulbourethral glands. These structures secrete fluids that help the survival of sperm cells. There are two external reproductive organs in the male, the testes, which are located in the scrotum.

DISEASES/DISORDERS OF THE MALE REPRODUCTIVE SYSTEM INCLUDE

Epididymitis

This condition is characterized by inflammation of the epididymis, a small, oblong structure located on and beside the posterior surface of the testes. The epididymis is a system of ductules that hold sperm for maturation. It is continuous with the vas deferens.

Erectile Dysfunction

This disorder is characterized by the inability of a male to develop or maintain an erection sufficient for penetrative sexual intercourse.

Hydrocele

The accumulation of serous fluid in the tunica vaginalis that surrounds the testes is known as a hydrocele.

Infertility

The inability or diminished ability to produce offspring is known as infertility. Infertility may be due to conditions such as substance abuse, infection, endocrine dysfunction, varicocele, and anomalies of the reproductive system.

Orchitis

This disorder is associated with inflammation of the testes. Orchitis may occur following a bacterial or viral infection such as the mumps.

Spermatocele

A spermatocele is a firm, painless cyst located in the epididymis. These cysts are typically removed surgically.

Testicular Cancer

Testicular cancers are tumors found in males typically between the ages of 20 and 40 years of age.

Varicocele

The dilation of the veins that drain the testes is known as a varicocele. This condition is associated with infertility.

GYNECOLOGICAL DISEASES/DISORDERS OF THE FEMALE REPRODUCTIVE SYSTEM INCLUDE

Benign Ovarian Tumors (Fibroids)

Fibroids are the most common benign tumor found in the female reproductive tract. The cysts themselves are painless; however, pain does occur where infection is involved or if twisting of the pedicle (the stem of a growth) occurs.

Cervical Cancer

The progression from normal cervical cells to dysplasia (abnormal development of tissue) and then to cancer may be related to repeated injuries to the cervix. Smoking is also associated with cervical cancer.

Cervical Polyps

Cervical polyps are best defined as fibrous or mucous tumors of the cervical mucosa. A polyp has a pedicle (stem) from which it grows. Where there is a possibility of polyps becoming cancerous, they should be removed.

Dysmenorrhea

Dysmenorrhea is best defined as pain (cramping) during menstruation. It is among the most frequent gynecological disorders. Approximately 50% of women experience this condition.

Endometriosis

Endometriosis occurs when endometrial tissue is present outside the endometrial cavity. Frequent locations are in or near the ovaries and the fallopian tubes. The pain associated with this condition can be incapacitating. This condition is also associated with infertility.

Infertility

Infertility is the inability or diminished ability to become pregnant after a minimum of 1 year of regular intercourse without contraceptives.

Pelvic Inflammatory Disease (PID)

Infection of the uterus, fallopian tubes, and surrounding pelvic structures that is not associated with surgery or pregnancy is known as pelvic inflammatory disease (PID). The condition is usually ascending, and the infection is spread from the vagina upward to the upper reproductive tract.

Vulvovaginitis

Vulvovaginitis is the simultaneous inflammation of the vulva and vagina, or of the vulvovaginal glands. This condition may be due to chemical irritation by medications, tight-fitting, nonabsorbent underclothing, poor perineal hygiene, and possibly by allergic reactions.

PREGNANCY-RELATED DISEASES/DISORDERS OF THE FEMALE REPRODUCTIVE SYSTEM INCLUDE

Abortion

Abortion is defined as the termination of pregnancy before the fetus reaches the point of viability. Symptoms include: Abdominal cramps, bleeding from the vagina (clots and pieces of tissue). Etiology includes: Faulty development of the embryo or placenta, endocrine imbalance, and infection. Approximately 50% of early abortions are associated with chromosomal disorders.

Abruptio Placenta

This condition constitutes a sudden untimely break-off or detachment of the placenta from the uterine wall. This is an emergency situation that threatens the lives of the mother and fetus.

Ectopic Pregnancy

Gestation (the development of a fetus) that occurs somewhere other than in the uterus is known as ectopic pregnancy. Within the fallopian tubes or within the peritoneal cavity are common sites.

Pregnancy-Induced Hypertension (PIH)

PIH is a complication of pregnancy associated with increasing hypertension, proteinuria, and edema. (PIH) occurs most typically in the last trimester.

Puerperal Infection

This condition is also known as puerperal fever and is the development of septicemia (the presence of pathogenic microorganisms in the blood) following childbirth.

BREAST-RELATED DISEASES/DISORDERS OF THE FEMALE REPRODUCTIVE SYSTEM INCLUDE

Galactorrhea

This condition is associated with continuation of milk secretions after breastfeeding has been discontinued. Galactorrhea is also associated with excessive secretions of milk.

Mastitis

Inflammation of the breast is known as mastitis. This condition occurs most often during breastfeeding in the second or third postpartum week. The usual cause of infection is introduction of disease-causing microorganisms through the nipple.

Practice Test 9

Questions

9 - 1

Should your pregnant client have an increase in femoral venous pressure, your assessment would most likely reveal:

1. varicose veins.
2. urinary frequency.
3. pain in the calf of the leg upon dorsal flexion of the foot when the leg is extended.
4. relatively painless contractions of the uterus that are not associated with labor.

9 - 2

Your client has just experienced a radical mastectomy. Which instruction should be given to the client to help to avoid complications associated with lymphedema?

1. Wear a tight elastic wrap on your arm during the day.
2. Keep your arm as immobile as possible.
3. Avoid any exposure to sunlight on your arm.
4. Gradually increase your arm's exercise, but avoid heavy lifting.

9 - 3

Your client says she felt a gush of fluid from her vagina. After determining that the client's membranes have ruptured, your first action would be to:

1. clean the client and provide a dry gown.
2. assist the client to the bathroom and help her clean up.
3. assess fetal heart tones.
4. assess maternal vital signs.

9 - 4

A 41-week gravida III comes to the labor and delivery unit crying and holding her abdomen. She has been having contractions for 8 hours at home with pain in her lower back. On palpation, her contractions are very intense and 5 minutes apart, but she is only dilated 2 cm. The physician prescribes intravenous oxytocin to:

1. increase duration of contractions.
2. increase resting tone.
3. decrease intensity of contractions.
4. increase uterine activity.

9 - 5

You are preparing a client in her twenty-third week of gestation for an amniocentesis during her next scheduled clinic appointment. You inform the client that prior to the amniocentesis, she should:

1. refrain from eating.
2. take an enema.
3. empty the bladder.
4. cleanse the abdomen.

9 - 6

Your client reaches 4 cm dilatation and asks for an epidural. Following administration of an epidural, the nurse will assess the client for the common side effect of:

1. hypotension.
2. hypertension.
3. headache.
4. dyspnea.

9 - 7

Upon reviewing the laboratory results of a client in her thirty-second week of pregnancy, you observe the hemoglobin to be 11.6 g/dl. Her pre-pregnancy hemoglobin is 13.6 g/dl. You know the decrease in the client's hemoglobin has occurred because:

1. the placenta destroys many maternal blood cells.
2. insidious blood loss is occurring.
3. the stress of pregnancy has probably caused a gastric ulcer to form.
4. the pregnant woman's plasma volume has increased, but the number of her red blood cells is probably the same.

9 - 8

The most typical sign of primary syphilis is:

1. painful, clustered vesicles on the genitalia.
2. rash and flu-like symptoms.
3. cardiovascular involvement.
4. painless chancre on the genitalia.

9 - 9

Your client's contractions are 5 to 7 minutes apart, she is dilated 2 cm, and the baby is at −1 station. This means the presenting part is:

1. 1 cm below the ischial spine.
2. in the pelvic outlet.
3. at the level of the ischial spine.
4. moving into the mid-pelvis.

9 - 10

Women who have had panhysterectomies, which include removal of both ovaries, may be encouraged to take:

1. estrogen.
2. calcium.
3. progesterone.
4. vitamin B_{12} by injection.

9 - 11

A pregnant client has chlamydia. The nurse will teach the client that:

1. chlamydia is not a sexually transmitted disease.
2. persons with chlamydia are carriers of the disease throughout their lives.
3. chlamydia is treated with antiviral medications.
4. the treatment of choice for chlamydia is erythromycin 250 mg po q 6 hours.

9 - 12

A client had a vasectomy at a local clinic. You are reviewing postoperative home care instructions with the client and his wife. Which of the following comments by the client's wife would indicate the need for a review of basic information regarding a post-operative vasectomy?

1. "I'm glad I didn't throw out your old athletic support."
2. "Having so much football on TV this week should help. He can rest on the couch and watch TV."
3. "It's lucky that golf tournament he wanted to play in is two weeks away. Maybe he won't have to miss it."
4. "Talk about nice timing. I just finished my last pack of birth control pills."

9 - 1 3

A client in her thirty-sixth week of gestation has premature rupture of the amniotic membranes. The nurse will give priority to which goal?

1. helping the client remain free of infection.
2. reaching the client's lecithin/sphingomyelin (L/S) ration of 2:1.
3. helping the client demonstrate effective coping abilities.
4. helping the client remain free of discomfort.

9 - 1 4

A client's Papanicolaou smear indicated the presence of dysplasia. You explain to the client that this indicates:

1. a decrease in the size or number of cells.
2. an increase in the size of cells.
3. an increase in the number of cells.
4. a change in the size, shape, and appearance of cells.

9 - 1 5

A client had a dilatation and curettage (D and C) under general anesthesia. The results of blood work drawn during surgery include a red blood count of 2,500,000 per cu/mm of blood. Which action should the nurse take?

1. Notify the nurse in charge about laboratory results.
2. Force fluids to 2000 cc per 24 hours.
3. Encourage the client to rest as much as possible.
4. Continue with the client's established plan of care.

9 - 1 6

Screening tests for cancer such as the Papanicolaou test or mammogram are considered to be which form of intervention?

1. acute
2. primary
3. secondary
4. tertiary

9 - 1 7

A 46-year-old male who has just had a routine pre-employment physical had the following laboratory results. Which laboratory finding warrants further and prompt investigation?

1. hemoglobin (Hgb) 14.8 g/dl
2. white blood count 7500/cm^3
3. prostate-specific antigen 19.6 ng/ml
4. bilirubin 0.6 mg/dl

9 - 1 8

Which of the following doses of ethinyl estradiol would be most appropriate to start with for an 18-year-old female experiencing dysmenorrhea?

1. 5 mcg
2. 35 mcg
3. 65 mcg
4. 5 mg

9-19

A postmenopausal client with no surgical history inquires about the benefits of taking daily estrogen versus an estrogen and progesterone combination. You know the reason for the combination is:

1. fertility is maintained with the combination.
2. estrogen alone will cause hirsutism and acne.
3. regular menstrual cycles resume with combination therapy.
4. progesterone will prevent hyper-proliferation of the uterus.

9-20

Which of the following is the most common cause of secondary amenorrhea?

1. gonadal dysgenesis
2. imperforate hymen
3. anorexia nervosa
4. pregnancy

9-21

The nurse has been teaching a prenatal client pelvic-tilt exercises. This intervention can be considered effective if the client experiences a decrease in:

1. leg cramps.
2. backaches.
3. hemorrhoids.
4. constipation.

9-22

You are teaching the mother of a term newborn how to care for the infant. Which statement made by the mother indicates a need for further teaching?

1. "My baby may have dark, tarry looking stools for a few days."
2. "My baby may have some peeling of the hands and feet."
3. "Diaper rash may be prevented by using protective ointments."
4. "I should hold and talk to my baby during feeding."

9-23

Which hormone is responsible for the ejection of breast milk?

1. oxytocin
2. follicle-stimulating hormone
3. glucagon
4. thyrotropin

9-24

Which of the following conditions would most likely be the cause of infertility in the adult male?

1. pertussis
2. mumps
3. varicella
4. pneumonia

9-25

Which manifestation is not an indication for a hysterectomy?

1. uterine prolapse repair
2. dysfunctional uterine bleeding
3. sterilization
4. uterine cancer

9-26

Postmenopausal hormone replacement therapy has which of the following effects on both high-density lipoprotein (HDL) and low-density lipoprotein (LDL)?

1. Hormone replacement therapy has an increase in HDL and decrease in LDL.
2. Hormone replacement therapy has an increase in HDL and increase in LDL.
3. Hormone replacement therapy has a decrease in HDL and decrease in LDL.
4. Hormone replacement therapy has a decrease in HDL and increase in LDL.

9-27

Which finding would interfere the most with the continuation of a pregnancy?

1. an increase in human chorionic gonadotropin
2. an increase in follicle-stimulating hormone
3. a decrease in alpha-fetoprotein
4. a decrease in progesterone

9-28

Teaching a client arm-strengthening exercises during the postmastectomy period is considered which of the following forms of intervention?

1. acute
2. primary
3. secondary
4. tertiary

9-29

A client at 12 weeks gestation has hyperemesis gravidarum. Which assessment will provide the most relevant information about the client's condition?

1. intake and output
2. fetal heart rate
3. activity level
4. emotional state

9-30

A client with genital herpes has been instructed concerning methods that will prevent transmission of that condition. Upon entering the client's room, the nurse observes the client's friend coming out of the bathroom. Which action would be essential for the nurse to take first?

1. Report the incident to the nurse in charge.
2. Record the incident in the nurses' notes.
3. Reinforce precaution instructions to the client and the client's friend.
4. Discuss precaution instructions with the client after the friend leaves.

9-31

A client is scheduled for a dilatation and curettage (D and C). Preoperative prescriptions include secobarbital po at bedtime. In addition to promoting sleep, the nurse understands that secobarbital is given to:

1. reduce the client's anxiety level.
2. lessen bronchial secretions.
3. decrease the muscle tone of the uterus.
4. minimize the need for postoperative analgesia.

9 - 3 2

A client with placenta previa had a cesarean section performed under spinal block anesthesia. A 4-pound (1814 g) infant was delivered and placed in an incubator in the premature nursery. Which action should be given priority when planning the client's postoperative care?

1. Instruct the client to lie flat in the bed for at least 6 hours.
2. Allow the client to see the infant as soon as possible.
3. Record the client's intake and output.
4. Assess for muscle fatigue.

9 - 3 3

A client who has recently experienced menopause approaches the nurse and says, "I want to continue breast self-examination but I don't know when to examine my breasts, since I am no longer having my period." Your best response would include the following information:

1. "It is no longer necessary to perform breast self-examination since you are not menstruating."
2. "You should perform breast self-examination on the first day of every month."
3. "You can examine your breasts on any day of the month, since you are no longer menstruating."
4. "You should select a day of the month and consistently perform breast self-examination on that date every month."

9 - 3 4

The nurse is caring for a client in a postpartum clinic. Which manifestations would indicate the presence of an abnormality?

1. a chill shortly after delivery
2. a pulse rate of 60 the morning after delivery
3. a urinary output of 3000 ml the second day after delivery
4. an oral temperature of 101°F the third day after delivery

9 - 3 5

Your client was hospitalized with a suspected incomplete abortion. She has abdominal pain and a moderate amount of vaginal bleeding. Which action would be most important to include in the client's nursing-care plan?

1. restriction of food and fluids
2. observation of amount and type of vaginal bleeding
3. instructions on birth control methods
4. limitation of activity until pain and bleeding cease

9 - 3 6

A client with a third-degree episiotomy and hemorrhoids is concerned that she might become constipated. You will advise the client to:

1. eat fruit with each meal.
2. increase intake of drinks with caffeine.
3. decrease intake of high-protein foods.
4. increase dairy product intake.

9-37

A 56-year-old client is on low-dose estrogen therapy to manage osteoporosis. Which of the following statements reflects the nurse's knowledge of the complications of estrogen replacement therapy?

1. The client needs to use contraceptives to avoid pregnancy.
2. The client needs to call her physician if she experiences any breathing difficulties.
3. It is important for the client to have regular gynecological checkups.
4. The client may need to consider plastic surgery for varicosities common with estrogen therapy.

9-38

A client in her twelfth week of gestation calls the physician's office and tells the nurse that she just had an episode of bleeding. The nurse determines that the client had a moderate amount of reddish-brown mucous discharge. Which action should the nurse take first?

1. Determine if the client has transportation and recommend that she see the physician.
2. Assure the client she has nothing to worry about and suggest she call if the bleeding gets worse.
3. Ask the client to lie down for an hour and then call to report what happens with the bleeding.
4. Tell the client that it sounds as though she has been too active and suggest she rest more throughout her pregnancy.

9-39

A mother is bottle-feeding her baby. On the third day postpartum, she develops engorgement in both breasts. The nurse should advise the mother to:

1. apply warm compresses to her breasts.
2. use an electric breast pump to empty her breasts.
3. apply a tight binder and ice packs to her breasts.
4. manually express the milk while taking a warm shower.

9-40

A 24-year-old gravida I with a history of mitral valve prolapse presents for delivery. Because of the rapid fluid shift that takes place following the delivery, the nurse would carefully observe for symptoms of:

1. endocarditis.
2. pulmonary embolism.
3. congestive heart failure.
4. pregnancy-induced hypertension.

9-41

A client with severe preeclampsia has been placed on the external fetal monitor. Moderate uterine contractions are occurring every 5 minutes, 50 to 60 seconds in duration. In view of the client's preeclampsia, which of the following should the nurse recognize as an ominous sign that must be monitored closely?

1. severe epigastric pain
2. urinary output of 60 cc per hour
3. 1+ protein in the urine
4. facial edema

9 - 4 2

A mother had a cesarean section and was transferred to the postpartum unit from the recovery room. Postpartum nursing management of this client includes administration of bromocriptine mesylate. The nurse should expect that this medication was prescribed to:

1. promote sodium retention.
2. suppress the production of chorionic gonadotropin.
3. inhibit secretion of the lactogenic hormone.
4. diminish lochial flow.

9 - 4 3

A client in her eighth month of pregnancy has been hospitalized with preeclampsia. One morning she tells the nurse she thinks her contractions are beginning. Which of the following approaches should the nurse use to fully assess the presence of uterine contractions?

1. Place the hands on opposite sides of the upper part of the abdomen and curve them somewhat around the uterine fundus.
2. Place the heel of the hand on the abdomen just above the umbilicus and press firmly.
3. Place the hand flat on the abdomen over the uterine fundus, with the fingers apart, pressing slightly.
4. Place the hand in the middle of the upper abdomen and then move the hand several times to different parts of the abdomen.

9 - 4 4

Your client has missed one menstrual period and comes to the physician's office for a pregnancy test. The client's pregnancy test is positive. You recognize this as a:

1. presumptive sign.
2. probable sign.
3. diagnostic sign.
4. subjective sign.

9 - 4 5

A 16-year-old high school student attends the antepartal clinic on a regular basis. She is a gravida I at 28 weeks gestation. The nurse assesses her to determine if she is retaining abnormal amounts of fluid. Which of the following findings would be indicative of a nursing diagnosis of alteration in fluid volume, excess?

1. She has gained 3 lbs (1361 g) during the past week.
2. She has gained 4.5 lbs (2041 g) over the past month.
3. She has gained 11 lbs (4990 g) in the second trimester of pregnancy.
4. She has gained 14 lbs (6350 g) since the onset of pregnancy.

9 - 4 6

A primigravida in her thirty-sixth week of gestation comes to the emergency department. The client is experiencing profuse painless vaginal bleeding. The primary nursing diagnosis at this time would be:

1. fear related to personal safety and safety of the fetus.
2. potential preterm delivery related to vaginal bleeding.
3. potential for infection related to loss of mucus plug.
4. altered tissue perfusion secondary to excessive blood loss.

9 - 4 7

Your client is 4 hours post cesarean section. Her vital signs are stable and she is receiving intravenous therapy. Interventions for the nursing diagnosis of altered perfusion related to excessive blood loss would include:

1. turn, cough, and deep breathe every 2 hours.
2. evaluate firmness and position of fundus.
3. administer analgesic medications.
4. massage uterus every 30 minutes.

9 - 4 8

Which of the following responses by the nurse reflects an understanding of the couvade syndrome, Mitleiden, or "suffering along" often experienced by expectant fathers?

1. "The symptoms that are felt will increase throughout the wife's pregnancy."
2. "Some men actually believe they are pregnant."
3. "Many expectant fathers have physical symptoms associated with their partner's pregnancy."
4. "You are getting an example of what happens to a pregnant woman."

9 - 4 9

A 19-year-old female is sexually active and has requested a prescription for the contraceptive Depo-Provera from her physician. You know this drug:

1. will need to be injected every ninety days.
2. should only be given to post-menopausal women.
3. can provide infertility for up to two years following the first injection.
4. is not a very reliable contraceptive.

9 - 5 0

Which instructions should the nurse plan to include when teaching a client how to perform perineal exercises?

1. "Press your knees against the mattress."
2. "Bear down using your abdominal muscles."
3. "Flex the muscles of your lower extremities."
4. "Tighten the muscles of your buttocks."

9 - 5 1

A newly married client wants to know how to prevent pregnancy by using the rhythm method. You teach her that pregnancy may be avoided by refraining from sexual intercourse around the time of ovulation. Ovulation usually occurs:

1. during the menstrual cycle.
2. 2 days after cessation of the menstrual cycle.
3. approximately 14 days after the start of the menstrual cycle.
4. immediately before the menstrual cycle begins.

9 - 5 2

Your male client is sexually impotent. You know that impotence may occur as a consequence of:

Select all that apply by placing a ✔ in the square:

❑ 1. inadequate blood flow to the penis.
❑ 2. side effects of drug therapy.
❑ 3. hypotension.
❑ 4. aging.
❑ 5. insufficient testosterone.

9 - 5 3

You are instructing a client who has received a penile implant about the care of the implant. You know he has a correct understanding if he says:

Select all that apply by placing a ✔ in the square:

- ❑ 1. "I will wear tight-fitting underwear."
- ❑ 2. "I will avoid contact sports."
- ❑ 3. "I will avoid lifting anything heavy for at least 3 weeks."
- ❑ 4. "I will report any persistent pain or swelling."
- ❑ 5. "I will abstain from sex for 2 weeks."

9 - 5 4

Should your client have testicular cancer, you would expect your assessment to reveal:

Select all that apply by placing a ✔ in the square:

- ❑ 1. a testicular lump that is soft.
- ❑ 2. an increase in the size of one testicle.
- ❑ 3. a feeling of heaviness in the scrotum.
- ❑ 4. a sharp pain in the groin or above the penis.
- ❑ 5. a heightened sensitivity to testicular pressure.

9 - 5 5

You are instructing a client how to use a condom. You know the client will need additional instruction if he says:

Select all that apply by placing a ✔ in the square:

- ❑ 1. "I will choose condoms that are lubricated with silicone."
- ❑ 2. "I will store my condoms in a cool, dry place."
- ❑ 3. "I will dispose of my condoms in a lined container."
- ❑ 4. "I will use a new condom each time I have sex."
- ❑ 5. "I will discard condoms that are over 7 years old."

Practice Test 9

Answers, Rationales, and Explanations

9 - 1

① Your assessment would most likely reveal varicose veins. Clients who are pregnant may have an increase in femoral venous pressure. An increase in femoral pressure will distend the veins and could cause varicose veins. Increased circulating volume and hormonal relaxation of the blood vessel walls contribute to vascular wall distention and elevated venous stasis or varicosities.

2. An increase in femoral pressure does not put pressure on the bladder.

3. Pain in the calf of the leg upon dorsal flexion of the foot when the leg is extended is known as Homans' sign. A positive Homans' sign is suggestive of venous thrombosis but may also be associated with conditions other than thrombosis. Also, absence of calf pain does not rule out thrombosis.

4. Braxton-Hicks contractions are painless and irregular. They may occur throughout pregnancy and may enhance placental blood flow.

Client Need: Health Promotion and Maintenance

9 - 2

④ Clients experiencing a radical mastectomy should gradually increase arm exercises. In addition to removal of the breast tissue, the axillary lymph nodes and some lymph channels are removed during a radical mastectomy. In order to promote the circulation of lymph in the compromised lymph system, moderate range of motion and exercise should be encouraged. Actions that compromise the circulation of lymph include lifting heavy objects and using a tight grip, such as the grip used to open a jar.

1 and 2. Compression and immobility tend to decrease, not increase, circulation to the affected area and would therefore be contraindicated.

3. There is no positive correlation between moderate exposure to light and compromise of lymph circulation.

Client Need: Physiological Integrity

9 - 3

③ **The nurse will assess the fetal heart tones to ensure that the umbilical cord has not pro-lapsed and compromised the fetus.**

1. The client can be cleaned up after determining fetal well-being.
2. Once the amniotic sac has ruptured, the mother should remain in bed to prevent the possibility of a prolapsed umbilical cord.
4. The maternal vital signs would be assessed after the fetal heart tones have been evaluated. Once the amniotic sac ruptures, it is the fetus, not the mother, who could be compromised.

Client Need: Health Promotion and Maintenance

9 - 4

④ **The physician prescribed oxytocin (Pitocin) intravenously to increase uterine activity and promote more effective contractions. The client is experiencing dystocia (ineffective uterine contractions) caused by dysfunctional labor.**

1. The problem is not duration of the client's contractions but the fact that the contractions are ineffective.
2. The frequency of the client's contractions is every 5 minutes. This suggests that there is enough resting tone between contractions for the uterus to relax and the placenta to be perfused. What is needed is increased uterine activity.
3. Oxytocin was prescribed to increase uterine activity, not decrease intensity of contractions.

Client Need: Physiological Integrity

9 - 5

③ **You will instruct the client to empty her bladder prior to the amniocentesis. Since the bladder lies in the anterior pelvic cavity, it should be emptied prior to the amniocentesis to prevent possible puncture or displacement of the uterine cavity and fetus. An amnio-centesis involves inserting a needle through the maternal abdomen and into the uterine cavity to collect a sample of amniotic fluid.**

1. It is not necessary to be npo for an amniocentesis. The procedure is performed using a local anesthetic.
2. It is not necessary to have an enema. The gastrointestinal tract is not involved.
4. The client will not need to cleanse her abdomen. The nurse will prep the abdomen with a cleansing agent immediately before the procedure.

Client Need: Safe, Effective Care Environment

9 - 6

① Following the administration of an epidural, the most common side effect is hypotension due to diminished vasomotor tone. During the post-block phase, the nurse will closely monitor the mother's cardiovascular and ventilatory integrity.

2. Hypotension, not hypertension, is the most common side effect.

3. Headaches will not occur because the epidural is in the dural space.

4. Some difficulty in breathing could occur, but this is not a common side effect.

Client Need: Physiological Integrity

9 - 7

④ A normal occurrence during pregnancy is an increase in plasma volume. As a result, a physiologic anemia occurs. A physiologic anemia is due to an increase in plasma volume, not a decrease in red blood cells. The opposite may be true of dehydrated clients; they may have elevated hemoglobin due to hemoconcentration.

1. The placenta does not destroy maternal red blood cells.

2. Blood loss is both uncommon and untoward during pregnancy.

3. Gastric ulcers are not known to occur due to the stress of pregnancy, although heartburn and reflux are common complaints.

Client Need: Health Promotion and Maintenance

9 - 8

④ The most typical sign of primary syphilis is a painless chancre on the genitalia. Syphilis is characterized by three distinct stages. Primary syphilis usually presents itself with a painless chancre on the genitalia, which may go unnoticed. Secondary syphilis is often flu-like in nature, involving generalized fatigue, rash, and fever. Latent syphilis, which may not present itself for years, involves the whole body and may present with confusion, muscle weakness, and cardiovascular involvement.

1. Primary syphilis usually presents with a painless chancre on the genitalia.

2. The rash and flu-like symptoms are more common to secondary syphilis.

3. The neurological and cardiovascular involvement of this disease is usually seen during the latent phase.

Client Need: Physiological Integrity

9 - 9

④   **When the presenting part is at the -1 station, the fetus is said to be moving from the pelvic inlet to the mid-pelvis.**

1.   The ischial spine would be zero station.

2.   If the fetus were in the pelvic outlet, the station would be positive.

3.   Since the fetus is at -1 station, it is actually 1 cm above the ischial spine.

Client Need: Physiological Integrity

9 - 1 0

①   **Women who have had panhysterectomies, including removal of both ovaries, are often encouraged to take estrogen. The decision to provide hormone replacement therapy (HRT) or estrogen with progestin is made on an individual basis. Estrogen is produced and secreted by the ovaries. A woman who has had a panhysterectomy may be encouraged to take HRT because it may help to maintain bone density and decrease certain cardiac risk factors.**

2 and 4. Calcium and vitamin B_{12} levels are not directly associated with ovarian function.

3.   Progesterone is important in preventing hyperproliferation of the uterus and in the onset of menses. In the absence of a uterus, this role wouldn't be applicable.

Client Need: Health Promotion and Maintenance

9 - 1 1

④   **The treatment of choice for pregnant women with chlamydia is erythromycin (Erythrozone) 250 mg po q 6 hours for 7 days. Chlamydia is a sexually transmitted disease caused by the bacterium *Chlamydia trachomatis*. It is highly contagious.**

1.   The nurse should teach the client that chlamydia is a sexually transmitted disease.

2.   Chlamydia can be treated successfully. People who have chlamydia and are treated effectively are not carriers of the disease.

3.   Chlamydia is not caused by a virus. It is caused by the bacterium *Clamydia trachomatis* and is treated by anti-infectives.

Client Need: Physiological Integrity

9 - 1 2

④ **The client's wife needs a basic review regarding postoperative home care for a vasectomy. Sperm remain in the semen beyond the point of occlusion of the vas deferens and only gradually disappear from the ejaculate. An alternate method of contraception should be used until semen analysis confirms absence of sperm from the ejaculate. It usually takes 15 to 20 ejaculations or 4 to 6 weeks before all sperm are removed from the proximal portions of the sperm ducts.**

1. A support for the scrotum is helpful following a vasectomy. Ice packs may also be applied to reduce swelling and relieve discomfort.

2. It is recommended that the client rest a few days following a vasectomy. Lying about on the sofa would probably be beneficial.

3. The client should be able to participate in a golf tournament 2 weeks post-surgically without any problem.

Client Need: Health Promotion and Maintenance

9 - 1 3

① **Keeping the client free from infection is essential, since bacteria may travel upward into the uterus and compromise the well-being of the fetus. Because of the break in the surface of the amniotic membranes, the client will be at risk for infection.**

2. At 35 weeks gestation, the lecithin/sphingomyelin (L/S) ratio should have already reached 2:1. Therefore, the (L/S) ratio will not be a consideration.

3. It is important for the client to cope effectively. However, keeping the mother and fetus free from infection is the primary goal.

4. Premature rupture of the amniotic membranes does not produce pain.

Client Need: Safe, Effective Care Environment

9 - 1 4

④ **You explain that dysplasia is bizarre cell growth that results in cells that differ in size, shape, and appearance from other cells of the same tissue.**

1 Atrophy is a decrease in the size or number of cells. It primarily affects skeletal muscle and secondary sex organs.

2. Hypertrophy is an increase in the size of cells and hence the size of the organs they form.

3. Hyperplasia is an increase in the number of cells in an organ or tissue. As the cells multiply, volume increases.

Client Need: Physiological Integrity

9 - 1 5

① The nurse should notify the nurse in charge. The normal range for red blood cells in a healthy adult female is 4,500,000 to 5,000,000 cu/mm. Since 2,500,000 is significantly lower than normal, this must be brought to the attention of the nurse in charge so further instructions for care may be obtained.

2. Forcing fluids may increase the client's circulating fluid volume, but the client needs the oxygen-carrying capacity of the red blood cells. Also, increasing fluids under the circumstances could cause nausea, vomiting, and possible aspiration.

3. Rest alone will not increase the number of red blood cells needed to prevent the development of hemorrhagic shock.

4. The plan of care should be modified to meet the client's immediate needs.

Client Need: Physiological Integrity

9 - 1 6

③ Secondary interventions are those that diagnose and treat illness. Because screening tests like the Papanicolaou (pap) test are done specifically to diagnose an illness and have no action in preventing the illness from occurring, they are considered to be secondary interventions.

1. Acute interventions are those that act immediately on a disease process.

2. Primary interventions, such as immunizations or wellness teaching, prevent disease.

4. Tertiary interventions, such as cardiac rehabilitation, are those that help in the recovery process.

Client Need: Physiological Integrity

9 - 1 7

③ Prostate specific antigen of 19.6 ng/ml would warrant prompt investigation. Prostate specific antigen (PSA) is a protease secreted by the prostate gland only. Serum PSA levels above 10 ng/ml are considered abnormally elevated. Elevations may be due to conditions such as benign prostatic hypertrophy, or may be due to a tumor in the prostate.

1. A hemoglobin of 14.8 g/dl is within the normal range for men (range is 14 to 18 g/dl).

2. A white blood cell count of 7,500/cm^3 is within the normal range (range is 5,000 to 10,000 cm^3).

4. A bilirubin of 0.6 mg/dl is within the normal range (range is 0.1 to 1.0 mg/dl).

Client Need: Physiological Integrity

9 - 1 8

② Ethinyl estradiol is a synthetic estrogen and a major component of most oral contraceptives presently on the market. The dosage of the pill is usually 35 mcg to 50 mcg. A young client usually is started on the smaller dose, and then the dose is increased as necessary.

1 and 3. There is no commonly marketed birth control pill containing 5 mcg or 65 mcg of ethinyl estradiol.

4. 5 mg represents 5,000 mcg, a grossly excessive dosage.

Client Need: Safe, Effective Care Environment

9 - 1 9

④ Progesterone will prevent hyperproliferation of the uterus. Estrogen hormone replacement therapy alone may cause hyperproliferation of the uterus, which increases the risk of uterine cancer markedly. As a general rule, only women without uteruses may take estrogen alone as their postmenopausal hormone replacement.

1. The intent of postmenopausal hormone replacement is not to resume fertility, but for cardiac protection and orthopedic benefits.

2. Estrogen therapy is not related to hirsutism and acne (the androgen hormones are).

3. Regular menstrual cycles do not resume with the combination therapy. That is more likely to occur with estrogen alone.

Client Need: Physiological Integrity

9 - 2 0

④ The most common cause of secondary amenorrhea is pregnancy. Secondary amenorrhea is the absence of menses after menstrual cycles have been established. Other causes may include infection, hormonal disturbance, and starvation.

1 and 2. Turner's syndrome (gonadal dysgenesis) and imperforate hymen cause primary amenorrhea (no history of menses).

3. Anorexia nervosa is a cause of secondary amenorrhea, but it is not as common as pregnancy.

Client Need: Physiological Integrity

9 - 21

② Pelvic-tilt exercises can be beneficial in preventing or relieving backaches in the pregnant woman. In the nonpregnant woman, pelvic tilting is useful in relieving menstrual cramps.

1. Leg cramps may be prevented or relieved by dorsiflexion and the plantar flexion of the foot in combination with ankle rotation.

3 and 4. To prevent or minimize hemorrhoids, one should avoid constipation by maintaining regular bowel habits, drinking plenty of fluids, and providing fiber in the diet.

Client Need: Physiological integrity

9 - 22

① A newborn should not have dark, tarry-looking stools for several days. Meconium stools usually last from 12 to 24 hours. The first meconium passed is sterile, but within hours, all meconium contains bacteria. The first passage occurs within 24 hours in 90% of normal infants.

2. Some peeling of the hands and feet is common in term newborns. However, thick, cracking, parchment-like skin is characteristic of the post-term newborn. The skin of the preterm newborn is smooth and thin enough to visualize blood vessels.

3. Diaper rash may be prevented by using protective ointment.

4. The infant should be held and "talked to" when feeding. This will promote socialization.

Client Need: Health Promotion and Maintenance

9 - 23

① The hormone responsible for the ejection of breast milk is oxytocin. Oxytocin is secreted by the pituitary gland and is responsible for the ejection of breast milk and contractions of the uterus. Prolactin, also secreted by the pituitary gland, plays a role in milk secretion.

2. Follicle-stimulating hormone (FSH) is responsible for the secretion of estrogen.

3. Glucagon increases blood sugar.

4. Thyrotropin stimulates the thyroid gland.

Client Need: Health Promotion and Maintenance

9 - 2 4

---

② The most likely cause of infertility in the male is mumps. Men who contract mumps during adulthood have a higher incidence of sterility. Mumps is a viral infection that typically affects the salivary glands (hence the classic swollen jaws associated with this disease). Its complications include central nervous system involvement, kidney infection, pancreas infection, and infection of the testicles.

1, 3, and 4. Neither pertussis (whooping cough), varicella (chickenpox), nor pneumonia is directly associated with male sterility.

Client Need: Physiological Integrity

9 - 2 5

---

③ Sterilization may be accomplished by hysterectomy, but it is not an indication for hysterectomy in the absence of pathology. The most appropriate surgical sterilization procedure for the female client is tubal ligation. Tubal ligation is a less extensive surgery and has a lower morbidity and mortality rate than hysterectomy.

1, 2, and 4. The removal of the uterus may be indicated in the instance of extreme uterine prolapse; dysfunctional uterine bleeding that doesn't respond to pharmacological measures; and uterine cancer.

Client Need: Physiological Integrity

9 - 2 6

---

① Estrogen replacement affects how the body metabolizes fats. High-density lipoproteins increase and low-density lipoproteins decrease. The overall effect is that the risk of heart disease may be decreased in postmenopausal women who are on hormone replacement.

2, 3, and 4. Hormone replacement therapy tends to increase HDL levels and decrease LDL levels.

Client Need: Health Promotion and Maintenance

9 - 2 7

---

④ A decrease in progesterone would interfere the most with the continuation of a pregnancy. Progesterone is needed to maintain a pregnancy.

1. Human chorionic gonadotropin (HGG) is a hormone of pregnancy and will increase.
2. Follicle-stimulating hormone (FSH) will increase.
3. A decrease in alpha-fetoprotein (AFP) may indicate a problem such as Down syndrome. A decrease in AFP is seen in high-risk pregnancy.

Client Need: Safe, Effective Care Environment

9 - 2 8

④ **Tertiary interventions, such as rehabilitation from a mastectomy, heart attack, or diabetes, are those that help in recovery from an illness or injury.**

1 and 3. Acute and secondary interventions, such as medication administration and screening, are used in the diagnosis and treatment of an illness.

2. Primary interventions, such as immunizations, are those that help to prevent illness.

Client Need: Health Promotion and Maintenance

9 - 2 9

① **Intake and output will provide the most relevant information about the status of a client with hyperemesis gravidarum. Hyperemesis gravidarum is characterized by intractable vomiting during pregnancy. It results in dehydration and electrolyte imbalance.**

2. The fetal heart rate would provide information about the status of the fetus but would not provide any information about the status of the client (mother) with hyperemesis gravidarum.

3 and 4. The activity level and emotional state of the client would provide some information about how the client is feeling generally, but it would not indicate the status of the client as regards hyperemesis gravidarum.

Client Need: Health Promotion and Maintenance

9 - 3 0

③ **The best way to handle the problem is to discuss it with the client and the client's friend. Toilet isolation is one way to prevent the spread of genital herpes.**

1 and 2. Reporting the incident to the nurse in charge and recording it in the client's chart can be done after reinforcing precautions that should be taken to prevent the spread of the client's illness or re-infection of the client.

4. The client's friend needs to be taught what precautions should be taken to prevent the spread of the disease.

Client Need: Safe, Effective Care Environment

9 - 3 1

① Secobarbital is given to reduce the client's anxiety. Secobarbital (Seconal) is a short-acting barbiturate that works as a central nervous system depressant. It is administered to a client scheduled for surgery to produce mild sedation, thus reducing the level of the client's anxiety.

2. Secobarbital (Seconal) is a short-acting barbiturate and does not affect bronchial secretions. Atropine, an anticholinergic, is a medication commonly administered shortly before surgery that decreases oral and respiratory secretions.

3. Secobarbital (Seconal) does not affect uterine muscle tone.

4. The effects of secobarbital (Seconal) will have worn off by the time the client has had the dilatation and curettage (D and C). The onset of po secobarbital (Seconal) is 15 minutes, peak effect 15 to 30 minutes, and the duration is 1 to 4 hours.

Client Need: Physiological Integrity

9 - 3 2

① The client should be instructed to lie flat in bed for at least 6 hours. Spinal anesthesia may cause a headache due to the potential for leakage of the cerebrospinal fluid through the needle tract in the dura. To prevent leakage, the client should remain flat in bed, preferably prone.

2. The client should see her infant as soon as possible. However, this is not a priority at this time.

3. A record of the client's intake and output will be maintained, but this is not the priority at this time.

4. Assessing the client's muscle fatigue is important, but it is not the priority at this time.

Client Need: Physiological Integrity

9 - 3 3

④ Once a woman experiences menopause, she should select a date of the month that is meaningful to her; i.e., her birthday, and consistently, every month, perform breast self-examination (BSF) on that date. All women should begin breast self-examination in adolescence and continue throughout their lives. Breast self-examination is an effective and economical tool in the fight against cancer.

1. All women should perform BSF as adolescents and throughout their lives. Women of all ages have been affected with cancer of the breast and should therefore perform BSF routinely throughout their lives. Experiencing menopause should not interrupt BSF.

2 and 3. The first day of each month, or any date of each month, would be an acceptable time; however, it is recommended that a date that has personal significance be adopted since that date would be easy to remember. Significant dates include birthdays and anniversaries. For example, if a woman was born on the 15th of March, she would perform breast self-examination on the 15th of every month.

Client Need: Health Promotion and Maintenance

9 - 3 4

④　**An oral body temperature of 101°F (38.3°C) on the third postpartal day indicates the probability of puerperal infection (septicemia following childbirth).**

1.　A chill shortly after delivery is not considered pathologic. It is associated with muscle exhaustion, a sudden release of pressure from nerves following the birth of the fetus, and a response to epinephrine, if it is has been administered.

2.　A heart rate of 60 beats per minute the morning after delivery is not abnormal. The reason for this slow pulse rate is thought to be due to the hypervolemia that occurs after birth.

3.　A urinary output of up to 3000 ml per day is normal following the delivery of a baby. This occurs as a consequence of an increase in the glomerular filtration rate and a decrease in progesterone, which has an antidiuretic effect.

Client Need:　Safe, Effective Care Environment

9 - 3 5

②　**The nurse should include in the client's care plan the amount and type of vaginal bleeding. Bleeding may continue and cause severe hemorrhage until all products of conception have been expelled. The number of pads used and the amount and type of drainage should be recorded.**

1.　There is no need to restrict food and fluids. The client needs nourishment and plenty of fluids.

3.　There is no indication that the client is interested in learning about birth control methods.

4.　Limiting the client's activity will be instituted. However, assessing the amount and type of drainage is most important, since severe hemorrhage could occur.

Client Need:　Physiological Integrity

9 - 3 6

①　**The client will be advised to eat fruit with each meal. Fruit will facilitate a normal bowel movement because of its fluid and fiber content.**

2.　Drinks with caffeine would not help to soften the stool and may cause stomach upset, nervousness, irritability, headache, and diarrhea.

3.　Whereas high-protein foods would help in healing the episiotomy, they do not soften stools.

4.　Dairy products contribute to constipation.

Client Need:　Physiological Integrity

9 - 3 7

③ **Women on low-dose estrogen therapy need to have regular gynecological checkups because they are at risk for uterine cancer; however, studies are unclear and further long-term studies are needed.**

1, 2, and 4. Low-dose therapy does not predispose a postmenopausal woman to pregnancy, respiratory difficulties, or varicosities.

Client Need: Health Promotion and Maintenance

9 - 3 8

③ **Many times, bleeding subsides with rest. The client needs to lie down for an hour and then call to report what is happening with the bleeding.**

1. Visiting the physician is unnecessary at this time.
2. Assuring the client there is nothing to worry about is belittling and blocks communication.
4. There is not enough evidence to support the need for bed rest throughout the pregnancy.

Client Need: Physiological Integrity

9 - 3 9

③ **The client should be advised to apply a tight binder and ice packs to the breasts. Management of breast engorgement in the bottle-feeding mother is directed toward comfort measures that do not stimulate further milk production.**

1. Applying warm compresses to the mother's breasts will stimulate further milk production.
2. Using an electric pump to empty her breasts would stimulate further milk production.
4. Manually expressing milk from the mother's breasts while taking a warm shower will stimulate milk production.

Client Need: Health Promotion and Maintenance

9 - 4 0

③ **This 24-year-old gravida I with a history of mitral valve prolapse needs to be observed for congestive heart failure. The rapid shift of fluids following delivery places a great workload on the heart.**

1. Endocarditis refers to the lining membrane of the heart. Endocarditis may be caused by microorganisms or an immune response.
2. Pulmonary embolism refers to an obstruction of the pulmonary artery or one of its branches, usually caused by an embolus from thrombosis in the lower extremities.
4. Pregnancy-induced hypertension (PIH) usually develops late in the second trimester or in the third trimester. The cause is unclear but seems to be associated with prenatal care, age, and parity.

Client Need: Physiological Integrity

9 - 4 1

(1) **The nurse will monitor the client for epigastric pain. Epigastric pain is a late sign in preeclampsia that may precede a seizure. The generalized edema that occurs in preeclampsia can also stretch the liver capsule and cause subcapsular hemorrhage and severe epigastric pain.**

2. Urinary output of 60 cc per hour is within normal limits.

3 and 4. Protein in the urine and facial edema are early signs of preeclampsia.

Client Need: Physiological Integrity

9 - 4 2

(3) **The nurse understands that bromocriptine mesylate (Parlodel) was prescribed to inhibit secretion of the lactogenic hormone. Bromocriptine mesylate (Parlodel) is a dopamine receptor agonist that acts on receptors in the anterior lobe of the pituitary to inhibit secretion of prolactin and interfere with lactogenesis.**

1. Bromocriptine mesylate does not directly affect sodium retention.

2. Bromocriptine mesylate does not suppress the production of chorionic gonadotropin. Chorionic gonadotropins are present in the urine of pregnant women. The detection of gonadotropins serves as a basis for the pregnancy test.

4. Bromocriptine mesylate does not diminish lochial flow (lochia refers to the discharge from the uterus of blood, mucus, and tissue during the puerperal period).

Client Need: Health Promotion and Maintenance

9 - 4 3

(3) **To assess for contractions and for changes in the intensity of contractions, the nurse will place the hand flat on the abdomen, over the fundus with the fingers apart and press lightly. Uterine contractions are initiated in the fundal portion of the uterus.**

1. Placing the hands on the opposite and upper part of the abdomen is an incorrect method for assessing contractions.

2. The heel of the hand is not used to assess contractions.

4. Placing the hands in the middle of the upper abdomen is not the correct way to assess contractions.

Client Need: Health Promotion and Maintenance

9 - 4 4

---

② A positive pregnancy test is a probable sign that is objective because it is a definite indicator of pregnancy but does not constitute diagnosis or confirmation. Other probable signs include enlargement of the abdomen, changes in the cervix, and Braxton-Hicks contractions.

1. Presumptive signs include menstrual suppression, nausea, vomiting, morning sickness, and pigmentation of the skin.

3 and 4. Positive signs and subjective signs are diagnostic and include fetal heart sound, fetal movement felt by the examiner, and roentgenogram outline of fetal skeleton.

Client Need: Physiological Integrity

9 - 4 5

---

① A sudden increase in weight may be indicative of fluid retention. Recommended weight gain in the second and third trimester for a pregnant adolescent is 0.4 kg (1 lb) per week. Because the client is an adolescent, she is at risk for developing preeclampsia. Edema is one of the primary signs of preeclampsia.

2. 4½ lbs over a period of 4 weeks is not excessive.

3. A weight gain of 11 lbs in the second trimester is not excessive. This is a little less than 1 lb per week.

4. A weight gain of 14 lbs since the onset of pregnancy is not excessive. This is about ½ lb per week.

Client Need: Physiological Integrity

9 - 4 6

---

④ The primary nursing diagnosis at this time would be altered tissue perfusion secondary to excessive blood loss. Hemorrhage can be life threatening and is therefore the first priority.

1. The client is probably very concerned about her personal safety and the safety of the fetus. However, the first priority should be placed on interventions that will treat the profuse bleeding that could be life threatening.

2. If action isn't taken to treat the hemorrhage, the lives of both the mother and fetus could be lost.

3. There is no indication that the mucus plug has been lost.

Client Need: Physiological Integrity

9 - 4 7

② **The nurse should evaluate the firmness and position of the fundus to prevent any further blood loss.**

1. The nurse will turn, cough, and deep breathe the client to prevent pneumonia and atelectasis, not to prevent excessive blood loss.

3. Administration of analgesics would help treat pain but would not affect blood loss.

4. The uterus should not be massaged routinely every 30 minutes. The client has had a cesarean section.

Client Need: Health Promotion and Maintenance

9 - 4 8

③ **The couvade, Mitleiden, or "suffering along" are terms that describe the behavior of expectant fathers who manifest many of the physical symptoms, such as morning sickness, weight gain, abdominal pain, backache, and leg cramps, associated with their partner's pregnancy.**

1. It isn't the increase in the severity of symptoms that is associated with couvade, but the fact that fathers may experience the physical symptoms of pregnancy.

2. The fathers do not believe they are pregnant. However, they do experience the physical symptoms associated with pregnancy.

4. Telling a father that the physical symptoms he is experiencing will let him know what happens to a pregnant woman indicates a lack of concern on the part of the nurse and is not appropriate.

Client Need: Physiological integrity

9 - 4 9

1 **Depo-Provera is a progesterone compound that, when used as a contraceptive, must be injected every ninety days.**

2. There is no need to prescribe Depo-Provera for post-menopausal women as a contraceptive. It is however, prescribed to treat abnormal bleeding caused by hormonal imbalance and secondary amenorrhea.

3. Fertility may occur after ninety days of the first infection of Depo-Provera if other injections of the drug are not given on a timely basis.

4. When taken as prescribed, Depo-Provera is a very reliable contraceptive.

Client Need: Physiological Integrity

9 - 5 0

④ **Tightening the muscles of the buttocks strengthens the pubococcygeus muscle in the perineal area.**

1, 2, and 3. Pressing the knees against the mattress, bearing down using the abdominal muscles, and flexing the muscles of the lower extremities will not strengthen or tighten the muscles of the buttocks. None of these muscles directly affect the perineal area.

Client Need: Health Promotion and Maintenance

9 - 5 1

③ **Ovulation usually occurs approximately 14 days after the start of the menstrual cycle. This is based on a 28-day cycle and can vary for a client who has shorter or longer cycles. To be most accurate with the rhythm method, the client should record her cycles for 8 months. Fertile days are calculated by subtracting 18 days from the length of the shortest cycle and 11 days from the longest cycle. These numbers are the days when intercourse should be avoided during each cycle. The rhythm method of birth control uses abstinence from sexual relations around the time of ovulation.**

1, 2, and 4. Ovulation usually occurs approximately 14 days after the start of the menstrual cycle.

Client Need: Physiological Integrity

9 - 5 2

① ② ④ and ⑤ **Impotence in the male (the inability to achieve or maintain an erection sufficiently rigid for sexual activity) may occur as a consequence of inadequate blood flow to the penis, the side effects of drug therapy, aging, insufficient testosterone, hypertension, complications of diabetes mellitus, and depression.**

3. Impotence may occur as a consequence of hypertension, not hypotension.

Client Need: Physiological Integrity

9 - 5 3

②③ and ④ Clients with penile implants should avoid contact sports because the force of physical contact could change the position or integrity of the implant. Straining while attempting to lift a heavy object can disrupt the internal sutures and the reconstructed tissue. It is important to report persistent pain and swelling, as they may be signs of infection.

1. The pressure of tight-fitting underwear can cause tissue erosion and curvature of the penis. Loose-fitting underwear is recommended.
5. A man who has received a penile implant should abstain from sex for 3 to 6 weeks. After 3 to 6 weeks, the healing is complete.

Client Need: Physiological Integrity

9 - 5 4

② and ③ Signs of testicular cancer include a testicular lump that is hard, an increase in the size of one testicle, a feeling of heaviness in the scrotum, a dull, aching pain in the groin or above the penis, and a diminished sensitivity to testicular pressure.

1. The testicular lump would be hard.
4. The pain would be dull.
5. There would be a diminished sensitivity to testicular pressure.

Client Need: Physiological Integrity

9 - 5 5

⑤ Condoms should be discarded if they are over 5 years old or beyond their expiration date.

1. A silicone lubricant is recommended because it will not deteriorate latex.
2. Keeping condoms stored in a cool, dry environment helps to maintain the integrity of the latex.
3. Condoms should be disposed of in a lined container to protect the public.
4. A new condom should be used each time sexual intercourse occurs.

Client Need: Health Promotion and Maintenance

Practice Test 10

Respiratory System and Acid-Base Imbalance

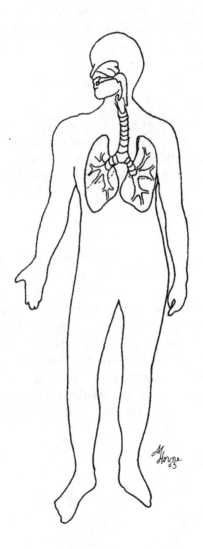

The Respiratory System

OVERVIEW

The respiratory system is composed of the nose and nasal cavities, throat (pharynx), larynx, trachea (a tube commonly known as the windpipe), bronchi, and lungs. The bronchi are subdivided into smaller bronchioles, and even smaller alveoli.

The respiratory system provides the body with oxygen and simultaneously removes carbon dioxide, a waste product of metabolism, from the body. This is accomplished through two types of respiration: external respiration and internal respiration.

EXTERNAL RESPIRATION

In external respiration, air containing 21% oxygen (O_2) is inhaled into the air spaces or sacs (alveoli) of the lungs, where it immediately passes into the small capillary blood vessels that surround these air sacs. At the same time another gas, carbon dioxide (CO_2), passes from the capillary blood vessels into the air spaces of the lungs and is exhaled. The air that is exhaled contains about 16% oxygen. External respirations occur between the outside environment and the capillary bloodstream of the lung.

INTERNAL RESPIRATION

At the same time external respiration is occurring, internal respiration is also taking place. Internal respiration is also known as cellular respiration. It occurs within all the organs of the body as oxygen passes out of the bloodstream and into tissue cells. At the same time, carbon dioxide passes from the tissue cells into the bloodstream, and the blood carries it back to the lungs to be exhaled.

ACID-BASE IMBALANCE

For body cells to function best, blood and body fluids must maintain a narrow acid-base range (pH of 7.35 to 7.45). Deviations from this range create conditions that interfere with cellular metabolism and can cause cell death. The normal acid-base range is maintained by respiratory and kidney functions. The respiratory system regulates the carbon dioxide (CO_2) concentration of the blood, while the kidneys regulate the bicarbonate (HCO_3) concentration. Increased amounts of CO_2 in the system lead to increased amounts of carbonic acid (water combines with CO_2 to produce this weak acid). The addition of carbonic acid to the blood lowers its pH, producing acidosis. The renal system responds by producing and releasing bicarbonate (HCO_3), a buffer that can raise the pH back into the normal range. If excessive amounts of HCO_3 are added to the blood (causing bicarbonate excess), or if CO_2 is deficient (causing carbonic acid deficit), a higher-than-normal pH is produced, resulting in alkalosis.

ACIDEMIA AND ALKALEMIA

Acid-base imbalances are classified according to whether the client is acidemic (blood pH <7.35) or alkalemic (blood pH >7.45), and by whether the cause is respiratory or metabolic. Both venous and arterial blood can be evaluated to determine acidemia or alkalemia, with the following normal value ranges:

	Arterial Blood	Venous Blood
pH	7.35–7.45	7.35–7.45
PO_2	80–100 mmHg	40–45 mmHg
PCO_2	35–45 mmHg	40–45 mmHg
HCO_3	20–30 mEq/l	20–30 mEq/l

RESPIRATORY ACIDOSIS (pH <7.35; PaCO$_2$ >45)

Respiratory acidosis (carbonic acid excess) is caused by alveolar hypoventilation (a limited volume of air in the lungs and/or limited air movement into and out of the alveoli, the small air sacs in the lungs) or decreased exchange of oxygen (O_2) and carbon dioxide (CO_2) in the capillaries that surround the alveoli. A variety of things can cause this limited air volume or movement, including: Cardiopulmonary, neuromuscular, skeletal, or airway diseases; acute infections; and the actions of drugs such as narcotics or sedatives. Laboratory findings in respiratory acidosis are as follows:

Plasma pH below 7.35
PCO_2 above 45 mmHg
HCO_3 normal if uncompensated, above 26 mEg/l if compensated

Any condition that decreases the number of functioning alveoli will interfere with the exchange of oxygen and carbon dioxide between the alveoli and the capillaries that surround them. Specific health conditions associated with respiratory acidosis and the mechanisms by which they produce carbonic acid excess are included in the following table:

Health condition	Causes acidosis by
Chronic obstructive pulmonary disease	Air trapping → ↑ inspired air volume → ↓ alveolar gas exchange → ↓ CO_2 → ↓ carbonic acid ↑
Barbiturate/sedative overdose	Depression of the respiratory center in the brain → ↑ respiratory rate → ↓ CO_2 → ↓ carbonic acid
Guillain-Barre syndrome	Paralysis of the respiratory muscles including the diaphragm → ↑ respiratory rate or apnea → ↓ CO_2
Pneumonia	Accumulation of infiltrates in the lungs → ↓ air in the alveoli → impaired gas exchange → ↓ CO_2 ↑
Atelectasis	Collapse of alveoli → ↑ number of functioning alveoli → ↑ gas exchange → ↓ CO_2 ↑

Any of these conditions can cause the partial pressure of arterial carbon dioxide (PaCO$_2$) to increase and the pH to fall. The body attempts to correct the acidosis by increasing the rate and depth of respirations, if the client's physical condition allows. This will increase the movement of CO_2 out of the body, thereby raising the pH. Additionally, the kidneys will release more hydrogen ions into the urine, lowering the hydrogen ion concentration of the blood. The higher the hydrogen ion concentration of the blood, the lower the blood pH. If the CO_2 concentration remains elevated for a long period of time (as in COPD), the kidneys will buffer the acidemia by adding increased amounts of bicarbonate (HCO_3) to the blood, and the pH will move into the normal range, despite continued high CO_2. This is referred to as compensated respiratory acidosis.

METABOLIC ACIDOSIS (pH <7.35; HCO₃ <22)

Metabolic acidosis (bicarbonate deficit) is caused in one of two ways: (1) the addition of an acid other than carbonic acid to the blood (as in diabetic ketoacidosis, DKA, when ketonic acid is produced by the incomplete breakdown of fatty acid for cellular energy); or (2) the loss of bicarbonate from blood and body fluids. Acid is also added to the blood in salicylate poisoning (aspirin overdose); renal failure (with the inability of the failing kidneys to remove hydrogen ions from the blood and concentrate them in the urine); and circulatory failure that produces a buildup of lactic acid. Recall that any increase/accumulation of hydrogen ions (H+), a component of all acids, in the blood results in a decrease in the serum pH and acidemic conditions. Laboratory findings in metabolic acidosis are as follows:

> Plasma pH below 7.35
> HCO₃ below 22 mEq/l
> PCO_2 normal if uncompensated, below 35 mmHg if compensated
> Urine pH <6 (caused by the body's attempt to raise the serum pH by secreting more hydrogen ions [H+] in the urine)

The following table lists health conditions (including those already mentioned) that can cause metabolic acidosis. The sequence of events whereby they either add acid to the system or cause the loss of bicarbonate is included.

Health condition	Causes acidosis by
Diabetic ketoacidosis	Production of ketones with breakdown of fatty acids → formation of ketonic acid → addition of ketonic acid to the blood → ↓pH
Uremia (renal failure) Renal tubular acidosis	↓ secretion of H+ into the renal tubules → ↓ secretion of H+ into the urine → H+ retention in the blood → ↓pH
Lactic acidosis	Anaerobic metabolism in muscles →↓ production of lactic acid → lactic acid added to the blood → ↓pH
Severe diarrhea	Loss of HCO₃ from the small and large intestine → ↓ available HCO₃ → ↓pH
Starvation	↓ available carbohydrates for glucose production → gluconeogenesis (production of glucose from fats and proteins) → incomplete metabolism of fats → production of ketones → formation of ketonic acid → addition of ketonic acid to the blood → ↓pH
Salicylate poisoning	Ingestion of aspirin → addition of ASA (acetylsalicylic acid) to the blood → ↓pH

In all of these conditions, bicarbonate is consumed (used up) in an attempt to buffer the acid, causing serum bicarbonate levels to be low. The respiratory system responds by increasing the rate and depth of respirations (for example, Kussmaul's breathing in DKA) in order to eliminate more CO_2, reduce the production of carbonic acid, and raise the blood pH. The kidneys respond by increasing the amount of bicarbonate released to the bloodstream, but this mechanism is slower in raising the pH. If the respiratory system is successful in raising the blood pH to the normal range, the condition is referred to as compensated metabolic acidosis.

RESPIRATORY ALKALOSIS (pH >7.45; PaCO$_2$ <35)

Respiratory alkalosis (carbonic acid deficit) occurs when excess amounts of carbon dioxide are exhaled. Alveolar hyperventilation (increased volume of air and/or increased air movement into and out of the alveolar sacs) decreases the PaCO$_2$ and increases the pH. Hyperventilation (increased depth and rate of breathing) occurs most commonly with anxiety, but also results from inappropriate mechanical ventilator settings (excessive oxygen concentration or excessively high ventilation rate) and from tachypnea associated with fever. Brain injury, brain infections like encephalitis, or brain tumors may also alter the respiratory rate by affecting the respiratory center in the brain. Laboratory findings in respiratory alkalosis are as follows:

> Plasma pH above 7.45
> PCO$_2$ below 35 mmHg
> HCO$_3$ normal if uncompensated, below 22 mEq/l if compensated

The following table shows the sequence of events in each of the conditions mentioned earlier, each of which leads to decreased CO$_2$ and carbonic acid deficit:

Health condition	Causes alkalosis by
Mechanical overventilation	↓ respiratory rate or ↓ O$_2$ concentration → ↓ "blowing off" CO$_2$ → ↑CO$_2$ in the blood
Hyperventilation due to anxiety	↓ rate and depth of breathing → ↓ "blowing off" of CO$_2$ → ↑CO$_2$
Encephalitis	Infection → stimulation of the respiratory center in the brain → hyperventilation → ↑CO$_2$
Fever	Increased body temperature → ↓ respiratory rate → ↑CO$_2$

The body attempts to correct the pH by decreasing the respiratory depth and rate (which will raise the PaCO$_2$ and increase the amount of carbonic acid); excreting bicarbonate and/or retaining hydrogen ions by adjusting their concentrations in the urine (decreasing serum bicarbonate levels and raising serum hydrogen ion levels); or by retaining chloride (normal serum chloride values range from 97 to 107 mEq/l). If any of these methods is successful in bringing the pH back to normal, the result is compensated respiratory alkalosis.

METABOLIC ALKALOSIS (pH >7.45; HCO$_3$ >26)

Metabolic alkalosis (bicarbonate excess) is caused by an increase in the bicarbonate level in or loss of acid from the blood and body fluids. This can occur as a result of either adding bicarbonate or removing acid from the system. Ingesting bicarbonate (as in individuals who treat indigestion with baking soda dissolved in water) or too much IV administration of bicarbonate during or following cardiopulmonary resuscitation can raise the pH of the blood. Acid is lost from the system with vomiting and with gastric suctioning. Likewise, diuretic therapy and a potassium deficit can cause metabolic alkalosis. The following table shows how these conditions cause either an increase in bicarbonate or a loss of acid:

Health condition	Causes alkalosis by
Severe vomiting	Loss of hydrochloric acid in digestive juices → removal of acid from the system → ↓ pH
Excess gastric suctioning	As above
Diuretic therapy	↓ excretion of H+ and chloride → ↑ H+ concentraton in the blood → ↓ pH
Potassium deficit	↓ blood potassium levels → ↓ K+ released from body cells → ↓ entry of H+ into cells (in exchange for K+ out of cells) → ↑ serum H+ levels → ↓ pH
Excess NaHCO₃	Addition of HCO₃ to the system → ↓ pH

Laboratory findings in metabolic alkalosis are as follows:

> Plasma pH above 7.45
> HCO_3 above 26 mEq/l
> PCO_2 normal if uncompensated, above 45 mmHg if compensated
> Urine pH >7 due to increased secretion of bicarbonate (HCO_3) into the urine in order to lower the serum pH

In all of these cases, the acid-base balance is shifted in the direction of "base" (alkalosis), and the pH rises. Although, theoretically, slowing the respiratory rate in order to conserve CO_2 would lower the pH, ventilatory drive (the normal and involuntary action of breathing in response to rising CO_2) generally prevents this. The kidneys are more effective in correcting metabolic alkalosis, by removing bicarbonate from the blood and conserving hydrogen ions, both of which will lower the pH. They do this by adjusting bicarbonate and hydrogen ion concentrations in the urine. More bicarbonate and less hydrogen are excreted. Since the body's effective mechanisms for lowering pH in conditions of metabolic alkalosis are by direct adjustment of the factor that leads to the problem—namely, bicarbonate levels—these adjustments would more accurately be called corrections than compensations.

NOTING PATTERNS

Although acid-base balance is complex and can sometimes be difficult to understand, there are two important patterns to note in relation to the pH and the CO_2 or HCO_3 in respiratory and metabolic acidosis and alkalosis. In the respiratory conditions, as the pH moves in one direction, the CO_2 moves in the other: acidosis occurs when pH falls and CO_2 rises, and alkalosis occurs when pH rises and CO_2 falls.

In the metabolic conditions, pH and HCO_3 move in the same direction: acidosis occurs when pH and HCO_3 fall, and alkalosis occurs when pH and HCO_3 rise.

DISEASES/DISORDERS OF THE RESPIRATORY SYSTEM INCLUDE

Upper Respiratory Infections

RHINITIS Rhinitis is characterized by inflammation of the nasal mucosa. This condition is often caused by nasal infections.

PHARYNGITIS Pharyngitis is associated with inflammation of the pharynx (throat). Symptoms include: Pain, redness, and difficulty swallowing.

LARYNGITIS This disorder is characterized by inflammation of the mucous lining of the larynx. Edema of the vocal chords results in hoarseness and loss of voice.

DEVIATED SEPTUM In this condition, the nasal septum strays far from the midline. Some people are born with this defect. A deviated septum can cause blockage of the airway in both nares. Surgical correction may be required.

EPISTAXIS Epistaxis (nosebleed) is most commonly caused by a blow or bump on the nose. Other causes include: Dry mucous membranes, infections, and hypertension. Treatments would include placing the client at 45 degrees and applying cool compresses.

CROUP Croup is characterized by obstruction of the larynx that produces a barking cough with stridor (a high-pitched sound). Croup may result from an infection, allergy, or foreign body in the larynx.

DIPHTHERIA Diphtheria is an acute infection of the throat and upper respiratory tract. It is caused by the organism *Corynebacterium diphtheriae*. The organism produces a leather-like opaque membrane in the pharynx and respiratory tract. A vaccine is available to prevent this disease.

PERTUSSIS The common name for pertussis is whooping cough. This is a serious bacterial infection of the pharynx, larynx, and trachea caused by *B. pertussis*, a bacteria that is highly contagious. A vaccine is available to prevent this disease.

Bronchial Tube Disorders

ASTHMA In this condition there is airway obstruction caused by spasms of the bronchi. The etiology (cause) of this condition includes: Allergy, infection, nervous tension, and/or emotional problems. It is usually treated with medications that dilate the bronchi.

BRONCHOGENIC CARCINOMA This condition is commonly referred to as lung cancer. There are several different types, namely: Squamous cell carcinoma, which comes from the lining of the bronchus; adenocarcinoma, which comes from the mucus-secreting cells; and small-cell or oat-cell carcinoma.

CHRONIC BRONCHITIS This condition is characterized by inflammation of the bronchi and bronchioles. The air passages may be blocked by edema and excessive mucus production.

CYSTIC FIBROSIS This is an inherited disease that affects the exocrine glands, which include the pancreas, sweat glands, and mucous membranes of the respiratory tract. It is a major cause of severe chronic lung disease in children. The parents of these children are taught to perform pulmonary chest physiotherapy, which is followed by deep breathing and coughing to help mobilize secretions.

Lung Disorders

ATELECTASIS In this condition, incomplete expansion of the air sacs (alveoli) occurs. Many of the alveoli are collapsed and cannot function. In atelectasis, the bronchioles and alveoli appear as deflated balloons.

EMPHYSEMA Emphysema is characterized by a loss of elasticity and breakdown in the alveolar wall (pulmonary parenchyma). This breakdown results in loss of movement in the air sacs. Chronic bronchitis is often associated with this disease.

PNEUMOCONIOSIS This is a condition caused by dust in the lungs and is accompanied by chronic inflammation (bronchitis). Different forms of this disease are associated with the specific particles inhaled. For example, coalworker's pneumoconiosis (black lung) is caused by the inhalation of carbon and silica that accumulates in the lungs; the inhalation of cotton, flax, and hemp causes byssinosis; and grinder's disease is caused by the inhalation of rocks and glass (silicosis).

PNEUMONIA Pneumonia is associated with acute infection and inflammation of the alveoli. It can be caused by pneumococci, staphylococci, fungi, and viruses.

PULMONARY ABSCESS This condition is characterized by a large collection of pus due to bacterial infection in the lungs.

PULMONARY EDEMA With pulmonary edema there is swelling and fluid in the alveoli and bronchioles. This condition is quite often caused by the inability of the heart to pump blood efficiently. The blood backs up in the pulmonary blood vessels and fluid seeps out into the alveoli and bronchioles.

PULMONARY EMBOLISM This disorder is characterized by clots and other material floating through the bloodstream. These substances may lodge in the vessels of the lung and cause a pulmonary infarction.

PULMONARY TUBERCULOSIS (TB) Pulmonary tuberculosis is highly contagious. It is caused by *Mycobacterium tuberculosis*. TB is transmitted through inhalation or swallowing the droplets contaminated with the tubercular bacillus. Pulmonary TB affects the lungs; however, the organism can invade any organ of the body.

Pleural Disorders

MESOTHELIOMA Mesothelioma is a malignant tumor that originates in the pleura. This rare tumor is associated with exposure to asbestos.

PLEURAL EFFUSION Effusion is the escape of fluid into a body part, such as the pleural cavity. Other examples of effusion are empyema (pyothorax), hydrothorax, and hemothorax.

PLEURISY (PLEURITIS) This condition is characterized by inflammation in the pleura (a serous membrane that enfolds both lungs and is reflected on the walls of the thorax and diaphragm).

PNEUMOTHORAX This condition is characterized by the accumulation of air or gas in the pleural space. A pneumothorax can be associated with trauma, perforation of the chest wall, tuberculosis, emphysema, and lung abscess.

Practice Test 10

Questions

10-1

An elderly client admitted to the hospital because of "confusion" has been taking baking soda several times a day for the past week for an upset stomach. Which of the following laboratory results would you expect to see?

1. bicarbonate elevation
2. low pH
3. low sodium
4. potassium elevation

10-2

Your client had a lobectomy of the left lung. The client returns to the unit with a chest tube in place attached to water-seal drainage. You observe fluid fluctuating in the chest tube with each respiration. Which interpretation of this observation is correct?

1. Oxygen is being lost through the client's chest tube with each respiration.
2. There is an air leak within the drainage system.
3. The apparatus is functioning properly.
4. Air is being drawn into the client's chest cavity.

10-3

For a client with multidrug-resistant tuberculosis to be considered no longer infectious, the client must:

1. remain afebrile for 5 days.
2. show a negative blood culture.
3. show negative daily sputum cultures for 3 consecutive days.
4. show a white blood cell count that is within normal limits.

10-4

An 82-year-old client has been admitted to the medical unit with a diagnosis of pneumonia. The client has an elevated temperature, respirations are rapid and shallow, and the client complains of chest pain. In order to decrease the client's chest pain, you would:

1. instruct the client to limit intake of air.
2. teach the client to increase the depth of respirations.
3. support the client's rib cage during coughing.
4. show the client how to relax the diaphragm.

10-5

A client with chronic obstructive pulmonary disease has been on prednisone for the past 2 years. The client is at risk for developing:

1. Cushing's syndrome.
2. Addison's disease.
3. Eaton-Lambert syndrome.
4. diabetes mellitus.

10-6

A client with chronic obstructive pulmonary disease is placed on a continuous aminophylline drip. The nurse knows that aminophylline may:

1. strengthen the heartbeat.
2. increase the heart rate.
3. dilate the coronary arteries.
4. decrease myocardial oxygen demand.

10-7

A client has had a bronchoscopy. Which of the following nursing observations would indicate possible complications?

1. The client coughs up small amounts of blood-tinged sputum.
2. The client complains of difficulty in breathing.
3. The client is very hoarse when speaking.
4. The client complains of a sore throat when swallowing.

10-8

Your client has a tentative diagnosis of severe acute respiratory syndrome (SARS). You expect your evaluation to reveal:

1. a low-grade fever.
2. a productive cough.
3. head and body aches.
4. constipation.

10-9

A client with chronic obstructive pulmonary disease enters the clinic experiencing shortness of breath, nausea, and dizziness. To assess the client's level of hypoxia, the nurse will:

1. obtain a throat culture.
2. obtain a sputum collection.
3. utilize an incentive spirometer.
4. utilize a pulse oximetry.

10-10

The nursing diagnosis of activity intolerance related to decreased oxygenation is established for a client. To promote activity tolerance in the client, the nurse will plan to:

1. have the client decide which activities will be completed for the day.
2. complete all care at one time to avoid disturbing the client later.
3. space nursing activities to allow the client frequent rest periods.
4. suggest ways in which the client can participate in performing care.

10-11

A 3-year-old is admitted to the hospital with a medical diagnosis of laryngotracheobronchitis. A mist tent with oxygen has been prescribed. Because the client is restless and crying, the nurse is unable to obtain an accurate respiration rate. Which action should the nurse take?

1. Ask another staff member to count the client's respirations.
2. Record an approximate respiratory rate.
3. Wait until the client is quiet before counting respirations.
4. Average the client's respirations per minute after taking them for 3 minutes.

10-12

A client who experiences severe asthma may develop life-threatening acid-base disturbances. Which of the following blood gas results would be most indicative of pending respiratory failure?

1. PO_2 of 90 mmHg
2. pH of 7.40
3. PCO_2 of 65 mmHg
4. O_2 saturation of 92%

1 0 - 1 3

The hallmark of chronic bronchitis is:

1. a daily productive cough.
2. dyspnea.
3. cyanosis.
4. right ventricular failure.

1 0 - 1 4

The nurse observes a client with tuberculosis putting a soiled disposable tissue in an ash-tray. Which response would be appropriate for the nurse to make?

1. "Let me get you a disposable bag for your used tissue."
2. "Let me get you an emesis basin to dispose of your used tissue."
3. "Did you receive instructions about disposal of soiled tissues?"
4. "Can I help you dispose of your soiled tissue?"

1 0 - 1 5

Oxygen is best delivered to the hypoxic client during meals by:

1. endotracheal tube.
2. facemask.
3. face tent.
4. nasal cannula.

1 0 - 1 6

The nurse begins resuscitation of a 4-year-old who has stopped breathing. To administer effective breaths for the child, the nurse should:

1. pinch off the child's nares and hyperextend the child's neck.
2. pinch off the child's nares and slightly extend the child's neck.
3. lift the child's jaw and breathe into the child's nares.
4. encircle and breathe into the mouth and nares of the child.

1 0 - 1 7

A client has a chest tube attached to water-seal drainage. Which of the following nursing measures is most important in preventing respiratory complications?

1. securing the tubing above the level of the incision
2. reinforcing the dressing over the insertion site
3. sealing the air vent on the suction control chamber of the drainage system
4. keeping the water-seal drainage system near the floor

1 0 - 1 8

Your client will receive atropine 0.4 mg intramuscularly 30 minutes before surgery. The nurse knows the purpose of this medication is to:

1. facilitate the effects of anesthesia.
2. prevent postoperative dehydration.
3. improve smooth muscle tone and prevent hemorrhage.
4. reduce oral and respiratory secretions during surgery.

10-19

A client who has adrenal insufficiency is to receive fludrocortisone acetate 0.1 mg by mouth. As you prepare to give this medicine, your client complains of dyspnea. You observe bilateral moist crackles in the lungs and a new S_3. You will:

1. give the dose as prescribed.
2. give the dose intravenously.
3. give twice the prescribed dose.
4. hold the dose and notify the physician.

10-20

Your 67-year-old client collapses while ambulating in the hall. The client is not breathing and does not have a palpable pulse. CPR is initiated. As soon as the client is connected to the monitor/defibrillator, you see that the EKG shows ventricular fibrillation. You know that the client requires defibrillation with a current dosage beginning at:

1. 2 joules.
2. 20 joules.
3. 200 joules.
4. 2000 joules.

10-21

Your client will have chest tubes attached to a water-seal drainage following surgery. During preoperative teaching, you will inform the client that the purpose of chest tubes is to:

1. allow for the removal of fluid and air.
2. make deep breathing and coughing easier.
3. prevent rapid reexpansion of the lung.
4. control internal hemorrhage.

10-22

Upon admittance to your intensive care unit, a client's laboratory work includes a serum glucose of 898 mg/dl, an arterial blood pH of 7.10, an arterial blood HCO_3 of 11 mEq/l, and an arterial blood PCO_2 of 37 mmHg. You anticipate the need to administer, in addition to insulin, the following treatment:

1. hetastarch 500 intravenously stat.
2. immediate intubation and hyperinflation to combat respiratory acidosis.
3. 1 unit of packed red blood cells given stat.
4. sodium bicarbonate infusion to combat metabolic acidosis.

10-23

An agitated client has diazepam prescribed, 5 mg intravenously every 2 hours as needed. After administering a dose, you notice that the client's respiratory rate has dropped from 20 breaths per min to 6 breaths per min. You know to administer:

1. fentanyl citrate.
2. fluorouracil.
3. fluconazole.
4. flumazenil.

10-24

This is your client's first postoperative day following a pneumonectomy. For evening nourishment, several beverages will be available. Which one will facilitate wound healing the best?

1. tomato juice
2. apple juice
3. orange juice
4. grapefruit juice

1 0 - 2 5

A client has bronchiectasis. In evaluating the effects of a prescribed expectorant, the nurse will anticipate:

1. cough suppression.
2. bronchial dilation.
3. reduced viscosity of respiratory secretions.
4. decreased production of respiratory secretions.

1 0 - 2 6

A full-term newborn is 1 day postoperative after a successful repair of a tracheo-esophageal fistula. The postoperative plan of care will include:

1. minimizing handling and stimulation.
2. gentle suctioning of oral secretions hourly.
3. frequent respiratory and abdominal assessment.
4. gastrostomy feedings every 2 to 3 hours.

1 0 - 2 7

Clients planning to use Nicoderm should be advised to:

1. start with a low dose and gradually increase the dosage.
2. change the patch weekly.
3. anticipate a lifetime of patch use.
4. rotate patch sites daily.

1 0 - 2 8

A mist tent has been prescribed for a 2-year-old client with bacterial pneumonia. When the mother of the client visits, she tells the nurse, "I just put my hand in the tent and my child's clothing is damp." Which action should the nurse take in response to the mother's comments?

1. Report the mother's conversation to the nurse in charge.
2. Encourage the client to drink fluids to replace those that were lost.
3. Take the client's body temperature and compare it with previous body temperatures.
4. Explain the purpose of humidity to the mother.

1 0 - 2 9

Your client is experiencing metabolic acidosis. A compensatory mechanism seen in clients experiencing metabolic acidosis is:

1. a deep, gasping type of respiration.
2. a marked, sustained inspiratory effort.
3. several short breaths followed by long irregular periods of apnea.
4. periods of apnea lasting 10 to 60 seconds, followed by gradually increasing depth and frequency of respirations.

1 0 - 3 0

The nurse delivers oxygen by hood to a preterm neonate. Which arterial blood gas indicates the intervention has been most effective?

1. pH 7.30, PCO_2 45, PO_2 45
2. pH 7.28, PCO_2 50, PO_2 40
3. pH 7.37, PCO_2 40, PO_2 80
4. pH 7.42, PCO_2 22, PO_2 100

10-31

A client with chest pain arrives on your unit. Prescriptions read: "Oxygen 2 to 4 liters per minute." There is history of chronic obstructive pulmonary disease. In addition to the oxygen saturation level, what other data must be considered when choosing an oxygen dosage?

1. hemoglobin
2. serum potassium
3. serum chloride
4. height

10-32

Which of the following symptoms would be the best indicator of a tension pneumothorax?

1. spitting up blood
2. sucking sounds made on inspiration
3. collapsed and flat-looking neck veins
4. deviation of the trachea

10-33

Your client had a radical neck dissection. In the immediate postoperative period, you detect the presence of stridor. You understand the most probable cause of stridor is:

1. laryngeal obstruction.
2. respiratory insufficiency.
3. mediastinal shifting.
4. congestive heart failure.

10-34

A client was admitted to the emergency department following a car accident. You note paradoxical movement of the chest wall and respiratory distress. What do you suspect is causing this?

1. pneumonia
2. flail chest
3. pneumothorax
4. cardiac tamponade

10-35

Your asthmatic client is being discharged home with the prescription "Beclomethasone dipropionate 2 puffs qid with spacer." When asked by your client about the use of this inhaler during status asthmaticus, you reply:

1. "It is for use during status asthmaticus; take 4 puffs."
2. "It is for use during status asthmaticus; remove the spacer prior to dosing."
3. "Status asthmaticus will never happen again."
4. "This is not to be used to treat status asthmaticus."

10-36

Your client is intubated and on mechanical ventilation. Pancuronium bromide has been prescribed. You know that this medication:

1. may cause marked bradycardia.
2. may be given even after your client is off of the ventilator.
3. is an analgesic with hypnotic effect.
4. should be given with sedation or analgesia.

10-37

You are concerned that your client may be developing adult respiratory distress syndrome (ARDS) following a motor vehicle accident. What early manifestations of this condition will you assess at this time?

1. dyspnea and tachypnea
2. cyanosis and apprehension
3. hemoptysis
4. diffuse crackles and rhonchi

10-38

A client has developed acute renal failure following a course of antibiotic therapy with the aminoglycoside tobramycin sulfate. Daily laboratory tests have been prescribed to monitor the progression of the disease. Which of the following arterial blood gas profiles is indicative of renal acidosis?

1. pH 7.35, PaO_2 95, $PaCO_2$ 35, HCO_3 20
2. pH 7.36, PaO_2 98, $PaCO_2$ 32, HCO_3 23
3. pH 7.40, PaO_2 78, $PaCO_2$ 50, HCO_3 38
4. pH 7.15, PaO_2 99, $PaCO_2$ 38, HCO_3 8

10-39

A client has been diagnosed with chronic obstructive pulmonary disease. Coughing has become increasingly productive. The sputum is thick and yellowish in color. The client is being treated with theophylline 100 mg po, qid. You know this drug is given to:

1. relieve bronchospasm.
2. decrease sputum production.
3. suppress coughing.
4. treat respiratory infection.

10-40

A client is experiencing Kussmaul respirations. These respirations:

1. act as a distraction for the client during painful episodes.
2. help the body rid itself of excess fluids.
3. enhance circulation by increased chest wall movement.
4. serve as a secondary defense in an attempt to get rid of hydrogen ions.

10-41

In addition to dehydration, elderly persons who experience prolonged diarrhea are at risk for which of the following disturbances?

1. hyperkalemia
2. respiratory acidosis
3. hypernatremia
4. metabolic acidosis

10-42

A client with multiple drug-resistant tuberculosis has been admitted to your unit. What do you expect your assessment to reveal?

1. crackles, cyanosis, and fever
2. fever, weight loss, and night sweats
3. sudden chest pain, hemoptysis, and tachycardia
4. nausea, diaphoresis, and severe chest pain

10-43

A client is admitted to the emergency department with multiple knife wounds to the chest. The knife is still in the client's chest. What should you do?

1. remove the knife
2. cleanse the chest wounds with saline
3. seal open chest wounds with an airtight dressing
4. place the client in a supine position

10-44

Two hours ago, a client's oxygen concentration was decreased to 40% oxygen by mask. The client's arterial oxygen pressure value also decreased by 20% to 50 mm Hg. Which of the following would you do initially?

1. Do nothing; the drop in arterial oxygen pressure is an expected outcome.
2. Increase the oxygen concentration to 60%.
3. Assess the client's situation and inform the physician of the changes.
4. Closely monitor the client's condition.

10-45

A client is receiving aminophylline to treat pulmonary emphysema that has been complicated by an upper respiratory infection. To evaluate the effectiveness of this drug, the nurse should monitor the:

1. amount and color of secretions.
2. rate and rhythm of respirations.
3. pattern of temperature elevations.
4. expansion of the chest cavity.

10-46

A client has chest tubes and needs to be transported to radiation therapy for treatment. Which of the following nursing actions is appropriate to provide safety during transport?

1. Keep the water-seal unit close to the client by taping it to the abdominal area.
2. Clamp the chest tube before disconnecting it from the water-seal unit.
3. Attach rubber-tipped forceps to the client's gown before transport.
4. Instruct the client to take deep breaths should the chest tube become dislodged.

10-47

A client with amyotrophic lateral sclerosis is brought to the emergency department in respiratory arrest. The best method to use when administering oxygen to this client would be:

1. positive pressure ventilation.
2. nasal cannula.
3. facemask.
4. oxygen tent.

10-48

Severe acute respiratory syndrome (SARS) is caused by a:

_____

Fill in the blank

10-49

A client is receiving oxygen therapy by face-mask. Which measures should the nurse include in the plan of care?

1. taking the body temperature rectally
2. giving a complete bed bath
3. encouraging additional fluids
4. assisting with coughing and deep-breathing exercises

10-50

A client with chronic obstructive pulmonary disease is in respiratory distress. To facilitate breathing, the nurse will place the client in which position?

1. supine and dorsal recumbent
2. dorsal with the head down and the feet elevated
3. upright at 90 degrees
4. semi-prone on the left side with right knee drawn up toward the chest

Practice Test 10

Answers, Rationales, and Explanations

1 0 - 1

① **You will expect to see bicarbonate elevation. Baking soda or sodium bicarbonate is used by some individuals as a home remedy for indigestion. This may, however, cause severe acid-base disturbances, an elevation in the serum bicarbonate level, and subsequent metabolic alkalosis.**

2 and 3. The nurse would anticipate a pH elevation with the ingestion of sodium bicarbonate and subsequent metabolic alkalosis, as well as an increase in serum sodium.

4.   The serum potassium would not be immediately or directly affected.

Client Need: Physiological Integrity

1 0 - 2

③ **You would understand that the apparatus is functioning properly. If fluctuations do not occur, something is plugging the tubing or the lung has reinflated.**

1.   Oxygen is not being lost through the client's chest tube with each respiration. The fluctuation indicates proper functioning. The purpose of chest tubes is to drain fluid and air from the pleural space and reestablish negative pressure. The fact that the fluid in the chest tube is fluctuating indicates the water-seal drainage is functioning properly.

2.   If there is an air leak within the drainage system, the nurse would observe a continuous (not intermittent) bubbling in the water-seal. This must be corrected by locating the source of the leak and repairing it.

4.   If air was being drawn into the client's chest cavity, the nurse would observe signs and symptoms of a collapsed lung or mediastinal shift such as dyspnea, anxiety, diaphoresis, and tachycardia.

Client Need: Physiological Integrity

1 0 - 3

③ **Sputum cultures must be negative on three consecutive mornings for a client to be considered no longer infected with the tubercle bacillus.**

1, 2, and 4. Remaining afebrile for five days, showing a negative blood culture, and showing a white blood cell count that is within normal limits do not confirm that clients with multidrug-resistant tuberculosis are no longer infectious. The sputum cultures must be negative (not contain tubercle bacillus) for three consecutive days.

Client Need: Physiological Integrity

10-4

③ **Supporting the rib cage during coughing will diminish pain and at the same time facilitate increased diaphragmatic movement.**

1. Instructing the client to limit intake of air is contraindicated.

2. Telling the client to increase the depth of respirations will help treat the pneumonia. However, this will not directly relieve the chest pain.

4. Showing the client how to relax the diaphragm will not relieve the pain.

Client Need: Health Promotion and Maintenance

10-5

① **The client is at risk for developing Cushing's syndrome due to long-term steroid use. This is the most frequent cause of Cushing's syndrome seen in clinical practice.**

2. Addison's disease occurs when the body secretes an inadequate amount of cortisol.

3. Eaton-Lambert syndrome is an autoimmune disorder caused by impaired presynaptic release of acetycholine at nerve synapses.

4. Steroids do alter carbohydrate metabolism. However, taking steroids does not increase the risk of developing diabetes unless the client is already predisposed to developing it.

Client Need: Physiological Integrity

10-6

② **The nurse knows that aminophylline increases the heart rate. Aminophylline dilates the bronchi but it also increases the heart rate. Tachycardia is a frequent side effect experienced by clients receiving this medication.**

1. Digitalis preparations frequently strengthen the heartbeat.

3. Nitrates dilate the coronary arteries.

4. Calcium channel blockers will decrease the myocardial oxygen demand.

Client Need: Health Promotion and Maintenance

1 0 - 7

② **Difficulty in breathing (dyspnea) would indicate a possible complication associated with a bronchoscopic examination. A serious complication following bronchoscopy would be swelling due to trauma from the procedure. The first symptom the client would experience is difficulty breathing. Other complications associated with a bronchoscopic examination include reaction to local anesthesia, aspiration, bronchospasm, pneumothorax, hemorrhage, and perforation.**

1. Coughing up small amounts of blood-tinged sputum could occur because of irritation to the mucous membranes during the procedure. This would not be considered a complication.

3. Bronchoscopy is the direct visual inspection of the larynx, trachea, and bronchi. Therefore, hoarseness could occur and would not be considered a complication.

4. A sore throat is not unusual because of the irritating effects of the examination.

Client Need: Physiological Integrity

1 0 - 8

③ **Head and body aches are among the symptoms associated with severe acute respiratory syndrome (SARS).**

1. Clients experiencing severe acute respiratory syndrome (SARS) are likely to have a high fever >100.4°F (>38.0°C) at the onset of the illness; chills may accompany the fever.

2. Clients with SARS develop a dry, nonproductive cough that may be accompanied by or progress to hypoxia.

4. Diarrhea, not constipation, may be experienced by 10% to 20% of clients.

Client Need: Safe, Effective Care Environment

1 0 - 9

④ **To assess the client's level of hypoxia, the nurse will use a pulse oximetry. A pulse oximetry is a noninvasive device that measures a client's arterial blood oxygen saturation and can detect hypoxemia before clinical signs appear.**

1. A throat culture is used to assess for the presence of disease-producing microorganisms.

2. A sputum collection is obtained to identify a specific microorganism and its drug sensitivities.

3. An incentive spirometer is a device that gradually increases airflow into the lungs. It does not assess for hypoxia.

Client Need: Physiological Integrity

10-10

③ **To promote activity tolerance in the client, the nurse will space nursing activities. Spacing activities diminishes the amount of oxygen needed at any one time and allows the oxygen reserves to be built up during periods of rest.**

1. Having the client decide which activities will be completed each day will not affect oxygen reserves.
2. Completing all care at one time would deplete all oxygen reserves and would be contraindicated.
4. There are energy-efficient methods that could be helpful for clients to learn in performing their care. However, it is the spacing of activities that allows for buildup of oxygen reserves.

Client Need: Physiological Integrity

10-11

③ **The nurse should postpone assessing respirations until the child becomes quiet. Every effort should be made to avoid further aggravation of the child's respiratory distress.**

1. Having another staff member attempt to count the child's respirations may upset the child further and is not recommended.

2 and 4. The child has a respiratory condition. Respirations should be counted 1 full minute, not estimated or averaged.

Client Need: Physiological Integrity

10-12

③ **A PCO_2 of 65 mmHg is indicative of impending respiratory failure. The normal pressure exerted by carbon dioxide gas in arterial blood (the PCO_2) is 38 to 44 mmHg. Pressures over 50 mmHg suggest there is excess PCO_2 in the blood, and acidosis is developing. Respiratory failure is a grave potential, should it occur.**

1. A PO_2 value of 90 mm Hg is within the normal range. The pressure exerted by oxygen (PO_2) in arterial blood is 80 to 105 mmHg.
2. The normal pH is between 7.35 and 7.45.
3. The normal O_2 saturation is > 90%.

Client Need: Physiological Integrity

10-13

① **The hallmark of chronic bronchitis is a daily productive cough that lasts about 3 months out of the year for 2 consecutive years.**

2, 3, and 4. Chronic bronchitis progresses to dyspnea, cyanosis, and right ventricular failure.

Client Need: Physiological Integrity

10-14

① It would be appropriate for the nurse to see that the client's soiled tissue is placed in a disposable bag. Clients with tuberculosis should place all soiled tissues into a disposable bag. Sputum-laden tissues should be confined to a closed container that can be disposed of in institutional incinerators. Proper handling of sputum prevents the organisms from becoming airborne.

2. Placing soiled tissues in an open emesis basin exposes others to the tubercle bacillus.

3. Assessing what the client knows concerning the disposal of contaminated materials should come after the soiled tissue has been disposed of properly.

4. Asking a client if you can help with the disposal of a soiled tissue might be answered in the negative.

Client Need: Safe, Effective Care Environment

10-15

④ Oxygen is best delivered to the hypoxic client during meals by nasal cannula. A prong is placed into each nostril, delivering low-flow oxygen without restricted mouth movement. Clients may talk, drink, and eat while receiving oxygen by nasal cannula without interrupting the oxygen flow.

1. Endotracheal tubes are taped in place until they are no longer needed to assist ventilation. During this time, clients are not fed through the mouth.

2 and 3. Facemasks and tents must be removed prior to eating.

Client Need: Safe, Effective Care Environment

10-16

② To administer effective breaths for a 4-year-old child, the nurse will pinch off the child's nares and slightly extend the child's neck.

1. A child's head should not be hyperextended during resuscitation because the trachea is soft and hyperextension could compress it.

3 and 4. Breathing into the nose (nares) and mouth simultaneously is appropriate only for infants.

Client Need: Physiological Integrity

10-17

④ Keeping the water-seal drainage system near the floor is the most important nursing measure the nurse can take to prevent respiratory complications. Maintaining the water-seal drainage system below the client's chest will prevent backflow of fluid and air into the client's pleural cavity.

1. Securing the tubing above the level of the incision will cause a backflow of air and fluid into the pleural cavity.
2. The dressing should not be reinforced unless there is a leak at the insertion site.
3. Water-seal drainage must have an air vent to provide an escape route for air passing through the water seal from the pleural space.

Client Need: Physiological Integrity

10-18

④ The purpose for administering atropine preoperatively is to prevent aspiration by reducing oral and respiratory secretions. Atropine is an anticholinergic that, when given properly, reduces oral and respiratory secretions.

1. A frequent side effect of atropine is drowsiness. However, drowsiness is not an expected outcome and atropine is not administered to produce drowsiness or to facilitate the effects of anesthesia.
2. Atropine does not affect hydration, nor does it contribute to dehydration postoperatively.
3. 0.4 mg of atropine does not affect smooth muscle tone.

Client Need: Safe, Effective Care Environment

10-19

④ You will hold the dose of fludrocortisone acetate (Florinef) and notify the physician if you auscultate bilateral moist crackles in the lungs and a new S sound. Florinef may cause sodium and water retention and is not to be given to those who manifest signs of pulmonary edema such as dyspnea and crackles.

1. Fludrocortisone acetate is contraindicated in clients suspected of pulmonary edema.
2. The route has been prescribed (po); however, the client has bilateral moist crackles and an S_3 sound. You would withhold the medication.
3. No amount of fludrocortisone acetate should be administered to this client because of bilateral crackles and the S_3 sound. The dosage should be withheld and the physician notified of the client's condition.

Client Need: Health Promotion and Maintenance

1 0 - 2 0

③ Two hundred joules is the recommended initial defibrillation dosage for an adult experiencing ventricular fibrillation.

1. Two joules is a neonate dosage.
2. Twenty joules is a pediatric dosage.
4. Two thousand joules is an overdose and unobtainable on a defibrillator.

Client Need: Physiological Integrity

1 0 - 2 1

① The nurse will inform the preoperative client that the purpose of chest tube insertion into the pleural space is to allow for the drainage of fluid and air and to reestablish negative pressure.

2. Deep breathing and coughing will become easier once fluid and air have been removed from the pleural space and negative pressure has been reestablished.
3. The lungs will expand as the fluid and air are removed from the pleural space.
4. Chest tubes do not have an impact on internal hemorrhage. However, a rising fluid level in the collection chamber, a drop in blood pressure, and rapid pulse are indicators of hemorrhage.

Client Need: Safe, Effective Care Environment

1 0 - 2 2

④ In addition to the insulin, the client should receive a sodium bicarbonate infusion to combat metabolic acidosis. This laboratory work suggests metabolic acidosis because a pH of 7.10 is less than the normal range of 7.35 to 7.45. The bicarbonate level (HCO_3) is low, also, at 11 mEq/l; the normal is 22 to 26 mEq/l. This combination of abnormals indicates metabolic acidosis. The treatment is sodium bicarbonate, an alkalyzing agent.

1. There is no evidence that fluid volume replacement is needed. Hetastarch (Hespan) is a volume expander usually used in shock due to burns, hemorrhage, sepsis, and trauma.
2. The client is in metabolic acidosis, not respiratory acidosis.
3. There is no indication that the hemoglobin is low. Therefore, there is no need for packed red blood cells.

Client Need: Physiological Integrity

1 0 - 2 3

④ **You will administer flumazenil. Flumazenil (Romazicon) is a benzodiazepine antagonist whose competitive inhibition of the receptor sites blocks the action of benzodiazepines. In this instance, the respiratory depression due to diazepam (Valium) administration would be corrected.**

1. Fentanyl citrate is an anesthetic agent.

2. Fluorouracil is an antineoplastic agent.

3. Fluconazole is an antifungal agent.

Client Need: Physiological Integrity

1 0 - 2 4

③ **Orange juice facilitates wound healing better than apple, tomato, and grapefruit juice. Orange juice contains high amounts of vitamin C. Vitamin C helps to form collagen, which plays an important role in wound healing.**

1. Tomato juice is higher in vitamin C than apple juice but not as high as orange or grapefruit juice.

2. Apple juice has the least vitamin C compared to tomato, orange, or grapefruit juice.

4. Grapefruit juice has the second-highest amount of vitamin C compared to orange, tomato, and apple juice.

Client Need: Physiological Integrity

1 0 - 2 5

③ **The nurse will anticipate an expectorant (mucokinetic agent) to improve the removal of respiratory secretions by thinning and decreasing the viscosity of the secretions in the client experiencing bronchiectasis.**

1. Antitussives are administered to provide symptomatic relief of coughing by suppressing the cough reflex.

2. Bronchodilators are administered to reverse airway obstruction and prevent bronchospasm.

4. Anticholinergics decrease production of respiratory and oral secretions.

Client Need: Physiological Integrity

10-26

③ Frequent respiratory and abdominal assessment of the infant with a repair of a tracheoesophageal fistula is necessary, since it is very likely that the infant aspirated prior to surgery and because the chest cavity was opened during surgery. Abdominal assessment would also verify the return of peristalsis and the presence of distension associated with peritonitis.

1. Periodic stimulation will encourage deep breathing and reinflation of the infant's lungs, and therefore should not be minimized.
2. Oral secretions should not need suctioning, since they are not copious and can be effectively swallowed.
4. Intravenous feeding can be used for several days to allow for initial healing of the esophageal repair.

Client Need: Physiological Integrity

10-27

④ Clients planning to use Nicoderm should be advised to rotate patch sites daily. Nicotine transdermal (Nicoderm) is a graduated nicotine patch designed to relieve withdrawal symptoms from tobacco cessation. Because the patches contain nicotine, they may be irritating to the skin and the sites should be rotated daily.

1. Administration of Nicoderm starts with a higher dosage and then the dosage is gradually decreased.
2. The Nicoderm patches should be changed daily, not weekly.
3. Nicoderm patches are designed to be used for 2 to 3 months and are then discontinued.

Client Need: Physiological Integrity

10-28

④ The nurse will explain to the mother that the function of the mist tent is to generate high humidity, which will help to liquefy respiratory secretions. The dampness on the child's clothing is due to condensation and is not harmful.

1. There is no need to report the mother's conversation, since the dampness of the child's clothing is an expected consequence of the humidity.
2 and 3. The dampness of the child's clothing is due to the humidity produced by the tent, not perspiration or an elevation of the child's body temperature.

Client Need: Physiological Integrity

10-29

① A compensatory mechanism seen in clients experiencing metabolic acidosis is a deep, gasping type of respiration called Kussmaul breathing. Kussmaul breathing is a compensating mechanism present in clients experiencing metabolic acidosis and renal failure. Kussmaul breathing is called air hunger and exceeds 20 breaths per minute.

2. Apneustic breathing is a marked, sustained respiratory effort associated with central nervous system disorders.

3. Biot's respirations are shallow breaths with apnea seen in clients with increased intracranial pressure.

4. Cheyne-Stokes respirations are rhythmic waxing and waning, deep to shallow breaths with temporary apnea. This type of respiration is pathological in adults but normal in children.

Client Need: Physiological Integrity

10-30

③ Arterial blood gases showing a pH of 7.37, a PCO_2 of 40, and a PO_2 of 80 indicate that the interventions have been effective. A pH of 7.37 is within the normal limits of 7.35 to 7.45. A partial pressure of carbon dioxide (PCO_2) of 40 is within the normal limits of 35 to 45 mmHg. A partial pressure of oxygen (PO_2) of 80 is within the normal limits of 75 to 95 mmHg.

1. pH 7.30, PCO_2 45, PO_2 45 = pH too low, PCO_2 almost too high, PO_2 too low.

2. pH 7.28, PCO_2 50, PO_2 40 = respiratory acidosis.

4. pH 7.42, PCO_2 22, PO_2 100 = respiratory alkalosis.

Client Need: Physiological Integrity

10-31

① In addition to the oxygen saturation level, hemoglobin data need to be considered when choosing an oxygen dosage. Oxygen is carried by hemoglobin; hemoglobin is the part of the blood to which oxygen binds and by which it is transported. A person with low hemoglobin has little capacity for oxygen transport. Supplemental oxygen would be indicated to maximize available oxygen transport.

2, 3, and 4. Serum potassium, serum chloride, and a client's height do not affect oxygen levels.

Client Need: Health Promotion and Maintenance

1 0 - 3 2

④ **Deviation of the trachea would suggest a tension pneumothorax. A tension pneumothorax is a lacerated lung that allows air to enter but not leave the pleural space. The air becomes trapped and builds pressure, which causes the lung on the injured side to collapse. When the lung collapses, mediastinal shifting to the other side of the body occurs.**

1. Spitting up blood (hemoptysis) is indicative of pulmonary emboli.
2. Sucking sounds made on inspiration are indicative of an open pneumothorax caused by an opening in the chest large enough to allow air to pass in and out freely during respirations.
3. Collapsed and flat-looking neck veins are indicative of dehydration.

Client Need: Safe, Effective Care Environment

1 0 - 3 3

① **The most probable cause of stridor following a radical neck dissection is laryngeal obstruction. Laryngeal stridor is identified upon auscultation of the trachea with a stethoscope. A coarse, high-pitched sound can be heard on inspiration. The most probable cause of stridor following a radical neck dissection is edema of the larynx. The surgeon should be notified immediately to prevent complete airway obstruction.**

2. Respiratory insufficiency is a condition in which respirations are not adequate to meet the body's need for oxygen following physical activity. Respiratory insufficiency is not associated with stridor.
3. Mediastinal shift occurs in response to severe trauma to the chest that traps air in the pleural space (tension pneumothorax). As the volume of trapped air increases, the lung collapses and organs shift to the opposite side of the chest. Symptoms include displacement of the trachea, dyspnea, cyanosis, and displacement of neck veins. Mediastinal shift is not associated with stridor.
4. Congestive heart failure (CHF) occurs when the heart is unable to meet the body's need for oxygen. When this occurs, sodium and water accumulate in the body. CHF is not a cause of stridor.

Client Need: Physiological Integrity

1 0 - 3 4

② **You will suspect flail chest. Flail chest is manifested by paradoxical movement of the chest wall and respiratory distress. The usual cause is fractured ribs, causing loss of chest wall stability. The flail segment will move paradoxically in with inspiration and out with expiration.**

1. Clinical manifestations of pneumonia include fever, chills, productive cough, and pleuritic chest pain.
3. Clinical manifestations of pneumothorax include diminished breath sounds on the injured side.
4. Clinical manifestations of cardiac tamponade are muffled and distant heart sounds, decreased blood pressure or pulse, steadily increasing central venous pressure, and possible distension of neck veins.

Client Need: Physiological Integrity

1 0 - 3 5

④   **The nurse will tell the client that beclomethasone dipropionate does not treat status asthmaticus. Beclomethasone dipropionate is not a bronchodilator but a steroid, and the full therapeutic anti-inflammatory action may take days.**

1.   Beclomethasone dipropionate medication does not treat status asthmaticus.
2.   Beclomethasone dipropionate medication does not treat status asthmaticus, and the spacer's function is to ensure accurate dosing.
3.   Status asthmaticus is a risk for every asthmatic client.

Client Need: Physiological Integrity

1 0 - 3 6

④   **You know that pancuronium should be given with sedation or analgesia. This paralytic agent does not affect pain sensation or anxiety levels and is very stressful to the client if given independently.**

1.   Pancuronium bromide commonly causes tachycardia, not bradycardia.
2.   Pancuronium bromide is a neuromuscular blocker.
3.   Pancuronium bromide does not affect pain threshold or consciousness.

Client Need: Physiological Integrity

1 0 - 3 7

①   **Early manifestations of adult respiratory distress syndrome (ARDS) are dyspnea and tachypnea. Other manifestations include cough and restlessness. ARDS is a sudden progressive disorder consisting of pulmonary edema of noncardiac origin, severe dyspnea, hypoxemia, reduced lung compliance, and diffuse pulmonary infiltrates.**

2.   Cyanosis and apprehension are later manifestations of adult respiratory syndrome.
3.   Hemoptysis refers to blood-tinged or bloody sputum. True hemoptysis is bright red and frothy, indicating bleeding in the respiratory tract.
4.   Diffuse crackles (rales) and rhonchi are later manifestations of ARDS.

Client Need: Physiological Integrity

10-38

④ **Arterial blood gases showing a pH of 7.15, a PaO₂ of 99, a PaCO₂ of 38, and a HCO₃ of 8 indicate renal acidosis. A pH of <7.35 generally indicates an acidosis, as is seen here. Low bicarbonate levels <22 mEq/l generally indicate that the acidosis is metabolic in origin, especially since the respiratory parameter (the PCO₂) is normal.**

1. This profile shows parameters that are within normal range.
2. This profile suggests hyperventilation; all parameters are within normal range except the PCO₂ (normal 35 to 45).
3. This profile suggests compensated respiratory acidosis: normal pH value with PaCO₂ retention and low PaCO₂ (hypoventilation). The high HCO₃ value is due to renal compensation.

Client Need: Health Promotion and Maintenance

10-39

① **Theophylline (Theo-Dur) is given to relieve bronchospasm. By relieving bronchospasm, theophylline allays airway obstruction.**

2. Theophylline does not decrease sputum production.
3. Theophylline does not suppress coughing.
4. Theophylline does not treat respiratory infections.

Client Need: Physiological Integrity

10-40

④ **Kussmaul respirations serve as a secondary defense mechanism in which the body attempts to rid itself of excess hydrogen ions (H+) that have accumulated due to conditions such as diabetic ketoacidosis. Kussmaul respirations are deep and often rapid respirations, present during times of metabolic acidosis.**

1. Clients experiencing Kussmaul respirations are not in pain.
2. The purpose of Kussmaul respirations is to rid the body of excessive hydrogen ions.
3. Kussmaul respirations do increase chest wall movement, but this is not the primary function of these respirations.

Client Need: Physiological Integrity

10-41

④ Elderly persons who experience prolonged diarrhea are at risk for metabolic acidosis. Bicarbonate is housed in gastrointestinal secretions. When copious amounts of these secretions are lost, such as through prolonged diarrhea, bicarbonate ions are lost. This loss affects the blood pH and causes an increase in the overall concentration of hydrogen ions, thus a decrease in pH, or acidosis.

1, 2, and 3. Potassium and sodium are excreted in diarrhea, thus placing these clients at risk for hypokalemia and hyponatremia, not hyperkalemia and hypernatremia. Metabolic, not respiratory, acidosis is also a risk, although respiratory compensation will eventually occur.

Client Need: Physiological Integrity

10-42

② The nurse would expect an assessment of a client experiencing multiple drug-resistant tuberculosis to reveal fever, weight loss, and night sweats. Other symptoms of tuberculosis include fatigue and cough.

1. Crackles, cyanosis, and fever are symptoms of pneumonia.

3. Sudden chest pain, hemoptysis, and tachycardia are symptoms associated with pulmonary embolism.

4. Nausea, diaphoresis, and severe chest pain are consistent with an acute myocardial infarction.

Client Need: Physiological Integrity

10-43

③ An open chest wound should be sealed (covered) with an airtight dressing to prevent pneumothorax from developing or becoming worse.

1. The knife should be stabilized with a bulky dressing but not removed. Removing the knife could cause additional injury. Surgery will be required to remove the knife.

2. Cleansing the wound is not a priority.

4. The client should be placed in a semi-upright position, not supine.

Client Need: Safe, Effective Care Environment

10-44

③ **Initially, the nurse should assess the client for signs and symptoms of oxygen lack, document findings, and notify the physician.**

1. A drop in arterial oxygen pressure (PaO_2) reflects changes in the client's oxygenation levels. 50 mm Hg is below the normal range of 90 to 100 mm Hg and may indicate deterioration in the client's condition.

2. The physician will need to prescribe any changes in the type of oxygen delivery and its concentration; therefore, you would not increase the oxygen concentration until consultation with the physician.

4. After the initial assessment for signs and symptoms of oxygen lack, the nurse should continue to closely monitor the client's condition and report any changes to the physician.

Client Need: Physiological Integrity

10-45

② **To evaluate the effectiveness of aminophylline, the nurse will monitor the rate and rhythm of the client's respirations. Aminophylline is a bronchodilator that relaxes the smooth muscle of the bronchi and relieves bronchospasm.**

1. Aminophylline does not affect the amount or color of secretions.

3. Aminophylline is not an antipyretic (agent that reduces fever).

4. Aminophylline does not expand the chest cavity. However, placing a client in an upright position will create more room for expansion of the diaphragm.

Client Need: Physiological Integrity

10-46

③ **To provide safety during transport of a client with chest tubes, a pair of rubber-tipped forceps should be attached to the client's gown. It is important for rubber-tipped forceps to be readily available should the chest tube become dislodged during the transport.**

1. The water-seal drainage should be kept upright and below the chest level.

2. Chest tubes should never be clamped for prolonged periods of time, and, unless essential, should not be disconnected from the water-seal drainage.

4. Deep breaths will not prevent complications following chest tube dislodgment.

Client Need: Safe, Effective Care Environment

10-47

① The best method to use when administering oxygen to a client with amyotrophic lateral sclerosis is positive pressure ventilation. Positive pressure ventilation would ensure oxygen flow despite absence of spontaneous respirations. Clients in respiratory arrest cannot move air on their own. Supplemental oxygen would be indicated to combat hypoxemia. Amyotrophic lateral sclerosis is a syndrome characterized by muscular degeneration and atrophy.

2, 3, and 4. Clients who are not breathing on their own do not benefit from oxygen without positive pressure ventilation.

Client Need: Physiological Integrity

10-48

Fill in the blank correct answer:

Virus

Severe acute respiratory syndrome (SARS) is caused by the coronavirus (SARS-CoV).

Client Need: Safe, Effective Care Environment

10-49

① Clients receiving oxygen therapy by facemask should have their body temperature taken rectally. The flow of oxygen and humidity will affect the reading of an oral temperature.

2. Receiving oxygen therapy by facemask will not interfere with a client's ability to participate in taking a bath.

3. Encouraging additional fluids is unnecessary, since receiving oxygen by facemask does not dehydrate clients.

4. Receiving oxygen by facemask does not necessitate coughing and deep breathing.

Client Need: Physiological Integrity

10-50

③ **The nurse will place a client with chronic obstructive pulmonary disease (COPD) in an upright position to facilitate ventilation. An upright position of 90 degrees causes organs in the abdominal cavity to fall away from the diaphragm by gravity, thus giving the lungs more room to expand.**

1. Lying on the back with the face upward is referred to as the supine (dorsal recumbent) position. This position is commonly used when examining a client's anterior chest and abdomen. It does not facilitate breathing.

2. A dorsal position with the head down and the feet elevated is contraindicated for clients experiencing respiratory distress because the abdominal organs press against the diaphragm and hinder breathing. This position may be used to treat clients in shock.

4. The left-side position is one in which the client is lying semi-prone on the left side with the right knee drawn up toward the chest. This position is commonly used when administering enemas. It does not facilitate breathing.

Client Need: Physiological Integrity

Practice Test 11

Mental Health Concepts, Communication, and Drug Abuse

OVERVIEW

Unlike the well-defined systems of the body, such as the cardiovascular system and the gastrointestinal system, the area of psychiatry is fraught with concepts, theories, sometimes-conflicting treatment modalities, and a cacophony of discourses, debates, and reviews. For these reasons, the following section on psychiatric and mental health nursing focuses on the concepts and principles that enjoy a degree of consensus and are basic to the beginning practitioner.

Nor ear can hear nor tongue can tell
the tortures of that inward hell.

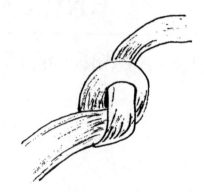

Byron, "The Giaour"
Best Quotations, Lewis C. Henry

Practice Test 11

Questions

11-1

For the past 6 weeks, you have administered chlorpromazine 50 mg tab. po, qid to your client. Today, as you approach the client with her medication, she says she feels weak and that her mouth, gums, and throat are sore. You determine that she has a fever of 102°F. You will suspect:

1. acute dystonia.
2. early manifestations of agranulocytosis.
3. neuroleptic malignant syndrome.
4. xerostomia.

11-2

A client was admitted to the hospital complaining of abdominal pain and weight loss. The client is scheduled for diagnostic tests to rule out cancer. The client tells the nurse, "I am scared." Which statement by the nurse would be most appropriate?

1. "What diagnostic tests are you going to have?"
2. "Tell me what you're afraid of."
3. "There is nothing to be afraid of; we won't hurt you."
4. "If cancer is diagnosed early enough, there is a good chance of a cure."

11-3

You are communicating with a newly admitted client. Which communication technique can interfere with the establishment of a therapeutic relationship?

1. clarifying
2. summarizing
3. giving an opinion
4. providing information

11-4

You are caring for a group of people who were trapped for 2 hours inside the elevator of a burning building. Which of the following understandings will be especially useful in meeting the needs of these people?

1. Encouraging those individuals to tell and retell the experience will help reduce its psychological impact.
2. Allowing them to break into groups to discuss the experience will reinforce the psychological impact on each individual.
3. Permitting them to keep talking about the experience will result in an increase in self-pity.
4. Discouraging any discussion of the experience will help these people to handle their anxiety.

11-5

A client goes into a coma and death seems imminent. Which of the following measures would be most important for the nurse to implement at this time?

1. Maintaining the client in positions of functional alignment.
2. Checking the client's vital signs every 15 minutes.
3. Giving the client skin and back care every hour.
4. Keeping the client comfortable and the room quiet.

1 1 - 6

When caring for a client who has recently lost a body part or valued function, it is essential for the nurse to include which of the following measures in the care plan?

1. Inviting the assistance of a person who has had a similar experience.
2. Encouraging an immediate independence in self-care.
3. Providing information to the client about how to contact community resources.
4. Allowing adequate time for the client to work through the grief.

1 1 - 7

A client has bulimia nervosa. During a binge, the client is most likely to consume:

1. fruits.
2. cakes and pies.
3. salads.
4. meats and breads.

1 1 - 8

Effective nursing management of clients who are dying requires the nurses caring for these clients to:

1. accept the inevitability of their own deaths.
2. recognize that loss and separation experiences are continual.
3. examine their own feelings and attitudes about dying.
4. understand that restoration of wellness is not possible.

1 1 - 9

A newly admitted client is unable to keep any schedule of activity due to an obsessive-compulsive handwashing ritual. Which of the following nursing actions would be most appropriate for the client at this point in the hospitalization?

1. Waking the client early enough to perform the handwashing rituals before scheduled activities begin.
2. Insisting that the client interrupt the rituals to attend scheduled activities.
3. Informing the client that ritualistic handwashing is interfering with scheduled activities.
4. Allowing the client to choose between completing the handwashing rituals and going to the scheduled activities.

1 1 - 1 0

The mother of an 8-year-old calls the mental health clinic and tells the nurse, "My child has suddenly become intensely afraid of getting into the tub to take a bath. He is standing in the living room screaming uncontrollably. What should I do?" Which of the following information should the nurse give the mother?

1. "Hold your child snugly and speak in a soft voice to him."
2. "Have your child lie down and rest for a few minutes."
3. "Bring your child to the clinic as soon as possible."
4. "Tell your child that nothing is going to happen to him if he gets into the tub."

1 1 - 1 1

A daughter admits her mother into a nursing home after it was determined that her mother has organic brain syndrome. On a subsequent visit, the mother will not speak to the daughter. The daughter calls the nurse to ask if she should come the next day. Which of the following responses by the nurse would be best?

1. Advise the daughter to wait until her mother gives some indication that she is ready to see her.
2. Suggest that the daughter come back the next day, since her continued interest will benefit the mother.
3. Tell the daughter that her mother will not miss her if she doesn't visit because she will become attached to staff members.
4. Tell the daughter that it is important for her mother to have visitors and suggest that she ask one of her friends to visit.

1 1 - 1 2

A client who was admitted to the medical-surgical unit with an acute gastrointestinal bleed is displaying a marked change in behavior. The client alternates between periods of talkativeness and stupor and frequently confabulates when talking. Because of the client's long history of alcohol abuse, you suspect:

1. Pick's disease.
2. Korsakoff-Wernicke syndrome.
3. Huntington's chorea.
4. epilepsy.

1 1 - 1 3

Which assessment finding is most likely to indicate child abuse?

1. parents who tell the nurse their 2-year-old seems ready for toilet training
2. parents who insist that their 2-year-old sit still for 30 minutes
3. an 18-month-old child with bruised areas on the forehead or knees
4. bluish-black areas on the buttocks of a newborn

1 1 - 1 4

The mother of a 6-year-old tells her child to put on his overshoes before going out into the rain. The child says, "No, they're too hard to put on." The mother turns to the nurse with a frustrated expression on her face. Which response by the nurse would be the most appropriate?

1. Say to the mother, "Maybe the overshoes are too small for the child's shoes."
2. Sit beside the child and say, "It's raining. You start pulling your overshoes on and I will help you with the hard part."
3. Hand the child the overshoes and say in a matter-of-fact manner, "If you will put the first one on, I'll put the second one on for you."
4. Say to the child, kindly but firmly, "You are trying to test your mother's authority. Put your overshoes on right now."

11-15

A client is experiencing alcohol withdrawal syndrome. The nurse should be alert for which of the following complications of this condition?

1. aphasia
2. hypotension
3. diarrhea
4. convulsions

11-16

Your client is hyperactive, euphoric, and demonstrates inappropriate impulsive behavior. Which nursing intervention will be most beneficial in channeling the client's hyperactivity?

1. Encourage projects that offer motor activity in moderation.
2. Suggest participation in competitive activities.
3. Set firm limits on unacceptable behaviors.
4. Help the client become aware of underlying anger.

11-17

A client's wife says to the nurse, "I'd do anything to help my husband stop drinking." The primary goal of the nurse's response should be to:

1. help the client's wife to clarify the problem as she sees it.
2. encourage the client's wife to join a support group such as Al-Anon.
3. tell the client's wife that she has done all she could possibly do to help her husband.
4. help the client's wife understand that alcoholism is a problem that only her husband can solve.

11-18

Because of chemotherapy, a client has lost all of his hair. The client appears distraught about his appearance and does not want to see anybody who comes to visit him. An appropriate nursing diagnosis for the client at this time is:

1. dysfunctional grieving related to hair loss.
2. defensive coping related to fear of rejection.
3. body-image disturbance related to body changes.
4. impaired adjustment related to perceived threat.

11-19

A 2-year-old has been hospitalized. The child's mother becomes upset when she comes to visit and the child turns his head away from her and holds his arms out to the nurse. The nurse will recognize that the most probable explanation for the child's behavior is:

1. He is angry with his mother for leaving him at the hospital.
2. He is testing the relationship between his mother and the nurse.
3. He now has a stronger emotional tie with the nurse than with his mother.
4. He is consciously trying to make his mother jealous.

11-20

A newborn is brought to the mother for the first time to be fed. The mother says to the nurse, "He's so little! I'm afraid I'll hurt him." Which of the following responses by the nurse would help to lessen the mother's fears?

1. "You can practice taking care of him while I am here."
2. "Is there someone at home who can help you care for him during the first few weeks?"
3. "You can watch me take care of the baby."
4. "The public health nurse can show you how to care for the baby when you get home."

11-21

Your client lost his job on New Year's Day. Since that time he has lost weight, cries frequently, and is unable to sleep. He says he is "worthless." The nurse will associate the information obtained in the assessment with which of the following conditions?

1. dysthymia
2. seasonal affective disorder
3. bipolar disorder—depression
4. major depression—single episode

11-22

Which one of the following medications will the nurse associate with the treatment of impulsive drinking?

1. naltrexone
2. disulfiram
3. chlordiazepoxide
4. fluphenazine

11-23

As you walk into your client's room, you notice the client is crying and seems to be distraught. An appropriate response to the client's behavior would be to say:

1. "I'm so sorry to have invaded your privacy. I will come back later."
2. "You look upset; would you like to talk about it?"
3. "I'm sorry you're upset; let me get a tissue for you."
4. "You seem distraught; have you received bad news?"

11-24

Your client is experiencing acute mania. The client is easily distracted, disorganized, and extremely restless. Which of the following nursing actions will be most helpful in meeting the nutritional needs of this client?

1. Tell the client, "You may become sick if you do not eat."
2. Provide high-calorie foods the client can hold in the hand while moving about.
3. Place the client in a quiet environment with a tray of favorite foods.
4. Tell the client, "Unless you eat, you will have to receive tube feedings."

11-25

A client who has recently recovered from alcohol withdrawal syndrome tells the nurse, "I know I'm not perfect, but I'm not an alcoholic." This nurse will recognize the client's comment as an example of:

1. projection.
2. rationalization.
3. repression.
4. denial.

11-26

A client was brought to the emergency department following a heroin overdose. The nurse's first intervention will be to:

1. administer a narcotic antagonist.
2. apply a hypothermia blanket.
3. establish a patent airway.
4. prepare to aspirate gastric contents.

11-27

It has become necessary to use physical restraints on an aggressive client. To ensure the client's comfort, the nurse will check the restraints every:

1. 15 minutes.
2. 30 minutes.
3. 45 minutes.
4. hour.

11-28

A client experiencing severe depression was hospitalized following a suicide attempt. The client has been scheduled for electroconvulsive therapy. Immediately before the treatment, the client will receive the neuromuscular blocking agent:

1. Atropair.
2. Pentothal.
3. Anectine.
4. Brevital.

11-29

A client with Alzheimer's disease is confused and disoriented. The client frequently asks the nurse, "Will you help me find my room? I must have taken a wrong turn." Which comment by the nurse would be most therapeutic?

1. "You lead the way and I'll be here to help if you make a wrong turn."
2. "Come with me, I'll take you to your room."
3. "Your room is the first one on the right past the dining room."
4. "It's time for your exercise. Come with me to the recreational room."

11-30

Your client is receiving lithium to treat a bipolar affective disorder. Blood samples will be drawn to monitor the client's serum lithium levels. The nurse understands that the therapeutic maintenance level of lithium ranges from:

1. 0.2 to 0.9 mEq/l.
2. 0.4 to 1.0 mEq/l.
3. 1.6 to 2.4 mEq/l.
4. 2.2 to 3.2 mEq/l.

11-31

A client is hospitalized with ulcerative colitis and scheduled for an ileostomy. Prior to surgery, the nurse is reinforcing the need to cough and deep breathe. The client says, "Don't treat me like a child. I know how to breathe." Which of the following responses would be the most appropriate for the nurse to make?

1. "Do you know the reason for doing this?"
2. "Do you feel I'm talking down to you?"
3. "You're overreacting."
4. "No one else has had that complaint."

11-32

You are changing your client's ileostomy bag. It is most important to take which of the following measures?

1. Refrain from showing distaste.
2. Maintain strict surgical asepsis.
3. Explain the details of the procedure.
4. Wipe the stoma with a mild antiseptic.

11-33

Your client is experiencing the manic phase of a bipolar disorder. The client is unkempt, profane, and hyperactive. Which nursing intervention would be the most therapeutic when the client's language becomes profane and abusive?

1. Let the client know the language being used is unacceptable.
2. Isolate the client from others until he stops his profane and abusive language.
3. Ignore the client's profane and abusive language.
4. Recognize the client's language as a part of the illness and set firm limits.

11-34

Your client is having delusions of persecution and refuses to eat. The client says the personnel are poisoning the food. Which one of the following responses by the nurse would be most appropriate initially in coping with this situation?

1. Permit the client to eat food that has been brought from home.
2. Tell the client, "No one is putting poison in your food."
3. Taste the client's food and say, "See, I told you there was no poison in your food."
4. Recognize the client's behavior as a symptom of the condition.

11-35

Your client has bulimia nervosa. Clients with bulimia nervosa attempt to maintain desired body weight by:

1. consuming a less-than-adequate amount of an otherwise well-balanced diet.
2. restricting high-calorie foods during binges.
3. premeditated binges.
4. self-induced vomiting along with laxative and diuretic abuse.

11-36

Your client is experiencing delusions of persecution. You are to administer the client's antipsychotic medication for the first time. Which one of the following actions would be most likely to ensure the client's acceptance of the medication?

1. Administer the medication when the client does not appear to be upset or delusional.
2. Request additional stand-by personnel in the event the client refuses to take the medication.
3. Explain the procedure for administering the medication prior to approaching the client.
4. Attempt to disguise the client's medication in food and drink.

11-37

Which one of the following nursing actions would be most effective in preventing a client who is a suicide risk from committing suicide?

1. administration of antidepressant medication
2. knowing the whereabouts of the client at all times
3. providing opportunities for the client to express thoughts and feelings
4. encouraging participation in ward activities

11-38

A client who is going to be discharged tells the nurse, "I'm afraid I won't be able to pay all my medical bills." Which comment by the nurse would facilitate further elaboration by the client?

1. "I'll introduce you to one of the social workers. They will be able to help you."
2. "I'll report your concern to the business office."
3. "I understand how you feel. The cost of health care is alarming."
4. "You seem worried about this situation."

11-39

A plan of care for an infant with fetal alcohol syndrome should place the most emphasis on overcoming problems involving:

1. fluid balance.
2. peripheral circulation.
3. nutrition.
4. airway clearance.

11-40

Your client has been diagnosed with hypochondriasis following a complete physical examination. The client was informed that no organic bases for the presenting complains were found. The client tells you, "I'm sure I have a terrible disease." Your best response would be to:

1. ignore the client's complaints.
2. reaffirm the medical findings.
3. ask the client, "Why do you think you are ill?"
4. tell the client she looks healthy.

11-41

A client was hospitalized following a suicide attempt after losing a job. One week later, you observe a sudden apparent improvement in the client. The nurse understands that the most probable reason for the apparent improvement is that the client:

1. has gotten some information about a new job.
2. has established supportive relationships with the personnel.
3. has been relieved of a stressful work environment.
4. may be committed to suicide and has a workable plan.

11-42

While watching the evening news on the television, a delusional client shouts, "You can't blame me for dropping that bomb." The nurse will recognize the client's behavior as a response to:

1. a hallucination.
2. a delusion of reference.
3. an illusion.
4. a delusion of persecution.

11-43

You are planning activities for a client who has an obsessive-compulsive disorder. You will choose times for the activities when the client is relatively anxiety-free. You understand the client's anxiety will be at its lowest:

1. immediately following the performance of the ritualistic behavior.
2. during the time the ritualistic behavior is being performed.
3. nearing the completion of the ritualistic behavior.
4. immediately before the performance of the ritualistic behavior.

11-44

A client with terminal cancer tells the nurse, "I'm dying." The most therapeutic response by the nurse would be:

1. "It must be frightening to know that you are dying."
2. "Tell me more about how you feel."
3. "There is always hope that a treatment will be available that might save your life."
4. "You really look much better."

11-45

An 8-year-old client has hemophilia. Which statement by the client would reflect the child's acceptance of the constant seriousness of the condition?

1. "I use a Water Pik for cleaning my teeth."
2. "I take Tylenol if I have pain."
3. "I wear a MedicAlert identification bracelet."
4. "I keep an emergency kit at my bedside."

11-46

A client is receiving haloperidol 5 mg po tid. To protect the client from a frequent side effect of this medication, the nurse will:

1. provide the client with a low-sodium diet.
2. instruct the client to rise slowly to a standing position.
3. restrict fluid intake to 1,000 cc daily.
4. provide a diet that is free of cheese products.

11-47

Prior to admission to the hospital, a child 2 years of age was partially bowel trained, but now defecates involuntarily. The nurse's approach to this situation should be based on which of the following assessments?

1. What is the child's reaction to the soiling?
2. How compulsive is the child about cleanliness?
3. Is the child too young for bowel training?
4. Is bowel training important to the child?

11-48

A client 45 years old is admitted to an alcoholic treatment center. He has been drinking a quart or more of liquor a day for 10 to 15 years. The client has been drinking up to the time of admission. In responding to long-term alcohol abuse, the nurse admitting the client would expect the immediate treatment to include which of the following prescriptions?

1. oral fluids and a narcotic
2. a cool bath, a barbiturate, and blood lithium levels
3. regular diet as tolerated, thiamine, and a tranquilizer
4. a spinal tap, bromides, and restraints

11-49

Your client has just awakened from an electroconvulsive therapy treatment. The most appropriate nursing action at this time would be to:

1. arrange for the client's diet to be served.
2. orient the client.
3. observe the client for signs of suicidal behavior.
4. provide the client with a quiet environment in which to rest.

11-50

A mother asks the nurse, "What are those little white spots all over my baby's face? None of my other babies had them." Which of the following responses would be best?

1. "They are called milia and will soon disappear."
2. "Most babies have them; there is no need to worry."
3. "You should not be concerned about such small cysts."
4. "Some babies have many more spots than your baby."

Practice Test 11

Answers, Rationales, and Explanations

1 1 - 1

② The nurse will suspect the early development of agranulocytosis (an acute disease characterized by a deficit or total lack of granulocytic white blood cells), a rare occurrence that is potentially fatal. Chlorpromazine (Thorazine) would be discontinued and reverse isolation instituted, along with stat bloodwork.

1. Dystonia is characterized by painful spasms of voluntary muscles affecting the neck, back, jaws, limbs, and eyes. Dystonia may be seen in the first 5 days of neuroleptic administration.

3. Neuroleptic malignant syndrome (NMS) is a rare, idiosyncratic reaction to neuroleptic agents, characterized by muscle rigidity, hyperthermia, and stupor. There is an increase in white blood cells.

4. Xerostomia is dryness of the mouth caused by reduction in the amount of saliva. Xerostomia is a common side effect associated with the administration of neuroleptic medications like Thorazine.

Client Need: Health Promotion and Maintenance

1 1 - 2

② The nurse's best response would include an open-ended statement such as, "Tell me what you're afraid of." This allows the client an opportunity to verbalize fears.

1. The client is not afraid of the diagnostic tests. The client is afraid the tests will indicate the presence of cancer.

3. Telling the client there is nothing to be afraid of is not realistic. It is the test results that are causing the fear.

4. Suggesting that early detection of cancer will give the client a "good chance" also suggests that if the cancer is advanced, the client won't have a "good chance."

Client Need: Physiological Integrity

1 1 - 3

③ Giving an opinion can be detrimental when a nurse is trying to build a relationship with a client. Giving an opinion takes decision making away from the client. It inhibits spontaneity, stalls problem solving, and creates doubt. Giving an opinion prevents the client from developing solutions.

1, 2, and 4.Therapeutic techniques of communication include clarifying, summarizing, and providing information. These techniques help to build a relationship.

Client Need: Psychosocial Integrity

1 1 - 4

① Repeated telling of a harrowing experience allows the people involved to reflect, recognize the importance of the experience in their lives, and begin the process of eventually mastering the experience.

2. Perpetuating a discussion of the experience should be done for the purpose of reducing the impact of the experience, not to reinforce the impact.

3. Self-pity should not be a goal but one of a series of stages that may be experienced by some individuals who have had a harrowing experience.

4. Avoiding the discussion of a terrifying experience prevents individuals from working through the trauma and coping effectively.

Client Need: Psychosocial Integrity

1 1 - 5

④ When the death of a client appears imminent, nursing measures should focus on the client's comfort and the preservation of a quiet environment.

1. Following the death of a client, the nurse should maintain the client's body in a position of functional alignment. This will assist in the preparation of the body for burial.

2 and 3. Taking the client's vital signs or giving back care serves no purpose under the circumstances.

Client Need: Psychosocial Integrity

1 1 - 6

④ When caring for a client who has lost a body part or valued function, the nursing-care plan should include measures that allow adequate time for the client to work through grief. Any loss, real or perceived, requires a period of time for grieving. Mourning is a well-defined psychological process by which grief is resolved. Encouraging the client's expression of feelings and listening are most important in caring for the grieving client.

1. Inviting the assistance of a person who has had a similar loss can be helpful once the client has worked through the grieving process.

2. Encouraging immediate independence and self-care may overwhelm the client.

3. Providing information about community resources should be done when the client has worked through the grieving process and is psychologically ready.

Client Need: Health Promotion and Maintenance

1 1 - 7

② **When binging, clients with bulimia nervosa will select high-calorie foods, such as cakes and pies, which require little chewing and are easily ingested. Bulimia is characterized by excessive food intake accompanied by purging.**

1. Fruits may be ingested during the phase of food restrictions, but during a binge, fruits would not be selected because they are not typically high-calorie or as easily ingested as cakes and pies.
3. Salads are not foods of choice during a binge. However, during the restrictive phase, these clients would likely select salads due to their low caloric value.
4. Meats and breads are not easily ingested and therefore are not selected during a binge. These foods require more chewing than items such as cakes and pies.

Client Need: Psychosocial Integrity

1 1 - 8

③ **To effectively care for dying clients, nurses must first examine their own feelings and attitudes about dying.**

1. Effective nursing care of dying clients requires more than an academic or intellectual acceptance of death.
2. Just recognizing that loss and separation are continual would not help nurses to care for dying client and their unique needs as they approach death.
4. Understanding that wellness is not possible for dying client is helpful to the extent that the nurse will be less likely to deny the needs of those clients. However, examining one's own feelings about dying is essential when caring for those who are dying.

Client Need: Psychosocial Integrity

1 1 - 9

① **Waking the client early enough to complete the handwashing ritual and still have time to attend scheduled meetings will help to involve the client in the milieu. Early on in the client's hospitalization, it would be important for the client to understand that no one is going to try to prevent the ritualistic handwashing.**

2. The purpose of obsessive-compulsive behavior is to relieve anxiety. Interrupting the rituals will only increase the client's anxiety.
3. Informing the client that the handwashing ritual is interfering with scheduled activities will not only increase anxiety but will place the client in a dilemma.
4. The client should not be placed in a position of choosing between performing a handwashing ritual and going to scheduled activities.

Client Need: Psychosocial Integrity

11-10

①   **The mother should be told to hold her child snugly and speak softly to him. The child is demonstrating behavior suggestive of a phobia. He is unable to control his anxiety and fears and needs someone to take control of him and the situation.**

2. A child who is out of control because of fear and anxiety is unable to lie down and rest.

3. Bringing the child to the clinic before helping him to gain control will only prolong the fear and anxiety he is experiencing.

4. Attempting to reason with a person who has a phobia is inappropriate, since a phobia is an irrational fear.

Client Need: Psychosocial Integrity

11-11

②   **The nurse should suggest that the daughter come back to see her mother, since the daughter's continued interest will benefit her mother. Consistent family contact is important in providing stability in the environment of a client with organic brain syndrome. Socializing can improve the client's quality of life.**

1. Clients with organic brain syndrome (pathological dysfunction of the brain) are not likely to initiate visits. It will be up to the client's daughter to plan and implement visits with the client.

3. The daughter's visit will be beneficial for her mother. The nurse should encourage socialization with family members.

4. Advising the daughter conveys the idea that the nurse knows best and that the daughter cannot think for herself. This approach fosters dependency and hinders problem solving.

Client Need: Psychosocial Integrity

11-12

②   **The nurse will suspect Korsakoff-Wernicke syndrome. Korsakoff-Wernicke syndrome, which involves disorientation, delirium, and inappropriate phrasing, is associated with long-term alcohol abuse.**

1. Pick's disease is a form of presenile dementia due to atrophy of the frontal and temporal lobes of the brain. The etiology is unknown.

3. Huntington's chorea is an inherited disease that is typified by involuntary face and limb movements.

4. Seizure activity is the hallmark of epilepsy.

Client Need: Physiological Integrity

11-13

② Parents who insist that their 2-year-old sit still for 30 minutes may attempt to enforce their demands in abusive ways. It is unrealistic for the parents of a 2-year-old to expect the child to sit still for 30 minutes.

1. It is appropriate for parents of a 2-year-old to expect the child to be ready for toilet training. A child cannot voluntarily control bowel and bladder sphincters until myelinization of the spinal cord occurs. Myelinization takes place between 12 and 18 months of age.

3. It would be appropriate for an 18-month-old to have bruised areas on the forehead and knees. At this age, children are falling often in their attempts to pull up and walk.

4. Mongolian spots (bluish-black areas on the buttocks and thighs of a newborn) are normally seen in 80% of nonwhite newborns and 10% of white newborns. The spots fade away with age.

Client Need: Psychosocial Integrity

11-14

② The nurse should let the child know that help will be given with the "hard part" of putting on overshoes. Children 6 years of age, like all children, need to have set limits. Compliance can be facilitated by giving the child an explanation for why the overshoes are needed. Also, limits are set and the child is not left without help if needed.

1. Suggesting that the overshoes may be too tight ignores the child's attempt to challenge his mother's authority.

3. Bargaining with the child puts the child in control and does not set limits on his behavior. If the child refuses to keep his end of the bargain, the situation is likely to escalate.

4. Even though the child is testing his mother's authority, it is not necessary for the nurse to verbalize the psychodynamics of the interaction. Challenging the child with a demand could escalate the situation unnecessarily.

Client Need: Psychosocial Integrity

11-15

④ The nurse should be alert for convulsions when clients are withdrawing from alcohol. Alcohol lowers the seizure threshold in vulnerable individuals. The sudden absence of alcohol from the system of an alcoholic may precipitate convulsions.

1. Aphasia is the absence or impairment of the ability to communicate by speaking, writing, or use of signs. It is due to dysfunction of the brain centers. Aphasia is a clinical manifestation of cerebrovascular accidents.

2. Clients who experience alcohol withdrawal are likely to have hypertension and tachycardia.

3. Nausea and vomiting may be experienced by clients in alcohol withdrawal. However, diarrhea is not a typical symptom.

Client Need: Physiological Integrity

11-16

① **Encouraging projects that offer motor activity in moderation can help diffuse hyperactivity.**

2. Competitive activities are harmful because they further stimulate the hyperactive client.

3. Setting firm limits is essential but does not defuse hyperactivity.

4. The attention span of the hyperactive client is extremely short and does not allow for interventions that focus on gaining insight.

Client Need: Safe, Effective Care Environment

11-17

① **The nurse's primary goal will be to help the client's wife clarify the problem as she sees it. This will help the nurse to know how to proceed.**

2. Suggesting a support group such as Al-Anon would be inappropriate before determining how the wife of the client views the problem.

3. Telling the client's wife that she has done all she could possibly do to help her husband is avoiding the wife's concern by attempting to placate her.

4. Alcoholics can be helped by others, but it is important for those who want to help to know how to help.

Client Need: Health Promotion and Maintenance

11-18

③ **An appropriate nursing diagnosis at this time would be body-image disturbance related to body changes. This diagnosis is evidenced by verbal and nonverbal responses to actual or perceived changes in the structure and function of the client's body.**

1. Grieving is an expression of distress at loss and is generally considered to be dysfunctional when it is prolonged or sustained (usually a year after the loss).

2. Defensive coping related to fear of rejection includes denial of problems, projection of blame onto others, and an attitude of superiority toward others.

4. Impaired adjustment related to the perceived threat includes the inability to modify lifestyle to accommodate change.

Client Need: Psychosocial Integrity

11-19

1. The nurse will recognize that the most likely explanation for the child's behavior is anger toward his mother for leaving him at the hospital. The client is unable to understand why his mother left him. A 2-year-old child has a strong attachment to his mother and needs to be close to her. Loss of contact will result in behavior that is manifested as fear and anger.

2. Testing relationships between adults will develop when the child is older. Children will test the relationship between their parents by pitting one parent against the other in an attempt to get their way about something, such as the purchase of a new toy.

3. The child does not have a stronger bond with the nurse. The child is only demonstrating his anger and fear by rejecting his mother at the moment.

4. A 2-year-old does not understand the abstract concept of jealousy.

Client Need: Psychosocial Integrity

11-20

1. Assuring the new mother that she can practice caring for her baby while under supervision may decrease her anxiety. The nurse's comment indicated her confidence in the new mother's ability to care for her baby.

2. Asking the new mother if someone at home can help her take care of her baby for a few weeks is inappropriate. The nurse should recognize the mother's concern and proceed to assess the client's strengths and weaknesses for caring for her baby.

3. Telling the new mother that she can learn how to take care of her baby by watching the nurse take care of the baby is placing the mother in a passive observer role. The mother should have the opportunity to actually participate in her baby's care while under supervision.

4. The client can be taught how to take care of her baby now. The nurse can teach her a great deal about taking care of her baby before she leaves the hospital. Waiting for a public health nurse to teach the mother is ignoring the mother's present need.

Client Need: Psychosocial Integrity

11-21

④ **The nurse will associate the information obtained during assessment with a major depression, single episode. There is evidence to suggest a great change from the client's previous functions. The client is unable to function socially or occupationally. The client is experiencing insomnia, weight loss, and is in constant emotional discomfort.**

1. Dysthymia occurs over a 2-year period and is considered mild to moderate in degree. Clients with dysthymia are at risk for developing major depression. Clients with dysthymia experience anhedonia (inability to find pleasure in anything).

2. Seasonal affective disorder (SAD) is characterized by hypersomnia, fatigue, weight gain, irritability, and difficulties with interpersonal relationships. This condition usually occurs in the winter and is effectively treated with 2 to 3 hours of bright light daily.

3. Bipolar disorders are mood disorders that include one or more manic episodes and one or more depressive episodes.

Client Need: Psychosocial Integrity

11-22

② **The nurse will associate disulfiram (Antabuse) with the treatment of impulsive drinking. It is usually given to alcoholics who have demonstrated the ability to stay sober. If clients drink alcohol while take this drug, they will experience the alcohol-disufiram reaction. Symptoms of this reaction include facial flushing, nausea, vomiting, hypertension, respiratory distress, and profuse sweating.**

1. The medication naltrexone (ReVia) is used to treat alcoholics by decreasing the client's craving for alcohol. This medication is not given to treat impulsive drinking.

3. Chlordiazepoxide (Librium) is administered to treat the symptoms of alcohol withdrawal, not impulsive drinking.

4. Fluphenazine (Prolixin) is an antipsychotic administered to treat acute and chronic psychoses. There is no association with this drug and the treatment of alcoholism.

Client Need: Psychosocial Integrity

11-23

② **It would be appropriate for the nurse to say, "You look upset; would you like to talk about it?" This response acknowledges that the client is upset and provides the client with an opportunity to express feelings.**

1. Leaving the room of a client who is crying and upset is inappropriate. The nurse who would do this is probably feeling incapable of relieving the client's emotional pain and is using the client's need for privacy as an excuse to leave.

3. Suggesting that you get a tissue for a client who is upset and crying is focusing on the physical aspects of the situation (runny nose and tears). It would be more therapeutic to focus on the underlying cause of the crying.

4. Instead of trying to guess what has upset the client, the nurse should acknowledge that the client seems upset and provide the client with an opportunity to talk about the problem.

Client Need: Psychosocial Integrity

11-24

② The nurse will provide hyperactive clients with high-calorie foods that can be held in the hand and eaten as the client moves about. Examples of high-calorie "finger-foods" include milk shakes and pastries. Constipation is also a concern; therefore, fiber and fluids are encouraged by providing fruits that can be eaten while the client is moving about.

1 and 4. It is not possible to reason with clients who are experiencing acute mania. They have a short attention span and are unable to concentrate.

3. Clients who are experiencing acute mania are unable to sit still. Simply placing them in a quiet, nonstimulating environment with favorite foods will not solve the problem.

Client Need: Physiological Integrity

11-25

④ The nurse will recognize that the client is using the defense mechanism (DM) of denial. Defense mechanisms are unconscious intrapsychic processes used by clients to ward off feelings of anxiety by preventing conscious awareness of threatening feelings. By using denial, the client is escaping the unpleasant realities of what it means to be an alcoholic.

1. Projection occurs when one attributes one's own intolerable attributes to another person, such as an alcoholic who accuses someone else of being an alcoholic.

2. Rationalization occurs when one attempts to present acceptable explanations for an intolerable attribute. An alcoholic might say, "If you had the job I have, you would drink too."

3. Repression occurs when traumatic events are pushed out of consciousness.

Client Need: Psychosocial Integrity

11-26

③ The nurse's first intervention when caring for a client who has had a heroin overdose is to establish a patent airway. Heroin overdose requires immediate intervention to prevent death.

1. Following the establishment of a patent airway, the nurse would anticipate administering the narcotic antagonist naloxone (Narcan). This medication quickly reverses central nervous system depression.

2. A hypothermia blanket would be appropriate for a client who had taken an overdose of stimulants, such as cocaine.

4. Aspirating gastric contents would be necessary when caring for a client who had taken an overdose of a sedative/hypnotic.

Client Need: Physiological Integrity

11-27

① If it becomes necessary to physically restrain a client, the nurse will know to check the restraints every 15 minutes. Frequent position changes, massaging the skin, and range-of-motion exercises are all helpful in preventing prolonged pressure against blood vessels and nerves.

2, 3, and 4. Waiting longer than 15 minutes to assess a client in restraints could place a client in jeopardy. The goal of restraints is safety for the client and others.

Client Need: Psychosocial Integrity

11-28

③ Immediately before an electroconvulsive therapy treatment, the nurse will administer the neuromuscular blocking agent succinylcholine (Anectine). Anectine is a neuromuscular blocking agent (muscle relaxant) used after induction of anesthesia to promote muscle paralysis. When administered intravenously immediately prior to electroconvulsive therapy (ECT), it relaxes muscles and prevents the risk of fractures and soft tissue injuries.

1. Approximately 30 to 60 minutes before electroconvulsive therapy, the nurse will administer atropine (Atropair) intramuscularly. Atropine is an anticholinergic that will decrease oral and respiratory secretions.

2 and 4. Methohexital sodium (Brevital) and thiopental (Pentothal) are both short-acting anesthetics, either of which may be given just prior to the neuromuscular blocking agent Anectine.

Client Need: Health Promotion and Maintenance

11-29

② The nurse should say, "Come with me, I'll help you to your room." Clients with Alzheimer's disease have progressive, irreversible memory loss and deterioration of intellect. They experience confusion and disorientation.

1. The client is confused and disorientated and unable to lead the way. Asking the client to lead the way is setting the client up for failure.

3. The client is unable to follow directions due to short-term memory loss, confusion, and disorientation.

4. Diverting the client's attention is avoiding the client's immediate need for orientation.

Client Need: Psychosocial Integrity

11-30

② The nurse knows that the therapeutic maintenance level of lithium (Lithotabs) ranges from 0.4 to 1.0 mEq/l. To prevent toxicity, lithium maintenance levels should not exceed 1.5 mEq/l.

1. In order to be therapeutic, lithium levels should fall between 0.4 and 1.0 mEq/l. A lithium level below 0.4 would not be therapeutic.

3. A lithium level between 1.6 and 2.4 could cause signs of advanced to severe lithium toxicity, such as mental confusion, lack of coordination, ataxia, stupor, and death.

4. A lithium level between 2.2 and 3.2 mEq/l could cause severe toxicity and death. Hemodialysis may be considered in such cases.

Client Need: Health Promotion and Maintenance

11-31

② It would be appropriate for the nurse to respond with, "Do you feel I'm talking down to you?" This response shows respect for the client's feelings and allows the client to calm down. The nurse should keep communications open despite the fact that the client is upset.

1. Asking the client, "Do you know the reason for this?" may put the client on the defensive and is not recommended.

3. Saying "You're overreacting" is minimizing the client's feelings and is judgmental.

4. Saying "No one else has had that complaint" is suggesting that the client's response is somehow out of the ordinary and therefore should be ignored.

Client Need: Safe, Effective Care Environment

11-32

① The nurse should not demonstrate an attitude of distaste when changing a client's colostomy bag. The client is likely to have feelings of embarrassment and a body image disturbance. Most clients with ileostomies worry about odor control and bowel excretion. They will take the attitude of the nurse as an example of the way other people will react. By not showing distaste when changing the client's ileostomy bag, the nurse is teaching the client not to be embarrassed about caring for the ileostomy.

2. There is no need to use sterile technique when changing a client's ileostomy bag. The gastrointestinal tract is not sterile.

3. There is no indication that the nurse is teaching the client how to change the ileostomy bag, only that the bag is being changed.

4. The stoma should be cleansed with gentle friction using mild soap and warm water. The skin should be patted dry. An antiseptic would be irritating to the skin.

Client Need: Psychosocial Integrity

1 1 - 3 3

④ **The nurse will recognize the client's language as part of the illness and will set firm limits. The client's offensive language is an outlet for uncomfortable hyperactive feelings that the client is unable to control.**

1. The client is not able to control the illness responsible for the profane and abusive language. Therefore, telling the client that the language is unacceptable is inappropriate.

2. The nurse should help the client to redirect the hyperactivity that underlies the use of profane and abusive language.

3. A manic client who is out of control should not be ignored. The nurse should provide structure and set limits that will help the client feel secure. Hyperactive clients want to know that someone is in control.

Client Need: Psychosocial Integrity

1 1 - 3 4

④ **The nurse should recognize the client's delusion as a symptom of the condition.**

1. Permitting the client to eat food that was brought from home is not therapeutic because it implies that the food served in the hospital is poisoned.

2. Delusions are false fixed ideas or beliefs. Simply telling a client that no one is poisoning the food will be totally ineffective.

3. A client who saw the nurse taste the food would not be convinced that the food wasn't poisoned. The client would reason that the nurse had tasted that part of the food that did not have poison in it.

Client Need: Psychosocial Integrity

1 1 - 3 5

④ **Clients with bulimia nervosa attempt to maintain their body weight by self-induced vomiting (purging), laxative and diuretic abuse, exercise, and avoidance of food (fasting) in between bouts of binging.**

1. Clients with bulimia do not eat a well-balanced diet. They have a pattern of fasting and then consuming large quantities of less-than-healthy, high-calorie foods.

2. During binges, these clients consume extremely large quantities of high-calorie, easily ingested foods such as milk shakes, cakes, and pies.

3. Binges are not always preplanned. In fact, binges may be associated with problems of impulse control.

Client Need: Psychosocial Integrity

11-36

③ **To facilitate compliance, the nurse should explain exactly what the procedure is for administering medications. An explanation may help to establish a therapeutic rapport based on mutual respect and trust.**

1. The nurse should not assume that because a client does not appear to be upset or delusional, the client is rational and calm.

2. Requesting additional stand-by personnel is likely to be interpreted by a suspicious delusional client as a threat.

4. Any attempt to deceive the client will compromise credibility and is inappropriate.

Client Need: Psychosocial Integrity

11-37

② **Knowing the whereabouts of clients who are suicidal should be the nurse's first consideration. It is an established fact that clients who have committed suicide have done so in very short periods of time. The nurse who knows the location of clients at all times can be assured of their physical safety.**

1. Whereas the administration of medication should not be minimized, the nurse should not think that clients who are at risk would not take their own lives simply because they are receiving medication. The fact that clients may need to take medications can be a contributing factor in their decision to attempt suicide.

3. Providing opportunities for suicidal clients to express their thoughts and feelings outwardly, as opposed to turning their anger inward, is therapeutic. However, it may not be sufficiently effective in deterring clients from taking their own lives.

4. Participation in ward activities does give clients who are at risk an opportunity to concentrate on something other than taking their own life. Physical activities can also be helpful in channeling potentially destructive behaviors. However, activities alone do not solve the underlying problems that contribute to the choice some clients make to take their lives.

Client Need: Psychosocial Integrity

11-38

④ **The nurse could facilitate further elaboration from the client by saying, "You seem worried about this situation." By identifying the client's feelings, the nurse opens the conversation for additional comments by the client.**

1 and 2. Telling the client that you will contact the business office or a social worker will bring the conversation to an abrupt end. The client will be left to worry about a problem that was not fully expressed.

3. Agreeing with clients doesn't leave them with an option to change their point of view or their feelings.

Client Need: Psychosocial Integrity

11-39

③ Poor feeding is usually a problem for infants with fetal alcohol syndrome. Feeding difficulties are related to a poor suck reflex, microcephaly, irritability, and later, hyperactivity. Other characteristics of infants with fetal alcohol syndrome are hypotonia, mental retardation, motor retardation, hearing disorders, and growth retardation, as well as facial features that include thin upper lip, hypoplastic maxilla, and short, upturned nose.

1, 2, and 4. Fluid balance, peripheral circulation, and airway clearance are not problems typically associated with fetal alcohol syndrome.

Client Need: Health Promotion and Maintenance

11-40

② The nurse should reaffirm the medical findings. Consistently reaffirming the medical findings is the most appropriate response to give clients who are experiencing hypochondriasis. This will expose the client to the facts.

1. Ignoring the client would convey a lack of interest and would be inappropriate.
3. Asking the client, "Why do you think you are ill?" will give the client an audience for verbalizing complaints.
4. Telling the client, "You look healthy" will provide an opportunity for the client to go through a list of complaints.

Client Need: Psychosocial Integrity

11-41

④ The most probable reason for sudden apparent improvement in a suicidal client is that the client may be committed to suicide and has a workable plan. A client who has decided to commit suicide will appear to the nurse to be improved. This sudden improvement comes about as a consequence of the client resolving all ambivalence about committing suicide.

1. There is no indication that the client has received any information about a new job.
2. There would be a gradual improvement in a client who developed a supportive therapeutic relationship with the personnel, not a sudden overall improvement.
3. Occasionally a client will show improvement when hospitalized and relieved of a stressful environment. However, when this happens the improvement is usually immediate, not a week after hospitalization.

Client Need: Psychosocial Integrity

11-42

② **The nurse will recognize the client's behavior as a response to a delusion of reference. Delusions of reference are false ideas (delusions) that outside occurrences have special meaning to oneself.**

1. A hallucination is a perception of the senses for which no external stimuli exists; for example, a person who hears people talking when no people are present.

3. An illusion is a misinterpretation of reality. For example, a client says there are bugs in an ashtray when in reality the ashtray is filled with cigarette butts.

4. A delusion of persecution is a false idea or belief that people are plotting against you. For example, a client says all of his coworkers are jealous of him and are trying to kill him.

Client Need: Psychosocial Integrity

11-43

① **Clients who have obsessive-compulsive disorders are the least anxious immediately after the ritualistic behavior has been completed.**

2 and 3. Interrupting an obsessive-compulsive client at any point during the performance of the ritualistic behavior will increase anxiety. Many clients feel they have to start the ritual all over again from the beginning if they are interrupted.

4. Clients are the most anxious immediately before the ritualistic behavior is performed.

Client Need: Psychosocial Integrity

11-44

② **A client who is dying can benefit from a broad opening statement that encourages expression of feelings, such as, "Tell me more about how you feel."**

1. Suggesting to a client, "It must be frightening to know you are dying" is based on the assumption that the client is frightened. This may not be the case.

3. Telling a dying client that a life-saving treatment might be found that will save her life is inappropriate and prevents the client from preparing for death.

4. Telling a dying client, "You really look better" is a barrier to further therapeutic communication. It signals the nurse's unwillingness to converse with the client about his impending death.

Client Need: Psychosocial Integrity

11-45

③ **Wearing a MedicAlert bracelet demonstrates a constant awareness of the seriousness of hemophilia. If clients with hemophilia are ever unconscious, it can still be determined that they have hemophilia.**

1. It is not necessary for clients with hemophilia to use a Water Pik. A soft-bristle toothbrush softened in warm water is acceptable for mouth care.

2. Tylenol for pain is an appropriate choice. However, it is less important than wearing a MedicAlert bracelet.

4. Keeping an emergency kit at the bedside is not likely to be of much use. Accidents are not likely to occur in bed.

Client Need: Psychosocial Integrity

11-46

② **Clients receiving haloperidol (Haldol) should be advised to make position changes slowly to minimize the potential for orthostatic hypotension.**

1. A low-sodium diet may be prescribed for a client who is experiencing hypertension, not hypotension.

3. Fluids should be encouraged, since clients have a tendency to become dehydrated.

4. Clients who are taking monoamine oxidase (MAO) inhibitors are to avoid foods with tyramine. Hypertensive crisis may occur with the ingestion of foods containing high amounts of tyramine. Foods containing tyramine include aged cheese, wine, pickled or smoked fish, overripe fruits, and foods containing aspartame.

Client Need: Health Promotion and Maintenance

11-47

① **The nurse's approach to this problem should be based on the child's reaction to the soiling. It is normal to expect some degree of regression with hospitalization.**

2 and 4. Overreacting and overanalyzing the child's behavior is not beneficial or relevant.

3. A 2-year-old is physically mature enough to be bowel trained and had demonstrated progress in that direction before hospitalization.

Client Need: Health Promotion and Maintenance

11-48

③ **The nurse would anticipate a treatment plan that includes a regular diet as tolerated, thiamine (B₁), and a tranquilizer. Nutritional deficiency is a major problem exhibited by individuals with a long history of alcohol abuse. Thiamine is used to retard peripheral neuropathy common in long-term alcohol abuse. A deficiency of thiamine may also lead to Korsakoff's syndrome. Tranquilizers may be used as a detoxification agent to prevent delirium tremens.**

1. Encouraging oral fluids is recommended, since the client is likely to be dehydrated. However, narcotics are contraindicated because they are central nervous system (CNS) depressants and potentiate the depressant effects of alcohol.

2. The client is not receiving lithium (Lithotabs). There is no need to draw blood for lithium levels. Also, barbiturates are central nervous (CNS) depressants and should not be taken because they potentiate the depressant effects of alcohol.

4. There is no indication that a spinal tap is needed.

Client Need: Physiological Integrity

11-49

② **The nurse should orient the client. Immediately after clients awaken following electroconvulsive therapy (ECT), they are confused and disoriented. The nurse's orientation should be brief, distinct, and easy to comprehend.**

1. Just because a client is awake does not mean that the gag reflex has returned. Until the client's gag reflex returns, nothing should be eaten. The client should not be served until orientated, coordinated, and able to manage the diet.

3. Clients are too confused immediately after awakening from ECT to contemplate suicide.

4. A quiet environment is helpful, but it would not be the first priority.

Client Need: Psychosocial Integrity

11-50

① **The nurse should tell the mother that the "little white spots" are called milia and that they will soon disappear. The white spots are due to retention of sebaceous material within the sebaceous glands. Milia are clinically insignificant and disappear during the neonatal period.**

2. Telling the client, "Most babies have them, don't worry," does not answer the mother's question.

3. Milia are not cysts. Telling a client not to be concerned without answering the question will block further communication and disregards the client's concerns.

4. Telling a mother that "Some babies have more spots than your baby" conveys that the client should not complain, since other babies are "worse off."

Client Need: Psychosocial Integrity

Practice Test 12

Miscellaneous Topics

OVERVIEW

The purpose of this section is to expose the student to questions that do not fall into any of the traditional body systems but that could appear on the NCLEX, including questions that relate to cultural diversity, and terrorism, and the influence of religious belief on health-care delivery.

Practice Test 12

Questions

1 2 - 1

When providing assistance at the site of an accident, the nurse should understand that the chief purpose of Good Samaritan laws is to:

1. discourage laypeople from giving first aid to accident victims.
2. encourage health professionals to give first aid at the scene of an accident.
3. require licensed health practitioners to provide first aid to persons in medical emergencies.
4. make it compulsory for the injured person to accept needed first aid.

1 2 - 2

According to Homeland Security, which of the following colors depicts a very high risk for a terrorist attack?

1. red
2. orange
3. green
4. yellow

1 2 - 3

At the scene of an automobile accident, which of the following actions is most appropriate to take prior to the arrival of the emergency services?

1. Identify the client.
2. Apply firm pressure over cuts and abrasions to stop bleeding.
3. Immobilize the victim in the position found at the site of the accident.
4. Keep the victim warm and calm.

1 2 - 4

A premature newborn with major deformities was just delivered. The infant has a grave prognosis, with Apgar scores <4. The mother of the infant is an active member of the Catholic Church. You will:

1. notify the pediatrician of the infant's condition.
2. document the findings.
3. provide the mother with emotional support.
4. initiate preparations for infant baptism.

1 2 - 5

Your client is a practicing orthodox Jew. Which of the following would be prohibited on this client's diet?

Select all that apply by placing a ✔ in the square:

❐ 1. Predatory fowl

❐ 2. Shellfish

❐ 3. Pork

❐ 4. Fish with scales

❐ 5. Milk

1 2 - 6

Which one of the following do you recognize as a nerve agent that could be used in chemical warfare?

1. VX
2. phosgene (CG)
3. cyanide
4. chlorine

1 2 - 7

Carcinoma of the pancreas is slightly more common among:

1. clients with black African or Eastern European Jewish ancestry.
2. clients of native Hawaiian ancestry.
3. clients with Mexican ancestry.
4. clients with Italian ancestry.

1 2 - 8

Immediately after the death of a client, which of the following actions would be important for the nurse to perform first?

1. Pad all orifices of the body.
2. Place the body in a normal anatomical position.
3. Assemble the personal effects for the family.
4. Put identification tags on the body.

1 2 - 9

Anthrax has been used in biological warfare. Which of the following information do you recognize as correct regarding this disease?

Select all that apply by placing a ✔ in the square:

❐ 1. Anthrax is caused by the spore-forming bacterium *Bacillus anthracis*.

❐ 2. Direct person-to-person spread of anthrax is extremely unlikely.

❐ 3. Persons infected with anthrax can be treated with antiviral agents.

❐ 4. There is vaccine for anthrax.

❐ 5. Anthrax occurs in animals such as cattle, sheep, and goats.

12-10

The nurse is recording the early morning care. An error is made while charting a narrative statement. The best way to correct this error is to:

1. cross out by making vertical and horizontal lines through the sentence.
2. tear out and rewrite the narrative.
3. erase completely and begin again.
4. draw a single horizontal line through the error and begin recording again.

12-11

Your client was exposed to smallpox during a biological warfare attack by terrorists. You know the incubation period for this disease is:

1. 3 to 4 days.
2. 5 to 9 days.
3. 10 to 14 days.
4. 2 to 3 weeks.

12-12

A 3-year-old presents to the emergency department with second-degree burns of the buttocks and lower extremities. The child's caretaker says, "I don't know how the child could have received these burns." The nurse has a responsibility to:

1. notify the Department of Social Services, Child Welfare.
2. notify the nursing supervisor.
3. notify the physician.
4. carefully document all findings.

12-13

The nurse is asked to be a witness when a client signs the consent form for a coronary artery angiography. Which of the following actions would be most important for the nurse to carry out?

1. Validate the client's understanding of the procedure, including the risks.
2. Inform the client of the risks involved in the procedure.
3. Give the client an explanation of the medical aspects of the procedure.
4. Have the client sign the consent immediately before the procedure.

12-14

Your client is a victim of a terrorist attack and has been poisoned with food containing the organism *Clostridium botulinum*. You know the toxins from this organism block chlorinergic synapses and can cause:

1. disorientation.
2. confusion.
3. flaccid paralysis.
4. fever.

12-15

The nurse receives a call from a parent stating her child ingested an unknown amount of kerosene that had been stored in a carbonated drink can. The immediate first-aid response will include:

1. giving ipecac to induce vomiting.
2. calling emergency 911.
3. contacting the poison control center.
4. observing the child's level of consciousness.

12-16

A Navajo woman was brought to the emergency department with a fractured femur. While the client was in the X-ray department, you asked her sister for information regarding the client's past medical history. You find the client's sister very reluctant to provide the information. You understand the most probably explanation for the sister's reluctance to share information about the client is because she:

1. mistrusts you.
2. does not feel she has the right to speak for her sister.
3. does not have information about her sister's past health history.
4. thinks it is not necessary to share this information.

12-17

Which one of the following religions prohibits meat in the diet?

1. Hinduism
2. Orthodox Judaism
3. Seventh-Day Adventism
4. Mormonism (the Church of Jesus Christ of the Latter-Day Saints)

12-18

You would like to suggest making changes in how nursing assignments are determined. The best approach to creating the necessary climate for change is to:

1. meet with the charge nurse and arrive at an agreement.
2. post a notice requesting signatures of those in favor of the idea.
3. gain the support of one peer at a time.
4. present the relevant facts to those affected.

12-19

The nurse is assessing a newborn for the first time. Which finding should the nurse report to the physician immediately?

1. temperature of 97.8°F, respirations 54 breaths per minute with periods of transient breathing, pulse rate of 142 beats per minute.
2. passage of a large black stool.
3. cyanosis of hands and feet.
4. widening of the nares with inspiration and respirations of 76 breaths per minute.

12-20

You are screening a client for lead poisoning. Due to developmental characteristics, which age group has the greatest need to be screened for lead poisoning?

1. toddlers
2. preschoolers
3. school-age children
4. adolescents

Practice Test 12

Answers, Rationales, and Explanations

---

1 2 - 1

---

② Good Samaritan laws have been enacted in almost every state and territory to encourage health-care professionals to assist in emergency situations. These laws limit liability and offer legal immunity for people who help in an emergency, providing they give the best possible care under the conditions of the emergency.

1. Good Samaritan laws were not enacted to discourage laypeople but to encourage health professionals to give first aid at the scene of an accident.

3. Health professionals are not required by law to give assistance at an accident.

4. Good Samaritan laws were not enacted to require injured persons to accept first aid.

Client Need: Safe, Effective Care Environment

---

1 2 - 2

---

① According to Homeland Security, red is the color that depicts a very high risk for a terrorist attack.

2. Orange is the color that depicts a high risk for a terrorist attack.

3. Green is the color that depicts a low risk for a terrorist attack.

4. Yellow is the color that depicts an elevated risk of a terrorist attack.

Client Need: Safe, Effective Care Environment

---

1 2 - 3

---

③ It is important to immobilize victims of a car accident at the scene before the emergency medical services arrive. Due to potential spinal cord injury, the victim should be immobilized prior to any attempts to move or transport.

1. Identification of the client is not the immediate concern.

2. Applying firm pressure over cuts and abrasions to stop bleeding could cause spinal cord injury when the client has not been immobilized.

4. Keeping the victim warm and calm should be done, but this would not be the first objective.

Client Need: Safe, Effective Care Environment

1 2 - 4

④ **Since the infant's prognosis is grave, and the mother wants the child baptized before death occurs, you should initiate preparations for baptism.**

1. This infant was born with major deformities. The pediatrician will have been on the scene at the time of the delivery and will be aware of the infant's condition and prognosis.

2. Documentation can come later. The nurse can demonstrate respect for the mother's beliefs by focusing attention on the preparation needed for the infant's baptism.

3. The best way to provide this mother with emotional support is to let her see you preparing for her infant's baptism.

Client Need: Psychosocial Integrity

1 2 - 5

① ② and ③ **Foods prohibited on the diet of a practicing orthodox Jew include predatory fowl, shellfish, and pork. Fish with scales and fins are not prohibited. Milk is not prohibited; however, it should not be mixed with meat or served with meat.**

4. Fish with scales or fins are not prohibited. Trout, bass, and brim are examples of fish that could be included in the diet. Catfish should not be included in the diet.

5. Milk is not prohibited; however, it should not be mixed with meat or served together with meat.

Client Need: Psychosocial Integrity

1 2 - 6

① **VX is a man-made, chemical warfare agent classified as a nerve agent. Nerve agents are the most toxic and rapid-acting of the known chemical warfare agents. Persons can be exposed via contaminated water, food, clothing, and vapors (gas).**

2. Phosgene is not a nerve agent. It is, however, a severe respiratory irritant that can be used in chemical warfare. Phosgene is a poisonous gas that causes suffocation when inhaled.

3. Cyanide is not a nerve agent. It is, however, an agent that can be used in chemical warfare. Cyanide inactivates respiratory enzymes and is rapidly lethal, producing drowsiness, tachycardia, coma, and death.

4. Chlorine is an agent that can be used in chemical warfare, but it is not a nerve agent. It is a highly irritating, very poisonous gas. Chlorine is capable of destroying the mucous membranes of the respiratory tract. Excessive inhalation may cause death.

Client Need: Physiological Integrity

1 2 - 7

① **Carcinoma of the pancreas is slightly more common among clients with black African or Eastern European Jewish ancestry.**

2.   There is a high rate of carcinoma of the pancreas among native Hawaiians but not as high as among clients with black African or Eastern European Jewish ancestry.

3.   There is a high rate of carcinoma of the pancreas among clients with Mexican ancestry but not as high as among clients with black African or Eastern European Jewish ancestry.

4.   There is a high rate of carcinoma of the pancreas among clients of Italian ancestry but not as high as among with black African or Eastern European Jewish ancestry.

Client Need: Physiological Integrity

1 2 - 8

② **Immediately after a death, the nurse should place the body of the deceased in a normal anatomic position. After death, the body undergoes many changes, including contraction of skeletal smooth muscle (rigor mortis). The care of the body should occur as soon as possible after death to prevent damage to tissues or disfigurement of the body parts.**

1.   It is not necessary to pad all body orifices. However, it may be necessary to place an absorbent pad under the buttocks of the deceased to take-up any feces or urine that may be released when sphincter muscles relax.

3.   All jewelry should be removed and personal effects gotten ready for the family; however, this is not the first priority.

4.   Two identification tags (one tied to the big toe and one tied to the hand or wrist) should be placed on the deceased. However, this is not the first priority.

Client Need: Physiological Integrity

1 2 - 9

① **Anthrax is caused by the spore-forming bacterium *Bacillus anthracis*.**

② **It is highly unlikely that anthrax would be spread by direct person-to-person contact.**

④ **There is a vaccine for anthrax, and those in the military, who are the most likely to become victims of this disease, could receive the vaccine.**

⑤ **Anthrax occurs in animals such as cattle, sheep, and goats. People who have jobs that place them in contact with these animals are at risk.**

3.   Because anthrax is caused by a bacterium, antiviral medications will not be effective as a treatment. Medications that are frequently prescribed include antibiotics such as penicillin, doxycycline, and ciprofloxacin.

Client Need: Health Promotion and Maintenance

1 2 - 1 0

④ **Draw a single horizontal line through the error and begin recording again.**

1. It is not necessary to make both horizontal and vertical lines through a charting error.

2 and 3. Tearing out a charting error or erasing errors is not responsible nursing and it could bring the nurse's credibility into question. Also, the charting of other health-care providers may be on the same page. In a lawsuit, the plaintiff's attorneys could use a single improper correction to compromise a nurse's credibility. One improper correction could cast doubt on the entire chart.

Client Need: Safe, Effective Care Environment

1 2 - 1 1

③ **The incubation period (the period of time from exposure to the onset of the first symptoms) is 10 to 14 days. The first symptoms of smallpox infection include an abrupt onset of chills, high fever, headache, backache, severe malaise, vomiting, possible delirium, stupor, and coma.**

1, 2, 4. The incubation period for smallpox is 10 to 14 days.

Client Need: Physiological Integrity

1 2 - 1 2

① **The nurse has the responsibility to notify the Department of Social Services, Child Welfare. It is mandatory in most states that the nurse report any suspected child abuse findings to child welfare.**

2. Notifying the nursing supervisor is proper protocol, but is not necessary.

3. Notifying the physician affords good communication and protocol, but is not required.

4. Documentation is important for legal investigation in relation to abuse, and the documentation should be specific and factual. This is second only to reporting suspected child abuse to child welfare.

Client Need: Health Promotion and Maintenance

1 2 - 1 3

① The nurse should validate that the client understands the procedure, including the risks. Before witnessing a client's signature on the consent form, the nurse should confirm that the client is well informed, including the risk of the procedure.

2 and 3. It is the physician's responsibility to inform the client of the benefits and risks of surgery and anesthesia.

4. The consent form should not be signed immediately prior to the procedure. It should be signed in an unhurried atmosphere after the procedure and risks are explained to the client's satisfaction.

Client Need: Safe, Effective Care Environment

1 2 - 1 4

③ Symptoms of botulism are muscle weakness and paralysis, and disturbance of vision, swallowing, and speech. This condition has a high mortality rate.

1, 2, and 4. Disorientation, confusion, and fever are not among the symptoms of botulism poisoning.

Client Need: Physiological Integrity

1 2 - 1 5

③ The parents should always call the Poison Control Center to ask for advice on how to proceed when a poisonous substance has been ingested, regardless of whether the amount of the substance is known or unknown.

1. To induce vomiting would be contraindicated, since kerosene (a petroleum-based substance) would burn as it comes up just as it did going down.

2. Emergency procedures outlined by the Poison Control Center may be implemented while awaiting a 911 response.

4. Pharyngeal edema (obstruction of the airway that may lead to respiratory distress) will need to be assessed, as well as the child's level of consciousness. However, calling the Poison Control Center is the first priority.

Client Need: Safe, Effective Care Environment

1 2 - 1 6

② The most probably explanation for the sister's reluctance to share information with the nurse is that she does not feel she has the right to speak for her sister. Navajos, as a general rule, do not think they have a right to speak for another person and may refuse to comment on a family member's health status.

1. Native Americans are generally very private and may hesitate to share much personal information. This is especially true if asked to share information concerning another person. Mistrust can be an issue, but it is more probable that the sister feels she does not have the right to speak for her sister.

3. It is unlikely that the client's sister does not have information about her past health history. She is more likely to feel that she does not have a right to speak for her sister.

4. It is unlikely that the client does not see the relevance in giving information about her sister's health history. However, because she feels she does not have a right to speak for another person, she may not provide the information.

Client Need: Psychosocial Integrity

1 2 - 1 7

① Hinduism prohibits all meat as well as foods cooked in animal shortenings.

2. Orthodox Judaism prohibits pork, predatory fowl, and shellfish. However, all meat is not prohibited.

3. Vegetarianism is encouraged among Seventh-Day Adventists.

4. Members of the Church of Jesus Christ of the Latter-Day Saints eat meat sparingly.

Client Need: Psychosocial Integrity

1 2 - 1 8

④ Change theory states that people who will be affected by a change need to have all relevant information presented to them for the change to occur. A meeting of all affected is a helpful way to discuss change. This way, all those affected will be present and able to discuss issues openly.

1. The charge nurse is only one person who could be affected by change. All the people who could be affected should be informed.

2. Posting a notice requesting signatures is not in keeping with proper protocol and may be interpreted as a threat.

3. When making changes, it is best for all involved to hear and discuss the issues in the same meeting. This leaves little room for misunderstanding and coercion.

Client Need: Psychosocial Integrity

1 2 - 1 9

④ **Widening of the nares with 76 breaths per minute indicates respiratory distress and should be reported to the physician immediately.**

1. A temperature of 97.8°F, respirations of 54 breaths per minute with periods of transient breathing, and a pulse rate of 142 beats per minute indicates that vital signs are within normal limits for this newborn.

2. Passage of one large black stool is normal meconium in the newborn infant.

3. Cyanosis of the hands and feet are normal findings in a newborn infant. Acrocyanosis means a dark blue color and is normal the first hour of life.

Client Need: Physiological Integrity

1 2 - 2 0

① **Toddlers have the greatest need to be screened for lead poisoning because of the possibility of brain damage. Lead poisoning is usually the result of pica (a perversion of appetite with ingestion of material not fit for food, such as clay, ice, starch, and plaster). Toddlers have a tendency to put substances into their mouths.**

2, 3, and 4. Preschoolers, school-age children, and adolescents are not as likely to put substances into their mouths as toddlers.

Client Need: Health Promotion and Maintenance

About the Authors

Linda Waide, MSN, MEd, RN, and Berta Roland, MSN, RN, are the founders of Contemporary Health Systems and Learning Made Easy, organizations dedicated to preparing nursing graduates to successfully pass the licensure examinations for both registered and practical nursing. They are the authors of **The Chicago Review Press NCLEX-PN and -RN Practice Tests and Reviews** and of **The Chicago Review Press Pharmacology Made Easy for NCLEX-PN and -RN Reviews and Study Guides**. Their organization Contemporary Health Systems offers review courses for nursing candidates nationwide.

Chicago Review Press Pharmacology Made Easy for NCLEX-RN Review and Study Guide

Chicago Review Press Pharmacology Made Easy for NCLEX-PN Review and Study Guide

Linda Waide, MSN, MEd, RN, and Berta Roland, MSN, RN

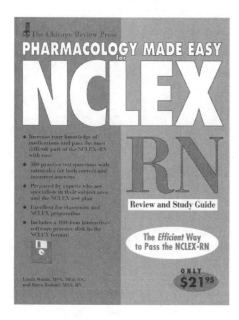
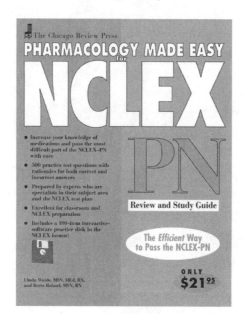

In a market dominated by lengthy tomes priced nearly double, the Pharmacology Made Easy study guides are the most efficient and economical review choices available. In each book, 295 carefully prepared written test questions cover drug actions, adverse reactions and side effects, contraindications and precautions, interactions, nursing considerations, and therapeutic benefits for more than 600 medications. Complete rationales for correct and incorrect answers are provided. Each book includes a 100-item interactive practice test on disk.

Paper, $21.95 (CAN $32.95)
8½ x 11
1-55652-392-0 (NCLEX-PN)
1-55652-391-2 (NCLEX-RN)

CHICAGO
REVIEW
PRESS

Distributed by Independent Publishers Group
www.ipgbook.com

Available at your local bookstore, or call (800) 888-4741.

The Chicago Review Press NCLEX-PN Practice Test and Review

Third Edition

Linda Waide, MSN, MEd, RN, and Berta Roland, MSN, RN

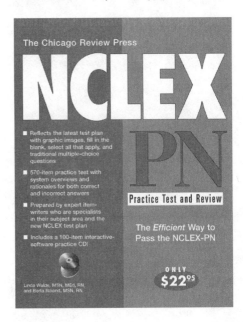

Fully revised to conform to the 2003 NCLEX test plan, this practice test and study guide includes "hot spot," fill-in-the-blank, and select-all-that-apply questions that reflect the new test format. In this book, 10 written practice tests covering all the body systems, plus two additional practice tests on mental health and miscellaneous topics, provide 570 carefully prepared test items and answers. Every practice test includes a system overview and complete rationales and explanations for both correct and incorrect choices. An Introduction offers advice on preparing for the exam and mastering the new question formats. It also includes a 100-item interactive-software CD that allows students to become comfortable with the on-screen exam. Candidates for licensure as practical nurses will find this book the most efficient, economical, and up-to-date test prep available.

Paper, $22.95 (CAN $33.95)
8½ x 11, 1-55652-528-1 (NCLEX-PN)

Distributed by Independent Publishers Group
www.ipgbook.com

Available at your local bookstore, or call (800) 888-4741.

How to use the Practice Test CD

1. To use the CD, you must have a PC with Windows 98 or higher.

2. Insert the CD in your computer's CD drive.

3. Click on start.

4. Go to Programs or All Programs.

5. Go to Contemporary Health Systems.

6. Click on the Learning Made Easy icon.

7. Follow the screen prompts to start the test.